Canadian Drug pocket

2006–2007

Con~~t~~ ~~Emergency~~

W9-CPY-326

www. media4u .com

Authors: Andreas Russ, M.D.
Klinikum Rosenheim
Pettenkoferstrasse 10
Rosenheim, 83022, Germany
russ@media4u.com

Carmine G. Nudo, M.D. C.M.
Royal Victoria Hospital
687 Pine Avenue West
Montreal, Quebec, H3A 1A1, Canada
nudo@media4u.com

Editor: Carla Maute, M.D.
Cover Illustration: Lucie Mikyna, Franka Krueger, Jaqueline Kühne-Hellmessen
Printer: Koesel GmbH & Co. KG, Am Buchweg 1, 87452 Altusried-Krugzell
Publisher: Börm Bruckmeier Publishing LLC, www.media4u.com

IMPORTANT NOTICE - PLEASE READ!
This book is based on information from sources believed to be reliable, and every effort has been made to make the book as complete and accurate as possible and to describe generally accepted practices based on information available as of the printing date, but its accuracy and completeness cannot be guaranteed. Despite the best efforts of author and publisher, the book may contain errors, and the reader should use the book only as a general guide and not as the ultimate source of information about the subject matter.
This book is not intended to reprint all of the information available to the author or publisher on the subject, but rather to simplify, complement and supplement other available sources. The reader is encouraged to read all available material and to consult the package insert and other references to learn as much as possible about the subject.
This book is sold without warranties of any kind, expressed or implied, and the publisher and author disclaim any liability, loss or damage caused by the content of this book.
IF YOU DO NOT WISH TO BE BOUND BY THE FOREGOING CAUTIONS AND CONDITIONS , YOU MAY RETURN THIS BOOK TO THE PUBLISHER FOR A FULL REFUND.

Printed in Germany
ISBN 1-59103-224-5

Preface

Drug therapy is the corner stone of the medical profession. As a medical student, resident, clinician, nurse, or pharmacist you are faced with a tremendous amount of information concerning drug therapy. In Canada it is often difficult to find a quick, convenient pharmaceutical reference that has relevant Canadian content.

I am proud to introduce the **Canadian Drug pocket**. This book is a pocket drug reference guide. A distinctly Canadian version of the already popular Drug pocket published in the US and Germany. The **Canadian Drug pocket** is unique among pocket reference guides. It includes information such as mechanisms of actions, effects, side effects and contraindications. As well as elimination half-lives, pregnancy risk categories and use during lactation. Most importantly it contains the active agents with their Canadian trade names and available forms, strengths, and recommended dosages.

I hope that this edition of the **Canadian Drug pocket** will be a useful clinical tool. It is a reference guide that is designed for the Canadian health professional. To assure continued improvement of the **Canadian Drug pocket**, any comments, criticisms, or additions would be greatly appreciated.

Carmine Nudo, M.D. C.M.   June 2005
nudo@media4u.com

Börm Bruckmeier Publishing LLC on the Internet:
www.media4u.com

Contents

Contents

6

8 Contents

1. Emergency

Adenosine	→38
Adenocard *Inj 3mg/ml*	**SVT** (not AF): 6mg rapidly IV, if no response, in 1-2min 12mg IV, then 12-18mg IV prn; **CH** ini 50mcg/kg IV, incr to 100mcg/kg, then to 200mcg/kg

Atropine	→80
Generics *Inj 0.1, 0.3, 0.4, 0.6, 1 mg/ml*	**Bradycardia, bradyarrhythmia:** 0.5-1.0 mg IV q3-5min, max 0.03-0.04mg/kg; **CH** 0.02mg/kg IV, minimum 0.1mg, max 0.5mg IV; **antimuscarinic:** 0.4-0.6mg IM/IV/SC q4-6h prn; **asystolic arrest:** 1mg IV, repeat q3-5min, max 0.04mg/kg; **organophosphate poisoning:** 1-2mg IM/IV q5-60min until symptoms disappear

Biperiden	→203
Akineton *Tab 2mg*	**Drug-induced extrapyramidal DO:** 2mg IM/IV q30min prn, max 8mg/24h; **CH** 0.04mg/kg/dose or 1.2mg/square meter/ dose IM, rep prn q30min, max 4 doses/d

Dextrose	→112
Generics *Inj 50mg/ml, 250mg/ml 2.5g/100ml, 5g/100ml, 10g/100ml, 20g/100ml, 30g/100ml, 40g/100ml, 50g/100ml, 60g/ 100ml, 70g/100ml*	**Hypoglycemia:** 25g (50ml of D50W) IV; **CH** >6mo: 0.5-1g/ kg (D25W 2-4ml/kg/dose) slowly IV, max 25g/dose, <6mo: 0.2-0.4g/kg (D10W 2-4ml/kg) slowly IV

Diazepam	→195 →209
Generics *Inj 1mg/ml, 5mg/ml*	**Seizures, status epilepticus:** 5-10mg IV, max rate 1mg/ min, rep prn q5min, max 30mg, or 10mg PR, rep prn; **CH** 1 mo-5 y: 0.2-0.5mg/kg slowly IV, rep prn q 5min, max 5mg, or 0.5mg/kg PR, rep prn in 4-12h, >5 y: 1mg IV, rep prn q5min, max 10mg or 0.3mg/kg PR, rep prn in 4-12h; **sedation:** 2-10mg IV/IM, rep prn in 4h; **muscle spasm:** 5-10mg IV/IM, rep prn in 4h

Digoxin →39

Digoxin pediatric
Inj 0.05mg/ml
Lanoxin *Tab 0.0625, 0.125, 0.25mg,*
Inj 0.05, 0.25mg/ml,
Ped elixir 0.05mg/ml
Generics *Inj 0.05, 0.25mg/ml*

AF, AF with tachyarrhythmia: ini 0.5mg IV, rep in 4h, 0.25mg PO in 8h + 12h

Diltiazem →28

Apo-Diltiaz *Inj 5mg/ml*
Generics *Inj 5mg/ml*

AF (rapid): 20mg (0.25mg/kg) IV x 2min, rep in 15min prn 30mg (35mg/kg) IV, then prn inf at 5-15mg/h

Diphenhydramine →227 →266

Generics *Inj 50mg/ml*

Anaphylaxis: 1mg/kg IV/IM, max 50mg single dose, rep prn q2-3h, max 400mg/d; **CH** 1.25mg/kg IV/IM qid, max 300mg/d

Dobutamine →18

Dobutrex *Inj 12.5mg/ml*
Generics *Inj 12.5mg/ml*

Low-output-failure: 1mg/ml (250mg in 250ml D5W) at 2.5-15mcg/kg/min, max 40mcg/kg/min

Dopamine →18

Intropin *Inj 40mg/ml*
Generics (dopamine + dextrose) *Inj 0.8mg/ml, 1.6mg/ml, 3.2mg/ml*

Acute hypotension: 400mg in 250ml D5W (1600mcg/ ml) a t 2-20mcg/kg/min IV, ini 2-5mcg/kg/min, incr by 1- 4mcg/kg/min q 10-30min, max 50mcg/kg/min

Epinephrine →18

Adrenalin *Inj 1mg/ml,*
Topical 1mg/ml
Epipen *Inj (IM)*
0.3m g/delivery
Epipen Jr. *Inj (IM)*
0.15mg/delivery
Generics *Inj 0.1mg/ml, 1mg/ml*

Cardiac arrest: 1mg (sol 1:10,000) IV/ET q3-5min prn; **CH** ini 0.01mg/kg IV, then prn 0.1mg/kg IV, max 0.2mg/kg IV (sol 1:10,000);
anaphylaxis: 0.3-0.5mg/kg IV/IM/SC, rep q10-15min prn

Esmolol →20

Brevibloc *Inj 10mg/ml, 250mg/ml* | **SVT:** ini 500mcg/kg IV x 1min, then 50mcg/kg/min IV x 4min, if response, do not change rate >25mcg/kg/min; if no response, rep 500mcg/kg IV x 1min, then 100mcg/kg/ min x 4min, prn rep 500mcg/kg IV x 1min, then incr inf by 50mcg/kg/min q4min, max 200mcg/kg/min

Fentanyl →187 →187

Generics *Inj 0.05mg/ml* | **Anaesthesia:** 50-100mcg IV/IM

Flumazenil →297

Anexate *Inj 0.1mg/ml* | **Benzodiazepine overdose:** 0.2-0.5mg IV x 30sec, rep q 60 sec, max 3mg

Furosemide →33

Lasix Special *Inj 10mg/ml* **Generics** *Inj 10mg/ml* | **Edema:** 20-40mg IV/IM, rep prn in 2h, then incr prn by 20mg >q2h until response; **CH** 1mg/kg/dose, prn incr by 0.25-0.5mg/dose q4-12h, max 10mg/kg/24h; **acute pulmonary edema:** ini 40mg slowly IV, prn incr in 1h by 40mg

Haloperidol →224

Haldol *Inj 5mg/ml* **Generics** *Inj 50mg/ml, 100mg/ml* | **Agitation:** 2-5mg IM, rep prn q1-8h

Heparin →48

Heparin Leo *Inj 100U/ml, 1000U/ml, 10000U/ml, 25000U/ml* **Heparin Lock Flush** *Inj 10U/ml, 100U/ml* **Hepalean** *Inj 1000U/ml, 10000U/ml, 25000U/ml* **Hepalean-LOK** *Inj 10U/ml, 100U/ml* **Generics** *Inj 2U/ml, 40U/ml, 50U/ml, 100 U/ml* | **DVT/pulmonary embolism:** ini 80U/kg IV, then 18 U/kg/ h, adjust by PTT testing; **CH** ini 50U/kg IV, then 10-25 U/ kg/h

Hyoscyamine →87 →274

Levsin *Tab 0.125mg, Tab ext.rel. 0.125mg, Gtt 0.125mg/ml, Inj 0.5mg/ml*

GI hypermotility/urinary spasm: 0.25-0.5mg IV/IM/SC prn q4h, max 4 doses/d; **CH** 2-12y: 0.0625mg-0.125mg/dose PO/SL, prn q4h, max 0.75mg/24h, >12y: 0.125-0.25mg/dose PO/SL, prn q4h, max 1.5mg/24h

Ketamine →188

Ketalar *Inj 10mg/ml, 50mg/ml*

Sedation + analgesia: 2-4mg/kg IM or 0.2-0.75mg/kg IV x 2-3min, then inf of 5-20 mcg/kg/min; **CH** 2-10mg/kg IM or 0.2-1mg/kg IV x 2-3min, then inf of 5-20 mcg/kg/min, 50% dose reduction in hypovolemia

Lidocaine →40 →191

Xylocaine CO$_2$ *Inj 17.3mg/ml*
Xylocaine *Inj 0.5%, 1%, 1.5%, 2.0%, 4.0%*
Xylocaine (with epinephrine) *Inj 0.5%, 1%, 1.5%, 2.0%*
Xylocaine Spinal *Inj 5.0%*
Generics *Inj 1%, 2.0%, Inj (with epinephrine) 1%, 2.0%*

VT/VF: ini 1mg/kg IV, then prn 0.5mg/kg IV q5-10min, max 3mg/kg, maint 1-4mg/min; **CH** 1mg/kg/dose IV q5- 10min, max 5 mg/kg, maint 10-50 mcg/kg/min; **local anesthesia:** 0.5-1% for infiltration, max 300mg

Lorazepam →197

Ativan *Inj 4mg/ml*

Status epilepticus: 4mg slowly IV, may rep after 10- 15min, max 8mg; **CH** 0.1mg/kg IV, max 4mg/dose

Magnesium Sulfate →95

Generics *Inj 500mg/ml*

Ventricular arrhythmia: 1-6g IV x 15min, then 3-20mg/min; **eclampsia:** ini 1-4g IV x 2-4min as 10-20% sol, maint 2-3g/h IV inf or 4-5g IM as 50% sol, rep prn q4h

Mepivacaine →191

Carbocaine *Inj 1%, 2%*
Isocaine *Inj 3%*
Isocaine (with levonordefrin) *Inj 2%*
Scandonest *Inj 3%*

Brachial nerve block: 50-400mg (1-2% sol.); **epidural nerve block:** 150-300mg (1-2% sol.); **local infiltration:** up to 400mg (0.5-1% sol.)

Scandonest (with epinephrine) *Inj 2%* **Polocaine** *Inj 3%* **Polocaine (with levonordefrin)** *Inj 2%*	
Methylprednisolone →106	
Depo-Medrol *Inj (M.-acetate) 20mg/ml, 40mg/ml, 80mg/ml* **Depo-Medrol with Lidocaine** *Inj 40mg (plus 10mg lidocaine)/ml* **Solu-Medrol** *Inj (M.-succinate) 40mg/vial, 125mg/vial, 500mg/vial, 1g/ vial* **Generics** *Inj 500mg/vial, 1g/vial*	**Status asthmaticus:** 1-2mg/kg IV; **anaphylaxis:** 125mg IV/IM or 2mg/kg IV/IM
Metoclopramide →83	
Generics *Inj 5mg/ml*	**Nausea:** 10mg IV q2-4h; **CH** 0.1-0.2mg/kg q6-8h
Morphine →181	
Generics *Inj 0.5mg/ml, 1mg/ml, 2mg/ml, 5mg/ml, 10mg/ml, 15mg/ml, 25mg/ml, 50mg/ml*	**Pulmonary edema:** 2-8mg IV; **pain:** 2-10mg IV, max 20mg prn q2-6h or 1-10mg/h IV inf, max 80mg/h or 5- 20mg IM/SC; **CH** 0.1-0.2mg/kg IV/IM/SC q2-4h, max 15mg/dose or 0.025-2.6mg/kg/h IV inf
Naloxone →183	
Generics *Inj 0.4mg/ml, 1mg/ml*	**Opioid reversal (after anesthesia):** 0.1-0.2mg IV q2- 3min prn; **CH** 0.01mg/kg IV, rep q2-3min; **opioid overdose:** 0.4-2mg IV, rep q2-3min, max 10mg; **CH** <20kg: 0.1mg/kg IV/IM/**ET** q2-3min, >20kg: 2mg IV, rep q2-3min

Nitroglycerin →36

Generic (NTG + dextrose) *Inj 0.1, 0.2, 0.4mg/ml*
Gen-Nitro *Spray metered SL 0.4mg/Spray*
Nitrolingual Pumpspray *Spray metered SL 0.4mg/Spray*
Nitrostat *Tab (SL) 0.3mg, 0.6mg*
Rho-Nitro Pumpspray *Spray metered SL 0.4mg/Spray*

Acute angina pectoris: 1-2 sprays SL, rep prn q5min, max 3 sprays or 0.4mg Tab SL, rep prn q5min, max 3 doses; **acute MI/angina pectoris:** ini 5mcg/min IV as inf of 50mg in 250ml D5W (200mcg/ml), incr prn by 5mcg/ min q3-5min to 20mcg/min, then incr prn by 10mcg/min

Norepinephrine →19

Levophed *Inj 1mg/ml*
Generics *Inj 1mg/ml*

Acute hypotension: ini 8-12mcg/min IV (4mg in 500ml D5W), maint inf at 2-4mcg/min

Oxytocin →291

Generics *Inj 10 U/ml*

Postpartum hemorrhage: 3-10U IM or 10U IV in 1L NS at 100-200ml/h

Pancuronium →190

Pancuronium *Inj 1mg/ml, 2mg/ml*
Generics *Inj 1mg/ml, 2mg/ml*

Paralysis (anesthesia): 0.04-0.1mg/kg IV

Phenobarbital →198

Barbilixir *Elix 4mg/ml*
Generics *Tab 15mg, 30mg, 60mg, 100mg,*
Elixir 5mg/ml,
Inj 30mg/ml, 120mg/ml

Status epilepticus: 10-20mg/kg IV, max rate 60mg/min, max 20mg/kg

Phenylephrine →19

Neo-Synephrin *Inj 10mg/ml*

Acute hypotension (mild-moderate): 200mcg IV, ini max 500mcg IV, rep prn q10-15min; **acute hypotension** (severe): inf 10mg in 500ml D5W, ini at 100-180mcg/min, prn decr to 40-60mcg/min

Phenytoin

Dilantin *Cap 30mg, 100mg, Susp (oral) 30mg/5ml, 125mg/ml*
Dilantin Infatabs *Tab (chew) 50mg*
Generics *Inj 50mg/ml*

Status epilepticus: ini 15-18mg/kg IV, max rate 0.5 mg/ kg/min, max 30mg/kg, rep 100mg PO/IV q6-8h; **CH** 15-20mg/kg IV, max rate 1-3mg/kg/min

Procainamide →41

Generics *Inj 100mg/ml*

VF (refractory)/ paroxysmal SVT with wide QRS: 20- 30mg/min or 100mg IV q5min, until max 17mg/kg, BP ↓ , dysrhythmia suppressed or QRS/PR widens >50%, maint inf of 2g in 250ml D5W at 2-6 mg/min

Propranolol →22

Inderal *Inj 1mg/ml*

SVT/AF/Af: 1-3mg IV, max 1mg/min, rep prn in 2min, rep third dose in >4h; **CH** 0.01-0.15mg/kg IV x 10min, rep prn q6-8h, max 1mg

Rocuronium →190

Zemuron *Inj 10mg/ml*

Paralysis (anesthesia): 0.6-1.2mg/kg IV

Salbutamol →61

Airomir *MDI 120mcg/dose*
Apo-Salvent *Resp. soln 5mg/ml, MDI 100mcg/dose, Sterules 1mg/ml, 2mg/ml, Tab 2mg, 4mg*
Ventolin *Sol (inhal) 1.25/2.5 ml, 2.5mg/ 2.5ml, 5mg/2.5ml, 5mg/ml*
Ventolin Diskus *Inhal 200mcg/blister*
Ventolin HFA *MDI 100mcg/dose*
Generics *MDI 100mcg/dose Sol (inhal) 5mg/ml, 0.5mg/ ml, 1mg/ml, 2mg/ml*

Asthma: 1-2puffs q4-6h prn

Sodium Bicarbonate

Sodium bicarbonate *Inj* 42mg/ml, 50mg/ml, 75mg/ml, 84mg/ml	**Metabolic acidosis:** 1mEq/kg IV, rep prn 0.5mEq/kg IV q 10min; **CH** 1mEq/kg IV, then 0.5mEq/kg prn q10min

Sodium Nitroprusside →32

Nipride *Inj* 50mg/vial	**HTN (malignant):** 0.3-10mcg/kg/min IV; max 70mg/kg within 14d; **CH** 0.3-10mcg/kg IV

Terbutaline →62, →290

Bricanyl Tablets *Tab* 2.5mg, 5mg	**Asthma:** 0.25mg SC q20min, max 3 doses; **preterm labor:** 0.25-0.5mg SC q2h

Theophylline →64

Generics *Inj* 0.8mg/ml, 1.6mg/ml, 4mg/ml	**Acute bronchospasm:** ini 4.6mg/kg IV x 6min, then inf at 0.5mg/kg/h

Thiopental →186

Pentothal *Inj (Sol)* 1g/vial, 2.5g/vial, 5g/vial, *Inj (Powder)* 250mg/syringe, 500mg/syringe, 500mg/vial, 1g/vial	**Anesthesia induction:** 3-5mg/kg IV; **convulsions:** 75-125mg IV (3-5ml of a 2.5% sol)

Verapamil →28

Generics *Inj* 2.5mg/ml	**SVT/AF/Af:** 5-10mg IV x 2min, rep prn 10mg IV in 30min; **CH** >2 y or >15kg (paroxysmal SVT): ini 0.1-0.3mg/kg IV x 2min, max 5mg/dose, rep prn in 30min, max 10mg

Advanced Life Support Algorithm

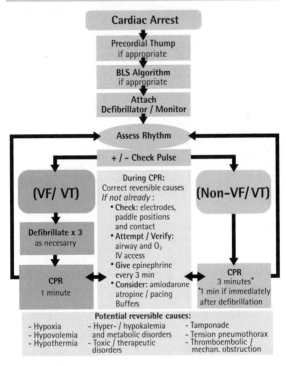

Cardiac Arrest

Precordial Thump
if appropriate

BLS Algorithm
if appropriate

Attach
Defibrillator / Monitor

Assess Rhythm

+ / − Check Pulse

(VF/ VT)

During CPR:
Correct reversible causes
If not already :
- **Check:** electrodes,
  paddle positions
  and contact
- **Attempt / Verify:**
  airway and O_2
  IV access
- **Give** epinephrine
  every 3 min
- **Consider:** amiodarone
  atropine / pacing
  Buffers

(Non-VF/ VT)

Defibrillate x 3
as necesarry

CPR
1 minute

CPR
3 minutes*
*1 min if immediately
after defibrillation

Potential reversible causes:

- Hypoxia
- Hypovolemia
- Hypothermia
- Hyper- / hypokalemia
  and metabolic disorders
- Toxic / therapeutic
  disorders
- Tamponade
- Tension pneumothorax
- Thromboembolic /
  mechan. obstruction

International Guidelines 2000 for CPR and ECC - a Consensus of Science, Resuscitation 2000, 46 (1-3), 3-447

2.   Cardiovascular System

2.1   Vasopressors

MA/EF (dobutamine): primarily beta-rec. agon., pos. inotropic, no vasoconstriction;
MA/EF (dopamine): dose-dependent dopamine-, beta-/alpha-rec. agon, renal vasodilation, cardiac output↓, vasoconstr.; **MA/EF (epinephrine):** primarily beta-rec. agonist, positive inotropic, chronotropic + bathmotropic effect, syst. BP↑, diast. BP↓, bronchodilation;
MA/EF (norepinephrine): primarily alpha-rec. agonist ⇒ syst./diast. BP↑;
MA/EF (midodrine): alpha-adren. agonism on arteriolar + venous rec. ⇒ vascular tone↑, venous pooling↓, BP↑; **AE:** headache, anxiety, fatigue, N/V, dyspnea, angina, hypertension/hypotension, arrhythmias, parasthesia, bradycardia, palpitati., hyperglycemia; **CI (dobutamine):** pheochromocytoma, idiopathic hypertrophic subaortic stenosis, hypersensativity to the drug; **CI (dopamine):** pheochromocytoma; **CI (epinephrine):** narrow angle glaucoma, anesthesia with halogenated hydrocarbons/cyclopropane, organic brain damage, labor, cardiac dilatation, corocary insufficincy; **CI (norepinephrine):** anesthesia with halogenated hydrocarbons/cyclopropane, vascular thrombosis; **CI (midodrine):** excessive supine hypertension, severe organic heart disease, acute renal disease, urinary retention, pheochromocytoma, thyrotoxicosis, hypersensitivity to the drug

Dobutamine	EHL 2min, Dur (1x dose) 10min, PRC B, Lact ?
Dobutrex Inj 12.5mg/ml **Generics** Inj 12.5mg/ml	**Cardiac decompensation:** ini 0.5-1mcg/kg/min IV, incr to 2-20mcg/kg/min, max 40mcg/kg/min

Dopamine	EHL 2min, Dur 10min, PRC C, Lact ?
Generics (dopamine + dextrose) Inj 0.8mg/ml, 1.6mg/ml, 3.2mg/ml	**Hypotension, heart failure:** ini 1-5mcg/kg/min IV, incr prn by 5-10 mcg/kg/ min increments, max 50mcg/kg/ min

Epinephrine	Dur 2min, PRC C, Lact ?
Adrenalin Inj 1mg/ml, Topical 1mg/ml **Epipen Jr.** Inj (IM) 0.15mg/delivery **Epipen** Inj (IM) 0.3mg/delivery **Generics** Inj 0.1mg/ml, 1mg/ml	**Cardiac arrest:** 0.5-1mg IV/ET, rep prn q 3-5min; **anaphylaxis:** 0.3-0.5 mg SC/IM, rep prn q10-15min; **CH:** 0.01mg/kg IV; 0.1mg/kg ET rep prn with 0.1mg/kg IV/ET q3-5min; **anaphylaxis:** 0.01mg/kg SC/IM (use 1: 1000 Sol), then 0.1mg/kg IV prn (IV: use 1:10.000)

Midodrine	EHL 0.5h, PRC C, Lact ?
Amatine Tab 2.5mg, 5mg	**Orthostatic hypotension:** ini 2.5mg PO tid, incr prn to max 40 mg/d; **DARF:** ini 2.5mgtid

Norepinephrine	Dur 1-2min, PRC C, Lact ?
Levophed Inj 1mg/ml Generics Inj 1mg/ml	**Acute hypotensive states:** ini 8-12 mcg/min IV, maint 2- 4 mcg/min
Phenylephrine	PRC C, Lact ?
Neo-Synephrine Inj 10mg/ml	**Acute hypotension:** 2-5mg SC/IM, max ini 5mg IV, rep prn q1-2h; 0.2-0.5mg slowly IV, max ini 0.5mg IV

Systemic Beta Adrenergic Agonists →61, α-β-Adrenergic Agonists →63

2.2 Beta Blockers

MA: competitive blockage of beta-receptors;
EF: neg. inotropic + chronotropic ⇒ cardiac output ↓, myocardial O_2 consumption ↓, renin secretion ↓, high-dose nonspecific membrane-stabilizing effect (quinidine-like);
AE: (acebutalol) congestive heart failure, bradycardia, bronchospasm, fatigue, dyspnea, nausea, dizziness, hypotension, rash (atenolol) congestive heart failure, AV block, bradycardia, bronchospasm, dizziness, vertigo, fatigue, diarrhea, nausea, dry mouth, (bisoprolol) arthralgia, dizziness, headache, insomnia, diarrhea, nausea, coughing, fatigue, edema, (carvedilol) congestive heart failure, syncope, bradycardia, hypotension, fatigue, dizziness, dyspnea (esmolo) hypotension, bradycardia, bronchospasm (labetalol) hypotension, jaundice, bronchospasm, dizziness, fatigue, headache, angina, nausea (metoprolol/nadalol) hypotension, bradycardia, congestive heart failure (AV block, bradycardia, hypotension, congestive heart failure, peripheral vasoconstriction bronchospasm, N/V, constipat., diarrhea, sexual ability ↓, insulin secretion ↓, glycogenolysis ↓, fatigue, insomnia, dizziness, drowsiness, weakness, nervousness, anxiety, mental depression (propranolol) chf, bronchospasm, anorexia, nausea, vomiting, diarrhea, abdominal pain;
CI (betablockers): bronchospasm, congestive heart failure, sinus bradycardia, second and third degree AV block, RV failure secondary pulmonary hypertension, cardiogenic shock, hypersensativity to drug;
CI (acebutalol/bisoprolol) anesthesia that produces cardiac depression;
CI (atenolol): sick sinus syndrome, severe PVD, pheochromocytoma without alpha-blockade, metabolic acidosis ;
CI (carvedilol): severe hypoten., hepatic impairment, mental incapacity,
CI (metoprolol): severe PVD, anesthesia that produces cardiac depress.,
CI (nadalol): allergic rhinitis,
CI (oxprenolol): alleric rhinitis, anesthesia producing cardiac depression,
CI (pindolol): anesthesia produc. cardiac depression **CI** (propranolol): allergic. rhinitis

		β_1	ISA
Acebutolol	EHL 3-4h, PRC B, Lact ?		
Monitan *Tab* 100mg, 200mg, 400mg **Sectral** *Tap* 100mg, 200mg, 400mg **Rhotral** *Tap* 100mg, 200mg, 400mg **Generics** *Tab* 100mg, 200mg, 400mg	**HTN:** ini 100mg PO bid, max 800mg/d PO qd or div bid; **Angina pectoris:** ini 200mg PO bid, maint 200-600mg PO div bid; DARF: GFR (ml/min) <50: 50%; <25: 25%	+	+
Atenolol	EHL 6-7h, PRC D, Lact ?	+	–
Apo, Novo, Nu-Atenol *Tab* 50mg, 100mg **Tenormin** *Tab* 50mg, 100mg **Generics** *Tab* 50mg, 100mg	**HTN:** ini 50mg PO qd, maint 50-100mg PO qd; **Angina pectoris:** ini 50 PO qd, maint 50-200mg/d PO qd or div bid; DARF: GFR (ml/ min) 15-35: max 50mg/d; <15: max 50mg/od PO		
Bisoprolol	EHL 10-12.4h, PRC C, Lact ?	+	–
Monocor *Tab* 5mg, 10mg	**HTN:** ini 5mg PO qd, max 20mg/d; **DARF/DAHF:** ini 5mg PO qd, caution with dose-titration		
Carvedilol	EHL 6-10h, PRC C, Lact ?	–	–
Coreg *Tab* 3.125mg, 6.25mg, 12.5mg, 25mg **Generics** *Tab* 3.125mg, 6.25mg, 12.5mg, 25mg	**Heart failure:** ini 3.125mg PO bid incr dose q2 wk as tolerated to max 25mg bid; DARF: not req; DAHF: contraindicated		
Esmolol	EHL 9min, PRC C, Lact ?	+	–
Brevibloc *Inj* 10mg/ml, 250mg/ml	**Periperative tachycardia/hypertension:** 1.5mg/kg (max 100mg) IV over 30sec then 0.15mg/kg/min , max 0.3mg/kg/min, **Atrial fibrillation/flutter:** ini 0.5mg/kg/min IV for 1min, then 0.05mg/kg/min IV for 4min; DARF: not req		
Labetalol	EHL 5-8h, PRC C, Lact +	–	(+)
Trandate *Tab* 100mg, 200mg **Generics** *Tab* 100mg, 200mg, *Inj* 5mg/ml	**Hypertensive emergency:** 20mg slow IV, then 40-80mg IV q10min prn, max 300mg total; **HTN:** ini 100mg PO bid, maint 200-400mg bid, max 1200mg/d; DARF: not req		

Metoprolol	EHL 3-7h, PRC C, Lact ?	β_1	ISA
Betaloc *Tab 50mg, 100mg, Inj 1mg/ml* **Betaloc Durules** *Tab ext.rel 200mg* **Lopresor** *Tab 50mg, 100mg, Inj 1mg/ml* **Lopresor SR** *Tab ext.rel 100mg, 200mg* **Novo-Metoprol** *Tab 50mg, 100mg* **Nu-Metop** *Tab 50mg, 100mg* **Generics** *Tab 50mg, 100mg*	**HTN, Angina pectoris**: ini 50mg PO bid or 50-100mg PO qd (ext.rel), incr prn max 400mg/d; **acute MI**: ini 5mg IV q2min up to 15mg, if tolerated give 50mg PO q6h for 48h, then 100mg PO bid; DARF: not req	+	−

Nadolol	EHL 20-24h, PRC C, Lact ?	−	−
Corgard *Tab 40mg, 80mg,160mg* **Apo-Nadol** *Tab 40mg, 80mg, 160mg* **Generics** *Tab 40mg, 80mg,160mg*	**HTN**: ini 80mg PO qd, maint 40-80mg/d, max 320 mg/d; **Angina pectoris**: ini 80mg PO qd, maint 40-80mg/d, max 240mg/ d; DARF: GFR (ml/min): >50: q24h, 31-50: q24-36h, 10- 30: q 24-48h, <10: q40-60h		

Oxprenolol	EHL 1.3-1.5h, PRC + Lact not rec	−	+
Trasicor *Tab 40mg, 80mg* **Slow Trasicor** *Tab ext. rel 80mg, 160mg*	**HTN**: ini 20mg PO tid, maint 120-320mg/d, max 480mg/d	−	+

Pindolol	EHL 3-4h, PRC B, Lact ?	−	+
Apo, Novo, Nu-Pindol *Tab 5mg, 10mg, 15mg* **Visken** *Tab 5mg, 10mg, 15mg* **Generics** *Tab 5mg, 10mg, 15mg*	**Angina pectoris**: ini 5mg PO tid, maint 15-40mg/d div tid; **HTN**: ini 5mg PO bid, maint 15-45mg/d, max 45 mg/d; DARF: not req	−	+

Propranolol	EHL 3-4h, PRC C, Lact ?	β_1	ISA
Inderal LA *Cap ext.rel 60mg, 80mg, 120mg, 160mg* **Novo-Pranol** *Tab 10mg, 20mg, 40mg, 80mg* **Generics** *Tab 10mg, 20mg, 40mg, 80mg, 120mg, Inj 1mg/ml*	**HTN:** ini 40mg PO bid, maint 120-240mg/d, max 640mg/d; ext.rel: ini 60-80mg PO qd, maint 120-160mg/d, max 640mg/d; **angina:** ini 10-20mg PO tid-qid, maint 160-240mg/d; **arrhythmias:** 1-3mg IV, rep after 2min prn; 10-30mg PO tid-qid; **MI:** 180-240mg/d PO div bid-qid; **migraine:** ini 80mg/d PO, maint 160-240mg/d; **essential tremor:** ini 40mg PO bid, maint 120mg/d; **pheochromocytoma:** preop. for 3 days 60 mg/d PO in div doses bid-tid in combination with an alpha blocking agent; **hypertrophic subaortic stenosis:** 20-40mg PO tid-qid; **CH** 2-4mg/kg/d PO div bid; DARF: not req	–	–
Timolol	EHL 2-4h, PRC C, Lact ?	–	–
Apo, Novo-Timol *Tab 5mg, 10mg, 20mg* **Generics** *Tab 5mg, 10mg, 20mg*	**HTN:** ini 10mg PO bid, maint 20-40mg/d, max 60mg/d; **MI:** 10mg PO bid; **migraine:** ini 10mg PO bid, maint 20mg/d qd; max 30mg/d; DARF: not req		

β1: selective blockage of β1-receptors;
ISA: intrinsic sympathomimetic activity = partial agonistic and antagonist activity

2.3   ACE Inhibitors
2.3.1   ACE Inhibitors - Single Ingredient Drugs

MA: competitive blockage of angiotensin converting enzyme ⇒ angiotensin II ↓, bradykinin ↑
EF: vasodilation ⇒ BP ↓, renal blood flow ↑, aldosterone ↓, catecholamines ↓, reversal of myocardial and blood vessel wall hypertrophy, protective in diabetic nephropathy
AE: acute RF, rash, dry cough, hair loss, angioedema, dizziness, fatigue, headache, hyperkalemia, hyponatremia, complete blood count changes, urticaria, hypotension
CI: angiodema, hypersensitivity to drug CI (cilazapril): ascites

Benazepril	EHL 0.6 h, PRC C(1), D(2nd, 3rd trim.), Lact +
Lotensin *Tab 5mg, 10mg, 20mg*	**HTN:** ini 10mg PO qd, maint 20-40mg PO qd or div bid, max 80mg/d; DARF: GFR (ml/min) <30: ini 5mg PO qd, max 10mg/d

Captopril	EHL 1.9h, PRC C(1), D(2nd, 3rd trim.), Lact +
Apo, Nu-Capto *Tab 6.25mg, 12.5mg, 25mg, 50mg, 100mg* **Capoten** *Tab 12.5mg, 25mg, 50mg, 100mg* **Generics** *Tab 6.25mg, 12.5mg, 25mg, 50mg, 100mg*	**HTN:** ini 25mg PO bid-tid, max 450 mg/d; **heart failure:** ini 12.5-25mg PO tid, incr to 150-300mg/d div tid, max 450mg/d; **LV dysfunction after MI**: ini 6.25mg po x 1, then 12.5mg PO tid, maint. 50mg PO tid; **Diabetic nephropathy:** maint 25mg PO tid; DARF: GFR (ml/min/1.73m2) 35-75: q12-24h; 20-34: q24-48h; 8-19: q48-72h; 5-7: q72-108h
Cilazapril	EHL 8.9h, PRC contraindicated, Lact +
Inhibace *Tab 1mg, 2.5mg, 5mg*	**HTN:** ini 2.5mg PO qd, maint 2.5-5mg qd, max 10mg/d; **heart failure:** ini 0.5mg PO qd, maint 1-2.5mg qd, max 2.5mg/d; DARF: GFR (ml/min) 10-40ml/min: ini 0.25-0.5mg qd max 2.5mg qd; <10ml/min 0.25-0.5mg qwk-biw
Enalapril/Enalaprilat	EHL 1.3h, PRC C(1st), D(2nd, 3rd trim.), Lact +
Vasotec *Tab 2.5mg, 5mg, 10mg, 20mg, Inj 1.25mg/ml*	**HTN:** ini 5mg PO qd, maint 10-40mg PO qd or div bid, max 40mg/d; 1.25mg IV q6h, max 5mg IV q6h; **heart failure:** ini 2.5 mg PO qd, maint 5-20mg/d PO div qd-bid, max 40mg/d; **CH** heart failure: 0.08mg/kg/d PO qd or div bid; DARF: GFR (ml/min) <30: ini 2.5mg PO qd, titrate prn, max 40mg/d; <30: 0.625mg IV q6h
Fosinopril	EHL 11.5h, PRC C(1st), D(2nd, 3rd trim.), Lact +
Monopril *Tab 10mg, 20mg*	**HTN:** ini 10mg PO qd, maint 20mg PO qd, max 40mg/ d; **heart failure:** ini 10mg PO qd, maint 20-40mg PO qd, max 40mg/d; DARF: not req

Minoxidil	EHL 2.3-28.9h, PRC C, Lact +
Loniten *Tab 2.5mg, 10mg*	**Severe HTN:** ini 2.5mg PO bid, incr to 10-40mg/d div bid, max 100mg/d; **CH** <12y:ini 0.2mg/kg/d PO^tdiv bid, incr q3d, max 50mg

Nitroprusside Sodium	EHL 3-4min
Nipride *Inj 50mg/vial*	**HTN emergencies:** ini 0.3-0.5mcg/kg/min IV, incr by 0.5mcg/kg/min, max 10mcg/kg/min; DARF: not req

2.8   Endothelin Receptor Antagonists

MA/EF (bosentan): specific and competitive antagonist at endothelin receptor types ETΛ and ETB ⇒ inhibition of endothelin-1 effects ⇒ pulmonary artery pressure ↓
AE (bosentan): headache, nasopharyngitis, hypotension, flushing, edema, liver injury
CI (bosentan): pregnancy, coadmin. with cyclosporine A, glyburide, moderate to severe liver impairment, known hypersensitivity

Bosentan	EHL 5h, PRC X, Lact -
Tracleer *Tab 62.5mg, 125mg*	**Pulmon. arteri. HTN** (WHO III-IV): ini 62.5mg PO bid for 4wk, then 125mgbid; DARF: not req

2.9   Diuretics
2.9.1   Thiazide Diuretics

MA: inhibition of the reabsorption of Na^+, Cl^- and H_2O in the distal convoluted tubule, secretion of K^+ ↑; **EF:** elimination of Na^+, Cl^-, H_2O and K^+ ↑, excretion of Ca^{2+} and PO_4^{3-} ↓
AE: hypokalemia, hypercalcemia, hyperuricemia, thrombosis, anemia, hyperglycemia
CI: anuria, renal insuff., sulphonamide hypersensitivity, hepatic coma

Chlorthalidone	EHL 40-89h, PRC B, Lact ?
Generics *Tab 50mg, 100mg*	**HTN:** ini 12.5mg PO qd, maint 12.5-50mg/d, max 50mg/d; **edema:** ini 25-100mg PO/d div tid-qid, max 200mg/d

Hydrochlorothiazide	EHL 10-12h, PRC B, Lact +
Apo-Hydro *Tab 25mg, 50mg, 100mg* **Novo-Hydrazide** *Tab 25mg, 50mg*	**Edema:** 25-100mg PO/d div qd-tid, max 200mg/d; **HTN:** ini 12.5mg PO qd, maint 12.5-50mg/d, max 50mg/d; **CH** 1- 2mg/kg/d PO qd or div bid

Indapamide	EHL 14–15h, PRC B, Lact ?
Lozide *Tab 1.25mg, 2.5mg* **Generics** *Tab 1.25mg, 2.5mg*	**HTN:** ini 1.25mg PO qd, incr prn, max 5mg/d; **edema:** ini 2.5mg PO qd, max 5mg/d

Metolazone	EHL 8–14h, PRC B, Lact +
Zaroxolyn *Tab 2.5mg*	**Edema:** 5–10mg PO qd, max 20mg/d; **HTN:** ini 2.5mg PO qd, max 10mg/d

2.9.2   Loop Diuretics

MA/EF: inhibition of the reabsorption of Na$^+$, Cl$^-$, K$^+$ and H$_2$O, primarily in the ascending limb of the loop of Henle ⇒ increased elimination of Na$^+$, Cl$^-$, K$^+$, H$_2$O, Ca^{2+} and Mg^{2+} **AE:** orthostatic hypotension, hypotension, thrombosis, appetite loss, diarrhea/constipation, N/V, headache, dizziness, hypokalemia, hypocalcemia, hyperuricemia, blurred vision, reversible hearing loss, skin photosensitivity; **CI:** severe electrolyte depletion, hypovolemia, oliguria/anuria, hepatic coma, hypersensitivity to the drug

Bumetanide	EHL 1–1.5h, PRC C, Lact ?
Burinex *Tab 1mg, 5mg*	**Edema:** 0.5–2mg PO qd, rep prn doses at 4–5h intervals, max 10mg/d; 0.5–1mg IV/IM, rep prn at 2–3h intervals, max 10mg/d; DARF: not req

Ethacrynic Acid	EHL 1–4h, PRC B, Lact -
Edecrin *Tab 50mg, Inj 50mg/vial*	**Edema:** 50–200mg/d PO div bid; 0.5–1mg/kg IV, max 100mg/d; **CH** ini 25mg PO, incr prn q2-3d by 25mg, max 2-3mg/kg/ d;

Furosemide	EHL 30–120min, PRC C, Lact ?
Lasix *Tab 20mg, 40mg, Sol (oral) 10mg/ml* **Lasix Special** *Tab 500mg, Inj 10mg/ml* **Novo-Semide** *Tab 20mg, 40mg, 80mg* **Generics** *Tab 20mg, 40mg, 80mg, Inj 10mg/ml*	**Edema:** ini 20–80mg PO, max 200mg/d or 20–40mg IV, incr by 20–40mg q6-8h prn, max 600mg/d; **HTN** ini 20–40mg PO bid, incr prn; **CH** ini 1–2mg/kg IV/IM/PO, incr by 1-2mg q6-8h until desired effect is achieved, max 6mg/kg/dose

2.9.3 Potassium-Sparing Diuretics

MA (amiloride, triamterene): inhibition of the reabsorption of Na^+, Cl^- and H_2O as well as inhibition of the K^+-secretion in the distal convoluted tubule
MA (spironolactone): competitive blockage of aldosterone receptor in late-distal tubule
EF: elimination of Na^+, Cl^- and H_2O ↑, K^+ elimination ↓
AE (amiloride): hyperkalemia, metabolic acidosis, megaloblastic anemia
AE (spironolactone): hyperkalemia, gynecomastia, impotence, amenorrhea, hirsutism, voice DO, skin DO
CI (amiloride): hyperkalemia, renal insufficiency, anuria, use of other antikaliuretics/ K-salts
CI (spironolactone): renal insufficiency, hyperkalemia, anuria

Amiloride	EHL 6-9h, PRC B, Lact ?
Generics *Tab 5mg*	**cirrhosis ascites, edema:** ini 5mg PO qd in combination with another diuretic or monotherapy ini 10mg PO qd or div bid, max 20mg/d; **cardiac edema/HTN:** ini 5-10mg PO qd, max 20mg/d

Spironolactone	EHL 1.3-1.4h, PRC D, Lact +
Aldactone *Tab 25mg, 100mg* **Novo-Spiroton** *Tab 25mg, 100mg*	**Edema with heart failure, cirrhosis, nephrotic syndrome:** ini 100mg PO qd or div bid, incr prn until diuretic effect is achieved, max 200mg/d; **HTN:** 50- 100mg PO qd or div bid; **CH** 1-3mg/kg/d PO

2.9.4 Potassium-Sparing Diuretics - Combinations

Amiloride + HCTZ	PRC B, Lact -
Apo, Nu-Amilzide *Tab 5 + 50mg* **Novamilor** *Tab 5 + 50mg* **Generic** *Tab 5 + 50mg*	**HTN, edema:** 50+5 - 100+10mg PO qd or div bid, max 4 tab/d

Spironolactone + HCTZ	PRC C, Lact ?
Aldactazide *Tab 25 + 25mg, 50 + 50mg* **Novo-Spirozine** *Tab 25 + 25mg, 50 + 50mg*	**Edema:** 25+25 - 200+200mg PO qd or div bid; **HTN:** 50+50 - 100+100mg PO qd or div bid

Triamterene + HCTZ	PRC D, Lact -
Apo, Nu-Triazide *Tab 50 + 25mg* **Novo-Triamzide** *Tab 50 + 25mg*	**HTN, edema:** 50+25mg PO qd

2.9.5   Diuretics - Carbonic Anhydrase Inhibitors

MA/EF: noncompetitive inhibition of the enzyme carbonic anhydrase $\Rightarrow$ urine volume $\uparrow$, urinary excretion of bicarbonate and sodium $\uparrow$ $\Rightarrow$ metabolic acidosis
AE: taste disturbances, paresthesia, metabolic acidosis, tinnitus; **CI:** hypersensitivity to drug, hyponatremia, hypokalemia, severe liver or renal impairment, hyperchloremic acidosis, suprarenal gland failure **CI** (methazolamide): severe pulmonary obsruction

Acetazolamide	EHL 4-8h, PRC C, Lact ?
Diamox *Cap sust. rel. 500mg* **Novo-Zolamide** *Tab 250mg* **Generics** *Tab 250mg*	**Acute angle closure glaucoma and pre-op:** 500mg IV q2-4h prn; 250mg PO q4h; **CH** 8-30mg/kg/d PO div tid; **Edema:** 250-375mg PO qd; **mountain sickness:** 0.5-1g PO div bid-tid, ini 48h before ascent, continue prn; DARF: 10-50ml/min: 250mg PO q12h
Methazolamide	EHL 14h, PRC C, Lact ?
Generics *Tab 50mg*	**Acute angle closure glaucoma:** ini 50-100mg PO bid-tid; **Chronic open angle:** 250mg/d in div doses, max 1g/d

2.10   Antihypertensive Combinations

Atenolol + Chlorthalidone	PRC D, Lact -
Tenoretic *Tab 50 + 25mg, 100 + 25mg*	**HTN:** 50+25 - 100+25mg PO qd; DARF: GFR (ml/min) 15-35: 50mg qd, <15: 50mg qod
Methyldopa + HCTZ	PRC B, Lact +
Apo-Methazide *Tab 250+15mg,250+25mg*	**HTN:** 250+15 - 750 + 45mg PO/d
Pindolol + HCTZ	EHL 3.5h, PRC D, Lact +
Viskazide *Tab 10 + 25mg, 10 + 50mg*	**HTN:** 10+25 - 20+100mg PO qd

Class IC antiarrhythmics (flecainide, propafenone)
MA: conduction and refractory time ↑ (AV node and ventricle), no vagolysis
AE: hypotension, AV block, nausea, pro-arrhythmias, cholestatic hepatitis
CI (flecainide): AV block II°-III°, shock, bi- or trifascicular block, **CI** (propafanone): sinus
or AV dysfunction, bradycardia, severe cardiac insufficiency, bronchospastic disease,
severe electrolyte imbalance or hepatic failure

Class II antiarrhythmics (Isoproterenol), see Beta Blockers →19

Class III antiarrhythmics (amiodarone, sotalol)
MA/EF: blockage of K⁺ channels ⇒ action potential length ↑
AE (amiodarone): corneal microdeposits, pulmonary fibrosis, hepatic damage,
photosensitivity, dysopias, erythema nodosum, hypo- and hyperthyroidism;
AE (sotalol): see Beta Blockers
CI (amiodarone): AV block II°-III°, bradycardia, thyroid diseases, iodine allergy,
acute hepatitis, thyroid dysfunction, pulmonary interstitial abnormalities
CI (sotalol): see Beta Blockers

Class IV antiarrhythmics see Calcium Channel Blockers - Non-Dihydropyridines
Other Antiarrhythmics (adenosine, atropine, digoxin , epinephrine)
MA/EF (adenosine): brief blockage of the AV node ⇒ termination of re-entry tachycardias,
neg. chronotropic at the sinus node
MA (atropine): competitive antagonism at muscarinic receptors
EF (atropine): tachycardia, antispasmodic, tear production ↓; sputum, sweat and bronchial
secretion ↓, mydriasis, blurred vision
AE (adenosine): flush, dyspnea, bronchospasm, nausea;
AE (atropine): decrease of sweat production, urinary retention, restlessness, hallucinations,
oral dryness, acute glaucoma
CI (adenosine): AV block II°-III°, sick-sinus, bradycardia
CI (atropine): narrow angle glaucoma, micturition disturbance, prostatic hypertrophy,
tachyarrhythmias, pyloric stenosis, thyrotoxicosis, GI obsruction, paralytic ileus, severe
ulcerative colitis, toxic megacolon, myasthenia gravis

Adenosine	Group IA, EHL < 10s, PRC C, Lact:?
Adenocard *Inj 3mg/ml*	**SVT:** 6mg IV as rapid bolus; if tachycardia persists after 1-2min then 12mg IV; **CH : SV arrhythmias conversion:** ini 0.05mg/kg IV as rapid bolus, then 0.05-0.1mg/kg IV, max 12mg/dose; DARF: not req

Amiodarone	Group III, EHL 28-107d, PRC D, Lact -
Cordarone *Tab 200mg, Inj 50mg/ml* **Generics** *Tab 200mg, Inj 50 mg/ml*	**Ventricular arrhythmias:** ini 150mg IV over 10min, then 360mg over 6h (1mg/min), hen 540mg IV over 18h (0.5mg/min); or 800-1600mg/d div qd-bid for 1-3 wk, then 600-800mg/d div qd-bid for 1 mo, then maint 200-400mg/d; DARF: not req

Atropine	EHL 4h, PRC C, Lact ?
Generics *Inj 0.1, 0.3, 0.4, 0.6, 1 mg/ml*	**Bradycardia, bradyarrhythmia:** 0.5-1.0 mg IV q3-5min, max 0.03-0.04mg/kg; **CH** 0.02mg/kg IV, minimum 0.1mg, max 0.5mg IV; **antimuscurinic:** 0.4-0.6mg IM/IV/SC q4-6h prn; **asystolic arrest:** 1mg IV, repeat q3-5min, max 0.04mg/kg; **organophosphate poisoning:** 1-2mg IM/IV q5-60min until symptoms disappear

Bretylium	EHL 7-11h, PRC C, Lact +
Generics *Inj 50mg/ml*	**Ventricular arrhythmias.:** ini 5 mg/kg IV over 1 min, if arrhythmia persists, 10 mg/kg IV over 1 min, and repeat PRN, max 30-35 mg/kg; maint 5-10 mg/kg q6-8 h IV/IM; **CH:** ini 5 mg/kg IV, attempt electrical defibrillation; if persists repeat PRN with 10 mg/kg, max 30 mg/kg; maint 5 mg/kg IM/IV q6 hours; DARF: CrCl 10-50 mL/min 25%-50% , ClCr <10 mL/min: 25% .

Digoxin	EHL 1.3-2.2d, PRC C, Lact +
Digoxin pediatric *Inj 0.05mg/ml* **Lanoxin** *Tab 0.0625, 0.125, 0.25mg, Ped elixir 0.05mg/ml* **Generics** *Inj 0.05, 0.25mg/ml*	**AF, heart failure:** ini 0.5mg IV, then 0.25mg q6h for 2 doses or ini 0.5-0.75mg PO then 0.125mg-0.375mg PO q6-8h until effect, maint 0.125-0.375mg PO/IV qd; **CH** 5-10 y: ini 20- 35mcg/kg PO div q6-8h, maint 25-35% of loading dose; DARF: GFR (ml/min) 10-50: 25-75% or q36h, <10: 10-25% or q48h

Sotalol	Group III, EHL 7-18h, PRC B, Lact ?
Sotacor *Tab 80mg, 160mg* **Generics** *Tab 80mg, 160mg*	**AF, ventricular arrhythmia:** ini 80mg PO bid, maint 160- 320mg/d div bid; DARF: CrCl 30-60: 50%, 10-30: 25%, <10: avoid

2.13   Cardiac Glycosides

MA: inhibition of active Na^+-K^+-transport into heart muscle cells $\Rightarrow$ intracellular $Na^+\uparrow$ $\Rightarrow$ Na^+-Ca^{2+} exchange $\Rightarrow$ intracellular $Ca^{2+}\uparrow$, vagal nerve activity$\uparrow$, sympathetic activity$\downarrow$

EF: pos. inotropic, stroke volume $\uparrow$, higher efficiency of the insufficient heart, tissue perfusion $\uparrow$, coronary perfusion $\uparrow$, neg. chronotropic and dromotropic, refractory time at S-A node $\uparrow$, at the myocardial $\downarrow$, $\Rightarrow$ activation of ectopic pacemakers, pos. bathmotropic

AE: AV block, arrhythmias, extrasystoles, allergic reaction, allergic dermatitis, skin rash, N/V, diarrhea, blurred vision, visual halos, confusion

CI: AV block II°-III°, WPW-syndrome, VT, carotid sinus syndrome, hypertrophic obstructive cardiomyopathy, myocardial ischemia, acute MI, pacemakers, hypercalcemia, hypokalemia, thoracic aortic aneurysm, V. fib.

Digoxin	EHL 1.3-2.2d, PRC C, Lact +
Digoxin pediatric *Inj 0.05mg/ml* **Lanoxin** *Tab 0.0625, 0.125, 0.25mg,* *Ped elixir 0.05mg/ml* **Generics** *Inj 0.05, 0.25mg/ml*	**AF, heart failure:** ini 0.5mg IV, then 0.25mg q6h for 2 doses or ini 0.5-0.75mg PO then 0.125mg-0.375mg PO q6-8h until effect, maint 0.125-0.375mg PO/IV qd; **CH** 5-10 y: ini 20- 35mcg/kg PO div q6-8h, maint 25-35% of loading dose; DARF: GFR (ml/min) 10-50: 25-75% or q36h, <10: 10-25% or q48h
Digoxin-Immune Fab	EHL 15-20h, PRC C, Lact +
Digibind *Inj 38mg/vial*	**Digoxin/digitoxin-intoxication:** **average-dose:** 400mg IV; 40mg will bind 0.5-0.6mg digoxin or digitoxin

2.14   Phosphodiesterase Inhibitors

MA: inhibition of phosphodiesterase ⇒ intracellular accumulation of cAMP ⇒ intracellular Ca^{++} ↑ ⇒ myocardial contractility ↑
EF: pos. inotropic effect (stroke volume, cardiac output ↑), pos. chronotropic effect, vasodilation (preload ↓, afterload ↓), bronchodilation
AE: cholestasis, nausea, hypotension, tachyarrhythmias, thrombocytopenia, splenomegaly, vasculitis, myositis, lung infiltration
CI: hypersensativity to drug

Milrinone	EHL 1-3h, PRC C, Lact ?
Primacor Inj 1mg/ml	**Heart failure:** ini 50mcg/kg IV over 10min, maint 0.375- 0.75mcg/kg/min; DARF: GFR (ml/min). 41-50: 0.43*, 31- 40: 0.38, 21-30: 0.33*, 11-20: 0.28*, 6-10: 0.23*, <5: 0.2* (* = mcg/ kg/min)

2.15   Antilipidemics
2.15.1   Bile Acid Sequestrants

MA/EF: intestinal binding of bile acids ⇒ interruption of the biliary cycle
⇒ bile acid production from cholesterol ↑ ⇒ serum cholesterol ↓; LDL-receptor activity ↑
⇒ LDL-resorption of the liver ↑ ⇒ serum cholesterol ↓
AE: constipation, abdominal discomfort/pain, nausea, diarrhea, resorption failure of drugs and fat-soluble vitamins
AE (colestipol): constipation, fat soluble vitamin deficiency, N/V, flatulence, abdominal distention; **AE (cholestyramine):** constipation, abdominal discomfort/pain, flatulence, N/V, bleeding tendencies due to hypoprothrombinemia
CI: bile duct obstruction
CI (colestipol): hypersensitivity to colestipol products, complete biliary obstruction, phenylketonurics
CI (cholestyramine): complete biliary obstruction, hypersensitivity to bile-sequestering resins

Colestipol	EHL no data, PRC , Lact +
Colestid Tab 1g, Granules (oral) 5g/pkt	**Hypercholesterolemia:** Tab: ini 2g PO qd/bid, max 16g/ d; Gran: ini 5g PO qd/bid, incr by 5g increments at 1-2 mo intervals, max 30g/d; DARF: not req

Cholestyramine	EHL no data, PRC C, Lact ?
Novo-Cholamine *Powder (oral) 4g/packet* **Novo-Cholamine Light** *Powder (oral)* *4g/packet* **Questran** *Powder (oral) 4g/9g* **Questran Light Sugar Free** *Powder (oral)* *4g/scoop* **Generics** *Powder (oral) 4g/packet*	**Hypercholesterolemia:** ini 4g PO qd, maint 4g 1-6 times/d, max 24g/d; DARF: not req

2.15.2 Cholesterol Absorption Inhibitors

MA/EF (ezetimib): inhibition of the intestinal absorption of cholesterol ad related phytosterols; **AE** (ezetimib): fatigue, pharyngitis, sinusitis, abd. pain, diarrhea, back pain, arthralgia, cough, viral infection; **CI** (ezetimib): hypersensitivity to e., hepatic dysfunction

Ezetimibe	EHL 22h, PRC C, Lact -
Ezetrol *Tab 10mg*	**Primary hypercholesterolemia, homozyg.** **fam. hyperchol., homozyg. sitosterolemia:** 10mg PO qd, may be administered with an HMG-CoA reducatse inhibitor; DARF: not req

2.15.3 HMG-CoA Reductase Inhibitors ("Statins")

MA: competitive inhibition of HMG CoA reductase; **EF:** intracellular cholesterol synthesis ↓, LDL↓, HDL ↑;
AE: skin reactions, myopathy, vasculitis, headache, abdominal pain, transaminases↑, dyssomnia; **AE** (atorvastatin): headache, liver enzymes↑, abdominal pain;
AE (fluvastatin): dyspepsia, diarrhea, abdominal pain, nausea, headache;
AE (lovastatin): headache, rhabdomyolysis, diarrhea, hepatotoxicity;
AE (pravastatin): GI disturbances, liver enzymes↑, headache, weakness, flu- like symptoms;
AE (simvastatin): headache, GI upset, rhabdomyolysis, transient hypotension, liver dysfunction
CI: hepatic diseases, pregnancy, lactation, hypersensitivity to product ingredients
CI (rosuvastatin): cyclosporine use

Atorvastatin	EHL 14h, PRC X, Lact ?
Lipitor *Tab 10mg, 20mg, 40mg, 80mg*	**Hypercholesterolemia, mixed** **dyslipidemia:** ini 10-20mg PO qd, maint 10-80mg PO qd, depending on lipid levels; DARF: not req

Fluvastatin	EHL < 3 h, PRC X, Lact ?
Lescol *Cap 20mg, 40mg*	**Hypercholesterolemia:** ini 20-40mg PO qd, max 80mg/ d, give 80mg in div doses bid

Lovastatin	EHL no data, PRC X, Lact ?
Mevacor *Tab 20mg, 40mg* **Generic** *Tab 20mg, 40mg*	**Hypercholesterolemia:** ini 20mg PO qd, maint 10-80mg/ d PO

Pravastatin	EHL 2.6-3.2 h, PRC X, Lact ?
Pravachol *Tab 10mg, 20mg, 40mg* **Generics** *Tab 10mg, 20mg, 40mg*	**Hypercholesterolemia:** ini 10-20mg PO qd, maint 10-40 mg/d; DARF: ini 10mg PO qd

Simvastatin	EHL no data, PRC X, Lact ?
Zocor *Tab 5mg, 10mg, 20mg, 40mg, 80mg*	**Hypercholesterolemia:** ini 20-40mg PO qd, maint 10-80mg/d; DARF: ini 5mg PO qd

Rosuvastatin	EHL 19h, PRC X, Lact ?
Crestor *Tab 10mg, 20mg, 40mg*	**Hypercholesterolemia:** ini 10 PO qd, maint 10-40mg/d

2.15.4 Fibric Acids

MA/EF: lipoprotein lipase activity↑ ⇒ triglycerides↓, LDL↓, HDL↑
AE: myalgia, rhabdomyolysis, N/V, transaminases↑, cholelithiasis, ventricular dysrhythmia, blood count changes; **AE** (clofibrate): diarrhea, flatulence, headache; **AE** (fenofibrate): rash, LFT↑; **AE** (gemfibrozil): epigastric pain, xerostomia, diarrhea, myopathy, hepatotoxicity; **CI:** primary biliary cirrhosis, great caution in children; **CI** (fenofibrate): severe hepatic or renal disease, gallbladder disease, hypersensitivity to fenofibrate; **CI** (gemfibrozil): hypersensitivity to gemfibrozil, gallbladder disease/biliary cirrhosis, severe liver/kidney disease, type I hyperlipoproteinemia
CI (bezafibrate): hepatic or renal impairment, PBC, lactation, type I hyperlipoproteinemia

Bezafibrate	EHL 1-2h, PRC X, Lact ?
Bezalip *Tab sust. rel 400mg* **Generics** *Tab 200mg*	**Hypercholesterolemia type IIa, IIb, mixed/Hypertriglyceridemia type IV, V:** 200mg PO bid-tid or sust. rel. 400mg PO qd; CrCl 40-60ml/min 200 bid, 15-40 200 qod to qd, <15 200mg q3d

Fenofibrate	EHL 20-22h, PRC C, Lact -
Apo-Feno-Micro *Cap 67mg, 200mg* **Generics** *Cap 100mg* **Gen, PMS-Fenofibrate Micro** *Cap 200mg* **Lipidil Supra** *Tab 100mg, 160mg* **Novo-Fenofibat** *Cap 67, 200mg*	**Hypertriglyceridemia:** ini 160mg PO qd, maint 100- 200mg PO qd

Gemfibrozil	EHL 1.5 h, PRC C, Lact -
Lopid *Cap 300mg, Tab 600mg* **Generics** *Cap 300mg, Tab 600mg*	**Hypertriglyceridemia:** 600mg PO bid

2.15.5 Nicotinic Acid

MA/EF: blockage of the triacylglycerol lipase $\Rightarrow$ lipoprotein lipase activity↑ $\Rightarrow$ triglycerides ↓, cholesterol ↓
AE: flush, a sensation of warmth in face, neck, and ears, GI disturbances, glucose tolerance↓, fasting blood sugar↑, pruritus, hepatotoxicity, feeling of restlessness, headache, hypotension, rash, tingling, itching, and dry skin
CI: acute CVS failure, hypersensitivity to niacin, active liver/peptic ulcer disease

Niacin	EHL 10h, PRC C, Lact ?
Niacin/Niacinamide *Tab 500mg* **Generics** *Tab 500mg*	**Hyperlipoproteinemia/hyperlipidemia:** ini 100mg PO tid incr slowly to 3g/d, max 6g/d; ext.rel.: 375mg PO qd for 1wk, then 500mg PO qd for 1wk, then 750mg PO qd for 1wk, then 1000mg PO qd; max 2g/d

3. Hematology

3.1 Plasma Expanders

MA/EF (dextran): high molecular weight polysaccharides with water-binding capability and intravascular retention ⇒ plasma volume↑
AE (albumin): hypersensitivity (shaking, chills, urticaria)
AE (dextran): allergic to anaphylactic reactions, great amounts of low-molecular-weight dextran can be nephrotoxic
AE (pentastarch): coagulopathy
CI (blood plasma substitutes): states of hyperhydration, hypervolemia, serious cardiac insufficiency, pulmonary edema, known allergy to active ingredients
CI (dextran): hypersensitivity to dextran or corn products, hemostatic defects, cardiac decompensation
CI (albumin): hypersensitivity to albumin, severe anemia, heart failure
CI (pentastarch): hypersensitivity to pentastarch, severe RF, CHF, bleeding DO

Albumin	EHL 15-20d, PRC C
Plasbumin *Inj (5%) 50ml vial, 250ml vial, 500ml vial, (25%) 20ml vial, 50ml vial, 100ml vial*	**Hypovolemia:** 0.5-1g/kg/dose, repeat prn, max 6g/kg/d, max 5ml/min for 5% and 1-2ml/min for 25%; **hypoproteinemia:** 0.5-1g/kg/dose, repeat q1-2d bases on loses

Dextran	EHL 41min, PRC C, Lact ?
Gentran 40 *Inj 100mg dextran 40/ml* **Gentran 70** *Inj 60mg dextran 70/ml*	**Shock, hypovolemia:** Dextran 40, 10% Sol: ini 10ml/kg IV as rapid inf, max 20ml/kg on the 1st d, thereafter 10ml/ kg/d for max 4d

Pentastarch	70% elimination in 24hrs, PRC C, Lact ?
Pentaspan *Inj 10g/100ml*	**Shock, hypovolemia:** 500-2000ml IV, max 28ml/kg/d

3.2 Anticoagulants

3.2.1 Unfractionated Heparin

MA/EF: forming complexes with antithrombin-III ⇒ inhibiting effect of antithrombin-III ↑ (by a factor of 1000) ⇒ inhibition of thrombin, factors Xa, XIa, XIIa, and callicrein ⇒ thrombin activated conversion of fibrinogen to fibrin ↓; activat. of the lipoprot. lipase

AE: hemorrhage complications, allergic reactions, anaphylaxis, osteoporosis, cutaneous necrosis, hair loss, thrombocytopenia

CI: heparin allergy, heparin induced thrombocytopenia (type II), active bleeding, imminent abortion, lumbar puncture, epidural anesthesia, hemophilia, ITP, severe liver damage

Heparin Sodium	EHL 2.13h, PRC C, Lact +
Heparin Leo Inj 100U/ml, 1000U/ml, 10000U/ml, 25000U/ml **Heparin Lock Flush** Inj 10U/ml, 100U/ml **Hepalean** Inj 1000U/ml, 10000U/ml, 25000U/ml **Hepalean–LOK** Inj 10U/ml, 100U/ml **Generics** Inj 2U/ml, 40U/ml, 50U/ml, 100 U/ml	**DVT, pulmonary vembolism Tx:** ini 80 U/kg IV, maint 18 U/kg/h IV, adjust dose based on PTT; **DVT PRO:** 5000 U SC q8-12h; **CH:** ini 50 U/kg IV, maint 10-25 U/kg/h IV, adjust dose based on PTT

3.2.2 Low-Molecular-Weight Heparins, Heparinoids

MA/EF (low-molecular-weight heparins): molecular weight ↓ ⇒ thrombin inhibition ↓, factor Xa inhibition ↑; effect on blood platelet function ↓, antithrombotic effect ↑, danger of hemorrhage ↓; neutralization ↓ through platelet factor 4; when used subcutaneously bioavailability ↑, half-life ↑;

MA/EF: (argatroban): specific and reversible direct thrombin inhibitor;

MA/EF: (danaparoid): = heparinoid, factor Xa inhibition;

MA/EF: (fondaparinux): selectivly binding to antithrombin III ⇒ activation of the innate neutralization of factor Xa;

MA/EF: (lepirudine): = recombined hirudin, direct inhibition of thrombin, prevention of thromboembolic diseases

AE/CI (low-molecular-weight heparins): see heparin →48

AE (argatroban): bleeding, hypotension, fever, cardiac arrest, ventricular tachycardia, diarrhea, nausea, allergic reactions;

AE (danaparoid): bleeding, tachycardia, chest pain, hyperkalemia, inj site hematoma;

AE (fondaparinux): bleeding, anemia, fever, edema, local irritation;

AE (lepirudine): bleeding, anemia, abnormal LFT, allergic reactions

CI (LMWH, dalteparin, enoxaparin, nadroparin, tinzaparin): uncontrolled active bleeding, severe HTN, hemmorhagic stoke, hypersensativity to pork, history of HIT;
CI (nadroparin): hypersensitivity to nadroparin, acute infectious endocarditis, severe hemorrhagic diathesis/states, Nadr induced thrombocytopenia
CI (argatroban): active major bleeding, hypersensitivity to argatroban
CI (danaparoid): hypersensitivity to danaparoid, severe hemorrhagic diathesis/states, IM route, bacterial endocarditis, major blood clotting disorder, active PUD, hemorrhagic CVA or retinopathy, severe HTN, surgery involving brain/spine/eyes/ears
CI (fondaparinux): severe renal impairment, endocarditis, weight <50kg, thrombocytopenia, bacterial endocarditis, active bleeding
CI (lepirudine): hypersensitivity to hirudin products

Argatroban	EHL 39-51min, PRC B, Lact ?
Argatroban *Inj 100mg/ml*	**DVT PRO and Tx in heparin-associated thrombocytopenia:** 2mcg/kg/min, adjust dose based on aPTT, max 10mcg/kg/min; DARF not req
Dalteparin	EHL 2-5h, PRC B, Lact ?
Fragmin *Prefilled syr. 2500 U/0.2ml, 5000 U/0.2ml, 7500U/0.3ml, 10000U/0.4ml, 12500U/0.5ml, 15000U/0.6ml, 18000U/0.72ml, Inj10000 U/ml, 25000U/ml*	**DVT PRO, hip replacement:** ini 5000 U SC night preop, then 2500 U 6h after first dose, then 5000 U SC qd for 14d; **DVT PRO, gen. surgery:** ini 2500 U SC 1-2h preop, then 2500 U qd postop for 5-7d; **hip surgery:** 5000 U SC night preop then phs for 5-7d or 2500 U SC 1-2h preop and 8-12h later, then 5000 U qam for 5-7d; **DVT tx:** 200U/kg SC qd, max 18000U/d; **unstable angina or NQWMI:** 120 U/kg max 10000 U SC q12h for 5-8d; **anticoagulation, dialysis:** 5000 U into the arterial line
Danaparoid	EHL 1h, PRC B, Lact ?
Organan-DVT *Inj 750U/0.6ml* **Organan-HIT** *Inj 750U/0.6ml*	**DVT PRO (ortho., thorac., major surg.):** ini 750 U SC 1-4h preop, then 750 U SC q12h upto 14d; **DVT PRO (stoke patient):** ini 1000 U IV bolus then 750 U SC bid for 7-14d; **DVT/PE Tx (HIT):** 2250-2500 IV bolus then 400 U/h for 4h, then 300 U/h for 4 h, then 150-200U/h for 5-7d; DARF req

Enoxaparin	EHL 4.5h (range 3-6h), PRC B, Lact ?
Lovenox *Inj 10mg/0.1ml, 30mg/0.3ml, 40mg/0.4ml, 60mg/0.6ml, 80mg/0.8ml, 100mg/ml, 120mg/0.8ml, 150mg/1ml*	**DVT PRO, hip/knee replacement:** 30mg SC q12h ini 12-24h postop for 7-14d; **DVT PRO abd., gyne surgery:** ini 40mg SC 2h preop, then 40mg SC qd for 7-10d; **Tx of DVT:** 1.5mg/ kg SC qd or 1mg/kg SC q12h, max 180mg/d; **unstable angina or NQWMI:** 1mg/kg SC q12h for 2-8d with ASA, max 100mg/dose; DARF req
Fondaparinux	EHL 17-21h, PRC B, Lact ?
Arixtra *Inj 2.5mg/0.5ml*	**DVT PRO, hip/knee replacement**: ini 2.5mg SC6-8h postop, then 2.5mg qd; DARF: GFR (ml/min) <30: contraind.
Lepirudine	EHL 1.3h, PRC B, Lact ?
Refludan *Inj 50mg/vial*	**Heparin-associated thrombocytopenia with VTE:** ini 0.4mg/kg bolus IV, max 44mg, maint 0.15mg/kg/h IV, max 16.5mg/ h; **ACS:** ini 0.4mg/kg IV bolus then 0.15mg/kg/h x 72h, max 40mg bolus, max 15mg/h infusion; DARF ini 0.2mg/kg bolus IV, then GFR (ml/min): 45-60: 0.075mg/kg/h; 30-44: 0.045mg/kg/h; 15-29: 0.0225mg/ kg/h; <15, dialysis: 0.1mg/kg IV qod
Nadroparin	EHL 6h, PRC B, Lact -
Fraxiparine *Inj 9500U/ml, 1900U/0.2ml, 2850U/0.3ml, 3800U/0.4ml, 5700U/0.6ml, 7600U/0.8ml, 9500U/ml* **Fraxiparine Forte** *Inj 19000U/ml, 11400U/0.6ml, 15200U/0.8ml*	**DVT PRO:** 2850U SC 2-4h preop then qd for atleast 7d; **DVT PRO, hip surgery:** 38U/kg SC 12h before and 12h after surgery then qd X 3d, then 57U/kg SC qd; **DVT tx:** 171U/kg SC qd, max 17100U/d; **UA,NQWMI:** 86 U/kg IV bolus, then 86 U/kg SC q12h with ASA

Tinzaparin	EHL 3-4h, PRC B, Lact ?
Innohep *Inj 10000U/ml, 20000 U/ml*	**DVT Tx with or without pulmonary embolism:** 175U/ kg SC qd; **DVT PRO, gen. surgery:** 3500U SC 2h preop then qd for 7-10d; **hip surg:** 50U/kg SC 2h preop then SC qd for 7-10d; **knee surg.:** 75U/kg SC qd postop for 7-10d; DARF req caution

3.2.3   Heparin Antidote

MA/EF: forming of a salt-like bond with heparin ⇒ inactivation of heparin
AE: hypotension, bradycardia, hypersensitivity reactions;
CI: hypersensitivity to protamine products; Note: severe hypotension/ anaphylactoid reaction with too rapid administration; allergic reactions in fish allergy, previous exposure to protamine (including insulin); risk of allergy unclear in infertile/vasectomized men with anti-protamine antibodies

Protamine	EHL no data, PRC C, Lact ?
Generics *Inj 10mg/ml*	**Heparin overdose (usual rule):** 1mg antagonizes approx. 90 U of beef heparin or 115U porcine heparin, max rate 50mg/10min; max 1x dose 50mg

3.2.4   Oral Anticoagulants

MA/EF (warfarin): inhibition of the vitamin K negotiated carboxylation of Ca^{2+} dependant blood clotting factors (II, VII, IX, X) in the liver
MA/EF (ancrod): thrombin-like enzyme from venom of the Malayan Pit Viper, enzymatically cleaves fibrinogen
MA/EF (AT-III): inactivation of thrombin, IXa, Xa, XIa, XIIa, and plasmin.
MA/EF (nicoumalone): inhibition of the vitamin K, inhibits formation of prothrombin, VII IX, X, protein C
AE: hemorrhage complications, skin necrosis, urticaria
CI: pregnancy, blood dyscrasias, recent CNS/eye surgery, hemmorhagic stroke, pericarditis/pericardial effusion, bacterial endocarditis, unsupervised patients, thrombocytopenia, GI ulcers, retinopathy, arterial brain aneurysms, severe HTN

Antithrombin III	EHL 2.5d, PRC B, Lact ?
Thrombate III *Inj 500U/vial, 1000U/vial*	**AT III deficiency:** individualized dosing

---

Warfarin

EHL 20-60h, PRC X, Lact +

Coumadin *Tab 1mg, 2mg, 2.5mg, 3mg, 4mg, 5mg, 6mg, 10mg, Inj 5.4mg/vial*
Generics *Tab 1mg, 2mg, 2.5mg, 3mg, 4mg, 5mg, 6mg, 7.5mg, 10mg*

Anticoagulation: ini 2-5mg PO qd for 2-4d, maint 2-10mg/d PO, adjust dose to PT/INR (PT: 1.2-2 times control)

3.3   Thrombolytics

MA/EF: activation of plasminogen ⇒ formation of plasmin ⇒ Plasmin proteolyses fibrin ⇒ dissolution of not yet fully organized blood clots (Streptokinase forms a streptokinase-plasminogen-complex ⇒ free plasminogen ⇒ plasmin);
AE: bleeding from wounds, gingival bleeding, hemorrhagic/thromboembolic stroke, internal bleeding, bruising, skin lesions, skin rash, hives, hypotension, fever, allergic reaction, head-/backache, arrhythmias;
Absolute CI (to fibrinolytic therapy): active internal bleeding, other thrombolytic use, CNS neoplasm, AV malformation, aneurysm, CNS procedure/trauma within 2 mo, SAH, intracranial hemmorhage, uncontrolled hypertension (over 180/110), bleeding diathesis, MI due to aortic dissection, allergy to streptokinase/anistreplase; (in acute stroke): seizure at onset of stroke, platelets <100,000/mm3, INR>1.7, PT>15 sec, heparin with 48h preceding onset;
Relative CI (to fibrinolytic therapy): age over 75, cerebrovascular disease, pregnancy or early postpartum, recent major surgery (< 10d), noncompressible vessel puncture, or organ biopsy, recent trauma, including CPR of over 2 min duration, recent GI bleeding, active ulcer disease (< 10d), acute pericarditis or subacute bacterial endocarditis, septic thrombophlebitis, high likelihood of left heart thrombus (e.g. mitral stenosis with atrial fibrillation), known coagulation defects, including anticoagulant therapy, significant hepatic dysfunction, conditions associated with bleeding risks (e.g. diabetic retinopathy), menstruation , terminal cancer or other end-stage disease, recent streptococcal infection, if streptokinase or anistreplase will be used, caution in known hypersensitivity to the drug

---

Alteplase

EHL 26.5-46min, PRC C, Lact ?

Activase rt-PA *Inj 50mg/vial, 100mg/vial*
Cathflo *Inj 2mg/vial*

Acute MI: >67kg: 15mg IV bolus, then 50mg over 30min, then 35mg over 1h; <67kg: 15mg IV bolus, then 0.75mg/ kg over 30min, then 0.5mg/kg over 1h; **acute ischemic stroke:** (within 3h of symptom onset) 0.9mg/kg, max 90mg, over 60min IV, with 10% of total dose admin as IV bolus over 1min; **thrombolysis of central venous device:** 2mg IV x 1

Anistreplase	EHL 70-120min, PRC C, Lact ?
Eminase *Inj 30 U/5ml*	**Acute MI:** 30 U IV over 2-5min
Reteplase	EHL 13-16min, PRC C, Lact ?
Retavase *Inj 10.4 U/vial*	**Acute MI:** 10 U IV over 2min, rep dose in 30min
Streptokinase	EHL 18-83min, PRC C, Lact ?
Streptase *Inj 250000 U/vial, 750000 U/vial, 1500000 U/vial*	**Acute MI:** 1.5 million U IV over 1h; intracoronary: 20,000 U bolus, then 2000-4000 U/min for 30-90min; **pulmonary or arterial embolism/arterial thrombosis:** 250,000 U IV over 30min, then 100,000 U/h IV for 24h; **deep vein thrombosis:** 250,000 U IV over 30min, then 100,000 U/h IV for 72h; DARF not req
Tenecteplase	EHL 17-20min, PRC C, Lact ?
TNKase *Inj 50mg vial*	**Acute MI:** single bolus IV: < 60kg: 30mg 60-69kg: 35mg; 70-79kg: 40mg; 80-89 kg: 45mg; > 90kg: 50mg
Urokinase	EHL < 20min, PRC B, Lact ?
Abbokinase *Inj 5000U/vial, 250000 U/vial*	**Pulmonary embolism:** 4400 U/kg IV over 10min, then 4400 U/kg/h for 12h; occluded IV catheter: 5000 U instilled into catheter, remove after 5min

3.4   Antiplatelets
3.4.1   Glycoprotein IIb-IIIa Inhibitors

MA/EF: antagonist of the glycoprotein IIb-IIIa-receptor on blood platelets ⇒ inhibition of platelet aggregation
AE (abciximab, tirofiban): hemorrhage complications, thrombocytopenia, nausea, fever, headaches;
AE (eptifibatide): bleeding
CI (abciximab, tirofiban): active bleeding, cerebrovascular complications during the last 2 years, operations and traumas during the last 6 wks., intracranial neoplasm, severe HTN, use of dextran, thrombocytopenia, vasculitis, aneurysm, AV anomalies, retinopathy of hypertensive or diabetic origin; **CI (tirofibin)**: pericarditis, cirrhosis
CI (eptifibatide): bleeding DO/surgery/CVA, hypersensitivity to eptifibatide products, severe renal dysfunction, platelet count < 100,000/mm(3);

Abciximab	EHL < 10min, PRC C, Lact ?
Reopro *Inj 2mg/ml*	**Percutaneous coronary intervention:** 0.25mg/kg IV over 1min 10-60min before procedure, then 0.125mcg/ kg/min, max 10mcg/min for 12h; **unstable angina not responding to conventional Tx:** 0.25mg/kg IV over 1min, then 10mcg/min for 18-24h concluding 1h after PTCA
Eptifibatide	EHL 1.13-2.5h, PRC B, Lact ?
Integrilin *Inj 0.75mg/ml, 2mg/ml*	**UA/NQWMI:** ini 180mcg/kg IV, then 2mcg/kg/min up to max 72h; **percutaneous coronary intervention:** ini 180mcg/kg IV before procedure, then 180mcg/kg bolus 10min after 1st bolus, then 2mcg/kg/min IV for 18-24h after the procedure; DARF serum-creatinine (mg/dl) <2: 100%; 2-4: ini 180mcg/kg IV, then 1mcg/kg/min
Tirofiban	EHL 90-180min, PRC B, Lact ?
Aggrastat *Inj 0.25mg/ml, 0.5mg/ml*	**Acute coronary syndrome:** ini 0.4mcg/kg/min IV for 30min, then 0.1mcg/kg/min for upto 48h or until 12-24h after coronary intervention; DARF GFR (ml/min) <30: 50%

3.4.2 Phosphodiesterase/Platelet Aggregation-Adhesion Inhibitors

MA (aspirin): inhibition of cyclooxygenase ⇒ synthesis of thromboxane A2 ↓ (aggregation activator for blood platelets), synthesis of prostacyclin ↓ (aggregation inhibitor in endothelium);
MA (clopidogrel, ticlopidine): blockage of the ADP-receptor of blood platelets;
MA (anagrelide, cilostazol, dipyridamole): inhibition of cAMP phosphodiesterase ⇒ cAMP in platelets ↑ ⇒ inhibition of platelet aggregation
EF: inhibition of platelet aggregation
AE (anagrelide): headache, thrombocytopenia, orthostatic hypotension;
AE (aspirin): allergic reactions, gastric ulcers, skin reactions, dizziness, tinnitus, dysopias, nausea, bronchospasm, alkalosis, acidosis;
AE (clopidogrel): dyspepsia, abdominal pain, constipation, bleeding;
AE (dipyridamole): dizziness, headache, rash, abdominal distress, exacerbation of angina pectoris; **AE** (ticlopidine): agranulocytosis, pancytopenia, allergic skin reactions
CI: hypersensitivity to the drug;
CI (clopidogrel): active bleeding, significant liver impairment, cholestatic jaundice;
CI (aspirin): GI ulcers, hemorrhagic diathesis, great caution with children
CI (ticlopidine): hematopoetic or bleeding disorders, severe liver dysfunction, active bleeding; **CI** (dipyridamole): IV in shock

Acetylsalicylic acid (ASA)	EHL 4.7-9h, PRC D, Lact ?
Asaphen *Tab* 80mg, 81mg **Asaphen E.C.** *Ent. coated tab* 80mg, 81mg **Aspirin** *Tab* 80mg, 325mg, 500mg, *Coated tab* 81mg, 325mg, 500mg *Cap* 325mg, 500mg, 650mg *Coated Cap* 325mg, 500mg, 650mg **Bufferin** *Cap* 325mg, 500mg **Novasen** *Tab* 325mg, 650mg **Generics** *Tab* 325mg	**Ischemic stroke, TIA:** 80-325mg PO qd; **PRO of recurrent MI, unstable angina pectoris:** 80-325mg PO qd; **Acute MI:** ini 160mg chewed/crushed; **Analgesic/antipyretic:** 325-650mg PO q4h prn, ch <12y: 10-15mg/kg PO q6h, max 2.4g/d; **Anti-inflammatory:** 975mg PO q4-6h, ch: 60-125mg/kg/d div q4-6h
Anagrelide	EHL 76h, PRC C, Lact ?
Agrylin *Cap* 0.5mg	**Essential thrombocythemia:** ini 0.5mg PO qid or 1mg PO bid, after 7d incr dose prn, do not increase by more than 0.5mg/d in any 1wk, max 10mg/d or 2.5mg as single dose
Aspirin + Dipyridamole	PRC D, Lact ?
Aggrenox *Cap ext.rel* 25mg + 200mg	**Prevention of stroke/TIA:** 1 Cap PO bid

Clopidogrel	EHL 7-8h, PRC B, Lact ?
Plavix *Tab 75mg*	**PRO of recurrent stroke, MI, peripheral arterial disease:** 75mg PO qd; **ACS:** ini 300mg PO, then 75mg PO qd; DARF not req

Dipyridamole	EHL alpha: 40min, beta: 10h, PRC C, Lact ?
Apo-Dipyridamole FC *Tab 25mg, 50mg, 75mg* **Persantine** *Tab 25mg, 50mg, 75mg, Inj 5mg/ml* **Generics** *Inj 5mg/ml*	**Prevention of thromboembolism after cardiac valve replacement:** 100mg PO qid 1h before meals, max 600mg/d

Ticlopidine	EHL 12.6h, PRC B, Lact ?
Ticlid *Tab 250mg* **Generics** *Tab 250mg*	**Prevention of stroke:** 250mg PO bid

3.5   Antifibrinolytics

MA/EF (aminocaproic acid, tranexamic acid): inhibition of plasminogen activation
AE (aminocaproic acid): hypotension, rash, weakness, myopathy, N/V;
AE (tranexamic acid): thromboembolic events, N/V, diarrhea, giddiness, hypotension;
CI (aminocaproic acid): disseminated intravascular coagulation, thrombosis prone;
CI (tranexamic acid): acquired defective color vision, subarachnoid hemorrhage, active intravascular clotting, SAH

Aminocaproic Acid	EHL 1-5h, PRC C, Lact ?
Amicar *Inj 250mg/ml, Tab 500mg*	**To improve hemostasis when fibrinolysis contributes to bleeding:** ini 5g IV/PO, then then 1-1.25g/h prn; DARF suggested

Tranexamic acid	EHL 3h, PRC C, Lact +
Cyklokapron *Inj 100mg/ml, Tab 500mg* **Generics** *Inj 100mg/ml*	**Conization of cervix:** 2-3 tabs PO q8-12h, 12d postop; **Epistaxis:** 2-3 tabs PO q8-12h for 10d; **Hyphema:** 2-3 tabs PO q8-12h for 7d; **Menorrhagia:** 2-3 tabs PO tid-qid; **Hereditary angioneurotic edema:** 2-3 tabs PO bid-tid; **CH** 25mg/kg, bid-tid

3.6   Hematopoietic Drugs

MA/EF: darbepoetin/erythropoietin ↑ ⇒ production of red cells in bone marrow ↑
MA/EF: filgrastim is a granulocyte colony-stimulating factor (G-CSF) ⇒ activation of hematopoietic elements;
MA/EF (ancestrim): recombinant-methionyl human stem cell factor;
AE (darbepoetin, erythrop.): HTN, headache, arthralgias;
AE (filgrastim) bone pain, flu-like symptoms;
AE (ancestrim): injection site reaction, bone pain, rash, respiratory symptoms
CI: hypersensitivity to the drug; **CI** (darbepoetin, erythropoietin): uncontrolled HTN, children < 2; **CI** (erythropoietin): pure red cell aplasia;
CI (ancestrim, filgrastim): hypersensitivity to E. coli derived proteins, ancestrim
Note: not for immediate correction of anemia; Monitor, control BP in chronic RF, monitor hematocrit twice weekly in chronic RF, once weekly in HIV-infected and CA patients until stable. Consider iron deficiency if no response

Ancestrim	EHL 2-5h, PRC B, Lact ?
Stemgen *Inj 1875 mcg/vial*	**Mobilization of peripheral blood progenitor cells:** 20mcg/kg/d sc, use in combination with filgrastim.
Darbepoetin Alfa	EHL 21h (IV), 49h (SC), PRC C, Lact ?
Aranesp *Inj 10, 20, 30, 40, 50, 60, 80, 100, 150mcg/syringe*	**anemia (CRF):** ini 0.45 mcg/kg IV/SC q week; titrate to hematologic response; **anemia in chemotherapy patients:** ini 2.25 mcg/kg SC q week; titrate to hematologic response
Erythropoietin/epoetin alfa	EHL IV: 4-13h in CRF; SC: 27h, PRC C, Lact ?
Eprex *Prefilled Syr 1000U, 2000U, 3000U, 4000U, 5000U, 8000U, 10000U, 40000U, Inj 20000 U/ml*	**Anemia (chronic RF):** ini 50-100 U/kg IV/SC 3x/wk, adjust dose to maintain target hematocrit (doses range 12.5-525U/kg 3x/wk) **anemia of zidovudine Tx:** 100 U/kg IV/SC 3x/wk x 8wk.; may be incr thereafter prn by 50-100 U/kg 3x/wk up to 300 U/kg 3x/wk; adjust dose based on AZT + hematocrit; **anemia in chemotherapy patients:** ini 150U/kg SC 3x/wk x 8wk, incr thereafter prn up to 300 U/kg 3x/wk DARF: see Prod Info

Filgrastim	EHL 2-7h, PRC C, Lact ?
Neupogen *Inj 300mcg/ml*	**Neutropenia – chemotherapy induced:** 5mcg/kg/d SC, incr prn in increments of 5mcg/kg/d for each cycle according to the duration and severity of the absolute neutrophil count (ANC) nadir; ch see Prod Info
Pegfilgrastim	EHL 15-80h, PCR C, Lact ?
Neulasta *Inj 6mg/syr*	**Neutropenia – chemotherapy induced:** 6mg SC per cycle of chemotherapy

3.7   Hemorheologics

MA/EF: blood viscosity ↓, erythrocyte flexibility ↑, microcirculatory flow ↑, tissue O₂ concentrations ↑; **AE:** GI disturbances, CNS depression, headaches; **CI:** hypersensitivity to pentoxifylline or xanthines, acute MI, severe CAD, PUD, bleeding diathesis

Pentoxifylline	EHL 0.4-1h, PRC C, Lact ?
Trental *Tab ext.rel 400mg* **Generics** *Tab ext.rel 400mg*	**Intermittent claudication:** ini 400mg PO bid-tid with meals

3.8   Other Hematologics

MA/EF, AE, CI (desmopressin): →117 ; **MA/EF** (aprotinin): proteinase (trypsin, chymotrypsin, cathespin, plasmin, kallikrein) inhibitor; **MA/EF** (drotrecogin alfa): recombinant activated protein C; inhibiting factors Va + VIIIa ⇒ antithrombotic effect; TNF-production ↓, leukocyte adhesion to selectins ↓, thrombin-induced inflammatory responses ↓ ⇒ antiinflammatory effect; **MA/EF** (thrombin): clots fibrinogen of blood
AE (aprotinin): allergic reaction, renal failure; **AE** (drotrecogin alfa): bleeding;
AE (thrombin): allergic reaction; **CI** (aprotinin/thrombin): hypersensitivity to drug
CI (drotrecogin alfa): active internal bleeding, hemorrhagic stroke within the last 3mo, intracranial or intraspinal surgery or severe head trauma within the last 2mo, trauma with an increased risk of life-threatening bleeding, presence of an epidural catheter, intracranial neoplasm or mass lesion, or evidence of cerebral herniation, known hypersensitivity, **CI** (desmopressin): Type 2B vWD, **CI** (factor IX): DIC, hyperfibrinolysis
Note (factor VIII, IX): risk of HIV/hepatitis transmission varies by product; factor VIII: reduced response with development of factor VIII inhibitors, hemolysis with large/rep.ed doses in A, B, AB blood type; factor IX: products that contain factors II, VII, and X may cause thrombosis in at-risk patients, stop infusion if signs of DIC

Antihemophilic factor (factor VIII)	EHL 15.8h, PRC C, Lact ?
Kogenate FS Inj 250IU/bottle, 500IU/bottle, 1000IU/bottle **Hekixate FS** Inj 250IU/bottle, 500IU/bottle, 1000IU/bottle **Recombinate** Inj 250IU/bottle, 500IU/bottle, 1000IU/bottle **ReFacto** Inj (moroctocog alfa) 250IU/vial, 500IU/vial, 1000IU/vial	**Hemophilia A:** individualize factor VIII dose; **CH** individualize factor VIII dose
Eptacog alfa (activated factor VII)	EHL 2.3h, PRC C, Lact ?
NiaStase Inj 1.2mg/vial, 2.4mg/vial, 4.8mg/vial	**Hemorrhage in patients with hemophilia A or B with inhibitors to factor VIII or IX:** 70-90 mcg/kg IV q 2h until hemostasis
Aprotinin	EHL 0.7h, PRC B, Lact ?
Trasylol Inj 10 000 KIU/ml	**Hemorrhage due to hyperfibrinolysis:** ini 200,000 to 500,000KIU IV, up to 1,000,000 KIU/d to control bleeding
Desmopressin	EHL IV 75.5min, PRC B, Lact ?
DDAVP Tab 0.1, 0.2mg, Spray (nasal) 10mcg/Spray, Inj 4mcg/ml **DDAVP Rhinyle Nasal Solution** Spray 100mcg/ml **Minirin** Tab 0.1mg, 0.2mg **Octostim** Spray (nasal) 150mcg/Spray Inj 15mcg/ml **Generics** Spray (nasal) 10mcg/Spray	**Hemophilia A, Type 1 von Willebrand's disease:** 10mcg/m2 IV 20-30min, max 20mcg; **CH** 0.3mcg/kg IV over 15-30min; **Diabetes insipidus:** 1-4mcg SC/IM/IV qd; 10-40mcg/d intranasal div qd-tid; 0.1mg PO tid, max 1.2mg/d; **Nocturnal enuresis:** 10-40mcg/d intranasal
Drotrecogin alfa	EHL no data, PRC C, Lact. ?
Xigris Inj 5mg/vial, 20mg/vial	**Severe sepsis:**24mcg/kg/h IV for96h;DARF: not req
Factor IX	EHL 12-17h, PRC B, Lact. ?
Immunine VH Inj 160IU/vial, 240IU/vial, 480IU/vial, 720IU/vial, 960IU/vial, 1440IU/vial	**Hemophilia B:** individualize factor IX dose, **CH** individualize factor IX dose

Gelatine, absorbable	EHL n/a,
Gelfoam *Powder 1g/envelope, Sponge 4cm², 12cm², 100 cm²* **Gelfilm** *Film 12.5cm2*	**Hemostasis**: apply to bleeding site until bleeding stops
Phytonadione (Vitamin K)	EHL 26-193h, PRC C, Lact +
Generics *Inj 2mg, 10mg/ml*	**Hypoprothrombinemia**: 2.5-25mg PO/IM/SC; **Anticoagulant-induced hypoprothrombinemia**: 2.5-10mg PO/SC/ IM; haemorrh. disease of the newborn: PRO: 0.5-1mg IM 1h after birth; Tx: 1mg SC/ IM

4.   Respiratory

4.1   Bronchodilators
4.1.1   Systemic Beta Adrenergic Agonists

MA/EF: (orciprenaline) nonselective beta-adrenergic agonists
MA/EF: stimulation of beta-2 receptors ⇒ relaxation of bronchial smooth muscles, mucociliary clearance ↑
AE: N/V, nervousness, tremors, dizziness, drowsiness, anxiety, headache, tachyarrhythmias, extrasystoles, hypertension, angina pectoris, N/V
CI: hypertrophic obstructive cardiomyopathy, cardiac arrhythmias; hypersensitivity to the drug

Orciprenaline	EHL 3-6 h, PRC C, Lact ?
Alupent *Syrup 10mg/5ml* **Orcipren** *Syrup 10mg/5ml* **Generics** *Syrup 10mg/5ml*	**Asthma/COPD:** Syrup 20mg PO tid or qid; **CH** 4-12yrs 10mg PO tid, >12yrs. 20mg PO tid
Salbutamol	EHL 4h, PRC C, Lact ?
Apo-Salvent *Tab 2mg, 4mg* **Ventolin** *Inj 500mcg/ml, 1000mcg/ml* *Oral soln 0.4mg/ml* **Ventolin Rotacaps** *Cap 200mcg, 400mcg* **Generics** *Tab 2mg, 4mg*	**Asthma/COPD:** 2-4mg PO tid-qid, max 16mg PO/d, IV: 5mcg/min, incr to 10mcg/min, max 20mcg/min, IM: 500mcg (8mcg/kg) q4h, max 20mg/d; **CH** asthma 2-6 y: 0.1mg/kg PO tid-qid, 6-12 y: 2mg PO tid-qid, max 8mg/d

4.1.2   Inhaled Alpha-Beta Adrenergic Agonists

MA/EF: stimulation of alpha- and beta-adrenergic receptors ⇒ relaxation of bronchial smooth muscles, mucosal vasoconstriction

Epinephrine racemic	EHL 4h, PRC C, Lact ?
Vaponefrin *Sol (inhal) 2.25%*	**Bronchospasm:** 0.5ml nebulized q3-4h; **Croup, CH** <4 y: 0.05ml/kg nebulized q2-4h, max 0.5ml/dose q1-2h

4.1.3   Inhaled Beta Adrenergic Agonists

MA/EF: selective stimulation of ß$_2$-receptors ⇒ bronchial muscles relax, mucociliar clearance ↑; **MA/EF:** (orciprenaline) nonselective beta-agonist;
MA/EF: see Systemic Beta Adrenergic Agonists →61;
AE: nervousness, dizziness, dry mouth/throat, tachycardia, tremors, headache, N/V;
AE: nervousness/tremors, tachycardia, coughing, nausea, headache;
CI: hypersensitivity to the drugs, hypertrophic obsructive cardiomyopathy, cardiac arrhythmias; **CI** (formoterol): lactose allergy, **CI** (salmeterol): hypersensitivity to lecithin, soya, lactose; **CI:** hypersensitivity to the drug
Note: salmeterol: long-acting ß$_2$-sympathomimetic, not for Tx of acute asthmatic reaction

Fenoterol	EHL 2-3h, PRC C, Lact ?
Berotec Inhalation Aerosol *MDI* *100mcg/dose* **Berotec Inhalation Solution** *Sol (inhal)* *1mg/ml, 0.625mg/ml, 0.25mg/ml*	**Asthma/COPD:** 1-2 puffs tid or qid, max 8 puffs/d; 0.5-1mg neb q6h
Formoterol	EHL 12h, PRC C, Lact -
Foradil *Cap 12mcg* **Oxeze Turbuhaler** *MDI 6mcg/dose,* *12mcg/dose*	**Asthma/COPD:** 6-12mcg bid, max 48mcg/d
Terbutaline	EHL 11-26h, PRC B, Lact +
Bricanyl Turbuhaler *MDI 0.5mg/dose*	**Asthma/COPD:** 1 puff prn, max 6 puffs/d
Salbutamol	EHL 4h, PRC C, Lact ?
Airomir *MDI 120mcg/dose* **Apo-Salvent** *Resp. soln 5mg/ml, MDI* *100mcg/dose, Sterules 1mg/ml, 2mg/ml,* *Tab 2mg, 4mg* **Ventolin** *Sol (inhal) 1.25mg/2.5 ml,* *2.5mg/2.5ml, 5mg/2.5ml, 5mg/ml* **Ventolin Diskus** *Inhal 200mcg/blister* **Ventolin HFA** *MDI 100mcg/dose* **Generics** *MDI 100mcg/dose* *Sol (inhal) 5mg/ml, 0.5mg/ml, 1mg/ml,* *2mg/ml*	**Asthma:** MDI: 1-2 puffs q4-6h, max 12 puffs/d; Sol (inhal): 2.5mg diluted in 3ml NS tid-qid; Cap inhal.: 200-400mcg q4-6h via Rotahaler; **PRO of exercise-induced asthma:** 180mcg (2 inhal) by MDI 15min prior to exercise; **CH asthma** MDI >4 y: 1-2 puffs q4-6h; Sol (inhal): 0.1mg/kg diluted in 3ml NS, max 2.5mg tid-qid; Cap inhal.: > 4 y: 200-400mcg q4-6h via Rotahaler
Salmeterol	EHL 5.5h, PRC C, Lact ?
Serevent *Diskhaler disks 50mcg/dose, MDI* *25mcg/dose, Diskus 50mcg/dose*	**Asthma/COPD:** 50mcg inhal bid

4.1.4   Alpha-Beta-Adrenergic Agonists

MA/EF : stimulation of alpha- and beta-adrenergic receptors ⇒ bronchodilation; vasoconstriction, cardiac output ↑ ⇒ BP ↑
AE (ephedrine): CNS stimulation, HTN, palpitations, tremor, N/V
AE (epinephrine): HTN, N/V, headache, arrhythmias
CI: (ephedrine): hypersensitivity to ephedrine, angle closure glaucoma, anesthesia with cyclopropane or halothane, thyrotoxicosis, DM, HTN (in pregnancy), other CVS DO
CI (epinephrine): cardiac dilatation/coronary insufficiency, narrow angle glaucoma, hypersensitivity to epinephrine, shock, intra-arterial injection, labor

Ephedrine	EHL 3-6h, PRC C, Lact ?
Generics *Tab 8mg, 15mg, 30mg, Inj 50mg/ml*	**Asthma:** 25-50mg q3-4h or 25-50mg SC or 5-25mg/dose slow IV, max 150mg/d

Epinephrine	PRC C, Lact ?
Adrenalin *Inj 1mg/ml, Topical 1mg/ml* **Epipen** *Inj (IM) 0.3mg/delivery* **Epipen Jr.** *Inj (IM) 0.15mg/delivery* **Generics** *Inj 0.1mg/ml, 1mg/ml*	**Asthma:** 0.2-0.5ml of 1:1000 Sol (0.2-0.5mg) SC q2h prn, rep q20min for a max of 3 doses. MDI: inhalation of 0.1% to 1% Sol prn

4.1.5   Inhaled Anticholinergics

MA/EF: anticholinergic ⇒ bronchodilating
AE: dry mouth, bitter taste, epistaxis, nasal dryness/congestion
CI: hypersensitivity to the drug, soya lecithin, soybean, peanut

Ipratropium	EHL no data, PRC B, Lact ?
Apo-Ipravent *Sol (inhal) 250mcg/ml, sterules 125mcg/ml, 250mcg/ml* **Atrovent** *MDI 20mcg/puff, Sol (inhal) 250mcg/ml, 125mcg/ml* **Novo-Ipramide** *Sol (inhal) 250mcg/ml* **Generics** *Sol (inhal) 125mcg/ml, 250mcg/ml*	**COPD, bronchospasms:** MDI: 40mcg inhal tid-qid, max 240mcg/d; Sol (inhal): 250-500mcg nebulized q4-6h prn, **CH** 5-12: 125-250mcg inh q4-6h prn

Tiotropium	EHL 5-7d, PRC B, Lact ?
Spiriva *Cap 18mcg*	**COPD:** 18mcg inhal qd

4.1.6   Xanthines/Theophyllines

MMA: inhibition of intracellular phosphodiesterase ⇒ cAMP ↑
EF: bronchial spasmolysis, central stimulation of respiration, positive inotropic and chronotropic, vasodilation (except for brain vessels), diuresis ↑
AE: N/V, tremors, convulsions, nervousness, gastroesophageal reflux, chest pain, tachycardia, palpitations, hypotension, rapid breathing, headache
CI: symptomatic coronary artery disease, PUD, **CI** (oxtriphylline): untreated seizure disorder

Aminophylline (85% theophylline)	EHL no data, PRC C, Lact ?
Phyllocontin *Tab sust. rel.* 225mg, 350mg **Generics** *Sol (oral)* 25mg/ml, 50mg/ml	**Bronchospasm, asthma:** ini 6mg/kg IV over 20-30min., maint 0.5- 0.7mg/kg/h IV inf; 16mg/kg/d PO div q6-8h, max 400mg/d

Oxtriphylline (64% theophylline)	PRC C, Lact +, serum level: 10-20 mcg/ml
Choledyl *Sol (oral)* 100mg/5ml **Generics** *Tab* 100mg, 200mg, 300mg	**Bronchospasm, asthma, COPD:** ini 200-400mg/d div q6-8h; maint 800-1200mg/d; **CH** (10-14 yrs.) ini 22mg/kg/d div q6h x 24h, maint 15-22mg/kg/d div q6h

Theophylline	PRC C, Lact +, serum level: 10-20 mcg/ml
Apo-Theo LA *Tab* 100mg, 200mg, 300mg **Novo-Theophyl SR** *Tab* 100mg, 200mg, 300mg **Theolair** *Sol (oral)* 80mg/ 15ml, *Tab* 125mg **Uniphyl** *Tab ext. rel.* 400mg, 600mg **Generics** *Elixir (oral)* 80mg/15ml, *Inj* 0.8mg/ml, 1.6mg/ml, 4mg/ml	**Asthma:** acute: ini 5mg/kg IV over 20-30min then maint 0.6mg/kg/h IV; 16mg/kg PO in div tid-qid; adjust dose based on serum level, max 400mg/d; DARF not req

4.2   Inhaled Corticosteroids

EF: suppression of inflammatory reactions ⇒ β$_2$-receptor sensitivity ↑
AE: hoarseness, oral and pharyngeal candidosis
CI: lung tuberculosis, fungal or bacterial respiratory tract infections, 1ry treatment of status asthmaticus,
CI (fluticasone): lactose allergy

Beclomethasone	EHL 3h, PRC C, Lact ?
QVar *MDI 50mcg/puff, 100mcg/puff* **Generics** *MDI 50mcg/puff*	**Asthma:** 50-400mcg inhal bid
Budesonide	EHL 2-3h, PRC C, Lact ?
Pulmicort Turbuhaler *Powder (inhal)* *100mcg/inhal., 200mcg/inhal. ,* *400mcg/inhal., Nebuamp 0.125mg/ml,* *0.25mg/ml, 0.5mg/ml*	**Asthma:** 200-400mcg inhal bid, max 2400mcg/d; 1-2mg neb bid; ch 6-12 y: 100-200mcg inhal bid; 0.25-0.5mg neb bid
Fluticasone	EHL 7.8h, PRC C, Lact ?
Flovent *MDI 50, 125, 250mcg/puff,* *Diskus (inhal) 50, 100, 250, 500mcg/inhal.*	**Asthma maint:** MDI/Diskus: 100-500mcg bid, max 1000mcg bid; **CH** 4-16 y: 50-100mcg bid, max 200mcg bid

4.3   Asthma/COPD Combinations

Budesonide + Formoterol	
Symbicort Turbuinhaler *MDI 100+6mcg/inhal, 200+6mcg/inhal*	**Asthma, COPD:** 100+6mcg - 200+6mcg q12h
Fluticasone + Salmeterol	
Advair Diskus *Powder (inhal)* *0.1+0.05mg/inhal., 0.25+0.05mg/inhal.,* *0.5+0.05mg/ inhal.*	**Asthma:** maint inhalation of 0.1-0.5 + 0.05mg q12h
Ipratropium Bromide + Fenoterol	
Duovent UDV *Sol (inhal)* *0.125mcg + 0.3125mg / ml*	**Asthma, COPD:** 4ml q6h prn
Ipratropium Bromide + Salbutamol	
Combivent *MDI 0.020 + 0.120mg/puff,* *Sol (inhal) 0.5 + 3mg/2.5ml*	**COPD:** 2 puffs qid; max 12 puffs/d

4.4   Leukotriene Inhibitors

MA: blockage of leukotriene receptors
EF: bronchial dilatation, decrease of bronchial hyperreactivity
AE: headache, fever, diarrhea, nausea, sinusitis

Montelukast	EHL 2.7-5h, PRC B, Lact -
Singulair Tab 10mg, Tab (chew) 4mg, 5mg, Granules 4mg/packet	**Asthma:** 10mg PO qhs; **CH** 2-5 y: 4mg PO qhs; 6-14 y: 5mg PO qhs
Zafirlukast	EHL 10h, PRC B, Lact -
Accolate Tab 20mg	**Asthma:** 20mg PO bid (1h ac or 2h pc)

4.5   Mucolytics, Expectorants

MA/EF (acetyl cysteine): splits disulfide bridges in protein part of mucus molecules
⇒ sputum viscosity ↓
AE (acetyl cysteine): allergic skin reactions, nausea, heartburn
AE (guaifenesin): dizziness, headache, N/V, rash, urticaria
CI (acetyl cysteine): restricted use in children < 1
CI (guaifenesin): hypersensitivity to guaifenesin products

Acetylcysteine	EHL 11min-2.27h, PRC B, Lact ?
Mucomyst Sol (inhal) 20% **Parvolex** Sol (inhal) 200mg/ml **Generics** Inj 200mg/ml	**Mucolytic:** nebulization of 1-10ml (20%) or 2-20ml (10%) q2-6h prn; intratracheal instillation: 1-2ml ET (10- 20%) prn up to qh
Guaifenesin	EHL 1h, PRC C, Lact ?
Balminil Expectorant Syrup 100mg/5ml **Benylin E Extra Strength** Syrup 200mg/5ml **Robitussin** Syrup 100mg/5ml	**Expectorant:** 100-400mg PO q4h or 600-1200mg PO q12h (ext.rel), max 2.4g/d; ch >12y: adult dose, 6-11y: 100-200mg PO q4h or 600mg PO q12h (ext.rel), max 1.2g/d, 2-5y: 50-100mg PO q4h or 300mg PO q12h (ext.rel), max 600mg/d

4.6   Mast Cell Stabilizers

MA/EF: stabilization of mast cell membranes ⇒ mediator release ↓
AE: bad taste, nausea, ocular burning, nasal congestion, cough
CI: hypersensitivity to the drug

Cromolyn Sodium	EHL 80-90min, PRC B, Lact ?
Intal *MDI 1mg/puff1 (inhal),* Spincaps *20mg/cartridge* **Nalcrom** *Cap 100mg* **Generics** *Sol (inhal) 1%*	**Asthma:** MDI: ini 2mg inhal. qid, maint 2mg q4-6h; Spincaps: 20mg inhal qid

Ketotifen	EHL 3-5h, PRC C, Lact +
Zaditen *Syrup 1mg/5ml, Tab 1mg* **Generics** *Syrup 1mg/5ml, Tab 1mg*	**Asthma:** ch >3 1mg PO bid, 6m-3y 0.05mg/kg bid

Nedocromil	EHL 1.5-3.3h, PRC B, Lact ?
Tilade *MDI 2mg/puff*	**Asthma:** 2 puffs qid, reduce dose after improvement; **CH** > 6 y: 2 puffs qid, reduce dose after improvement

4.7   Antitussives – Single Ingredient Drugs

MA/EF (dextromethorphan): acts on cough center in medulla oblongata ⇒ threshold for coughing ↑
AE (dextromethorphan): restlessness, hallucination, GI symptoms and skin reactions
AE (chlophedianol): excitation, hyperirritability, nightmares,
AE (hydrocodone): respiratory depression, HTN, sedation, nausea, vomiting
CI (dextromethorphan): advanced respiratory insufficiency, use of MAO inhibitors
CI (codeine): hypersensativity, acute asthma/COPD, resiratory depression, cor pulmonale, acute alcoholism, delerium tremens, severe CNS depression, use of MAO inhibitors, increased ICP, convulsion disorder, **CI** (hydrocodone): intracranial lesion, increased ICP

Codeine phosphate	EHL 2.5-3.5h, PRC C, Lact +
Linctus codeine *Liq (oral) 0.2%* **Generics** *Syrup 5mg/ml, Tab 15mg, 30mg*	**Cough:** 10-20mg PO/ SC q4-6h prn; **CH** > 2y: 0.5-1mg/kg/dose PO/SC/IM q4-6h, 2-6y: 1mg/kg/d PO div qid, max 30mg/ 24h; 6-12y: 5-10mg PO q4-6h prn; max 60mg/24h; DARF: GFR (ml/min) > 50: 100%, 10-50: 75%, <10: 50%

Hydrocodone	EHL 3.8h, PRC C, Lact ?
Hycodan *Syrup 5mg/5ml, Tab 5mg*	**Cough**: 5mg po q4h prn, max 30mg/d, **CH** 2-12y 2.5mg po q4h prnmax 15mg/d, <2y 1.25mg po q4h prn, max 7.5mg/d

Chlophedianol	PRC C, Lact ?
Ulone *Syrup 25mg/5ml*	**Cough**: 25mg po 3-4x/d, **CH** 6-12y 12.5-25mg 3-4x/d, 2-6y 12.5mg po 3-4x/d

Dextromethorphan	EHL 1.5-4h, PRC C, Lact +
Balminil DM *Syrup 15mg/ml* **Benylin DM** *Syrup 15mg/5ml* **Koffex DM** *Syrup 15mg/5ml* **Novahistex DM** *Syrup 15mg/5ml* **Novahistine DM** *Syrup 7.5mg/5ml* **Triaminic Softchew Cough** *Tab (chew) 7.5mg*	**Cough**: 10-20mg po q4h or 30mg po q6-8h prn, max 120mg/d

4.8 Antitussives – Combinations

Ammonium chloride + Codeine + Diphenhydramine

Balminil Codeine Night-Time + **Expectorant** *Syrup 125 + 3.3 + 12.5mg/5ml*	**Cough**: 5-10ml PO q6-8h PRN; **CH**: 6-12y: 2.5-5ml PO q6-8h PRN; max 4 doses/d

Acetaminophen + Diphenhydramine + Pseudoephedrine

Benadryl Total Allergy Regular Strength *Cap 500 + 12.5 + 30mg* **Benadryl Total Allergy Extra Strength** *Cap 500 + 25 + 30mg*	

Acetaminophen + Dextromethorphan + Pseudoephedrine

Triaminic Cough & Sore Throat *Syrup 160 + 7.5 + 15mg/5ml* **Triaminic Softchew Throat Pain & Cough** *Tab (chew) 160 + 5 + 15mg*	**Cough**: (Robitussin) 15ml PO q6-8h PRN; **CH**: (Triaminic) 6-12y: 2 tabs or 10ml PO q6h PRN, 2-6y: 1 tab or 5ml PO q6h PRN; max 4 doses/d

Acetaminophen + Chlorpheniramine + Dextromethorphan + Pseudoephedrine

Triaminic Cold, Cough & Fever *Syrup 160 + 1 + 7.5 + 15mg/5ml*	**Cough**: **CH** 6-12y: 10ml PO q6h PRN, max 4 doses/d

Chlorpheniramine + Dextromethorphan + Pseudoephedrine

Triaminic Cold & Cough *Syrup 1 + 5 + 15mg/5ml* **Triaminic Cold & Night Time Cough** *Syrup 1 + 7.5 + 15mg/5ml* **Triaminic Softchews Cold & Cough** *Tab (chew) 1 + 5 + 15mg*	**Cough: CH** 6-12y: 2 tabs or 10ml PO q6h PRN, max 4 doses/d

Dextromethorphan + Pseudoephedrine

Robitussin Honey Cough & Cold *Syrup 10 + 20mg/5ml* **Triaminic Cough** *Syrup 7.5 + 15mg/5ml* **Triaminic Cough & Congestion** *Syrup 7.5 + 15mg/5ml*	**Cough**: (Robitussin) 15ml PO q6-8h PRN, **CH**: 6-12y: 7.5ml PO q6-8h PRN, 2-6y: 3.75ml PO q6-8h PRN; (Triaminic) **CH**: 6-12y: 10ml PO q6h PRN, 2-6y: 5ml PO q6h PRN; max 4 doses/d

Guaifenesin + Acetaminophen + Dextromethorphan + Pseudoephedrine

Balminil Cough & Flu *Syr 100 + 325 + 15 + 30mg/15ml* **Benylin 1 Cold and Flu** *Cap 100 + 500 + 15 + 30* **Robitussin cough, cold & flu liqui-gels** *Cap 100 + 250 + 10 + 30mg* **Sudafed cold & flu** *Cap 100 + 250 + 10 + 30mg*	**Cough/nasal congestion:** 2 caps PO q4h prn, max 8/d

Guaifenesin + Bismuth

Bismutal *Rectal supp 250 + 150mg*	**Sore throat:** 1 supp prn

Guaifenesin+ Brompheniramine + Codeine + Phenylephrine +Phenylpropanolamine

Dimatane expectorant-C *Syrup 100 + 2 + 10 + 5 + 5mg /5ml* **Dimatane expectorant-DC** *Syrup 100 + 2 + hydrocodone 1.8mg + 5 +5mg /5ml* **Dimatane expectorant (no codeine)** *Syrup 100 + 2 + 0 + 5 + 5mg /5ml*	**Cough:** 5-10ml PO q6h prn; **CH** 6-12y 2.5-5ml PO q6-8h prn

Guaifenesin + Codeine + Pheniramine

Robitussin AC *Syrup 100 + 10 + 7.5mg / 5ml* **Robitussin with codeine** *Syrup 100 + 3.3 + 7.5mg /5ml*	**Cough:** 5-10ml PO q4-6h prn; **CH** 6-12y 2.5-5ml PO q4-6h prn

Guaifenesin + Codeine + Pseudoephedrine

Balminil Codeine + Decongestant + Expectorant *Syrup 100 + 3.3 + 30mg/5m* **IBenylin codeine** *Syrup 100 + 3.3 + 30mg /5ml* **Calmylin with codeine** *Syrup 100 + 3.3 + 30mg /5ml*	**Cough:** 10ml PO q4h prn, max 40ml/d

Guaifenesin + Codeine + Pseudoephedrine + Triprolidine

CoActifed expectorant *Syrup 100 + 10 + 30 + 2mg /5ml* **ratio-Cotridin expectorant** *Syrup 100 + 10 + 30 + 2mg/5ml*	**Cough:** 10ml PO q4-6h prn, max 40ml/d

Guaifenesin + Dextromethorphan

Balminil DM + expectorant *Syrup 200 + 15mg/5ml* **Benylin DM-E** *Syrup 100 + 15mg/5ml* **Dimetapp Cough & Cold** *Syrup 100 + 15 + 30mg/5ml* **Koffex DM + expectorant** *Syrup 200 + 15mg/5ml* **Robitussin DM** *Syrup 100 + 15mg /5ml*	**Cough:** 10ml PO q4h prn, max 60ml/d or 1-2 Tab PO q12h, max 4 Tab/d, 1-2 cap PO q6h PRN; **CH** >12y: adult dose, 6-11y: 5ml PO q4h, max 30ml/d or 1 Tab PO q12h, max 2 Tab/d, 2- 5y: 2.5ml PO q4h, max 15ml/d or ½ Tab PO q12h, max 1 Tab/d

Guaifenesin + Dextromethorphan + Pseudoephedrine

Balminil DM + decongestant + expectorant *Syrup 200 + 15 + 30mg /5ml* **Benylin DM-D-E** *Syrup 200 + 15 + 30mg /5ml* **Koffex DM + decongestant + expectorant** *Syrup 200 + 15 + 30mg /5ml* **Novahistine DM + decongestant + expectorant** *Syrup 100 + 15 + 30mg /5ml* **Robitussin cough & cold** *Cap 200 + 10 + 30mg*	**Cough:** 10ml PO q6h prn, max 40ml/d

Guaifenesin + Mepyramine + Potassium iodide + Theophylline

ratio-Theo-bronc *Syrup 50 + 6 + 80 + 35mg /5ml*	**Bronchospasm:** 10ml PO qid prn; **CH** >6y 2.5-5ml PO tid prn

Guaifenesin + Oxtriphylline	
Choledyl expectorant *Syrup 50 + 100mg / 5ml*	**Bronchospasm:** 10ml PO qid prn
Guaifenesin + Phenylpropanolamine	
Entex LA *Tab 600 + 75mg*	**Nasal congestion:** 1 tab PO bid prn; **CH** 6-12y half tab PO bid prn
Chlorpheniramine + Pseudoephedrine	
Triaminic Cold and Allergy *Syrup 1mg + 15mg/5ml* **Triaminic Softchews Cold and Allergy** *Tab (chew) 1mg + 15mg*	**Nasal congestion: CH** 6-12: 10ml or 2 tab PO q4-6h PRN, max 4 doses/d
Pseudoephedrine + Ibuprofen	
Sudafed Sinus Advance *Cap 30mg + 200mg*	**Sinus congestion:** 1-2 cap PO q4h PRN, max 6 doses/d
Codeine + Pseudoephedrine + Triprolidine	
CovanSyrup *10mg + 30mg + 2mg/5ml* **Ratio-Cotridin** *Syrup 10mg + 30mg + 2mg/5ml*	

4.9   Other Respiratory Drugs

MA/EF: cholinergic (parasympathomimetic) analogue of acetylcholine ⇒ stimulation of muscarinic, parasympathetic receptors ⇒ smooth-muscle contraction of airways, tracheobronchial secretions ↑
AE: cough, dyspnea, throat irritation, headache, lightheadedness
CI: hypersensitivity to methacholine

Methacholine	EHL no data, PRC C, Lact -
Provocholine *Sol (inhal) 100mg/vial, 160mg/vial, 320mg/vial, 1280mg/vial*	**Diagnosis of bronchial airway hyperreactivity:** inhalation of incr serial conc (0.025mg/ml - 25mg/ml)

5.   Gastroenterology

5.1   Antiulcer Drugs
5.1.1   H₂ Antagonists

MA: competitive antagonism at H_2-receptor on parietal cells
EF: inhibition of basal and histamine-stimulated acid secretion
AE: exanthema, headache, dizziness, confusion, agranulocytosis, gynecomastia, cholestasis, transaminases↑
CI: hypersensativity to drug

Cimetidine	EHL 2h, PRC B, Lact +
Novo-Cimetine *Tab 200mg, 300mg, 400mg, 600mg, 800mg* **Nu-Cimet** *Tab 200mg, 300mg, 400mg, 600mg* **Peptol** *Tab 200mg, 400mg, 800mg* **Generics** *Tab 200mg, 300mg, 400mg, 600mg, 800mg, Sol (oral) 300mg/ 5ml*	**Active ulcers:** 800-1200mg/d div qd-bid, x 4-6wk; **ulcer (maint):** 400mg qhs or 300mg PO bid; **GERD:** 1200mg/d PO x 8-12wk; **hypersecretory conditions:** 300mg qid, max 2400 mg/d; **NSAID lesion:** 800mg/d div qd-bid, **PRO NSAID:** 400mg PO qd, DARF: GFR (ml/min) >50: 100%, 10-50: 75%, <10: 50%

Famotidine	EHL 2.59-4h, PRC B, Lact ?
Pepcid *Tab 20mg, 40mg, Inj 10mg/ml* **Pepcid AC** *Tab 10mg, Tab (chew) 10mg* **Generics** *Tab 10mg, 20mg, 40mg, Inj 10mg/ml*	**Active ulcers:** 20mg bid PO/IV or 40mg PO qhs x 4-8wk; **ulcer (maint):** 20mg PO/IV qhs; **GERD:** 20 PO bid; **esophagitis (due to GERD):** 20-40mg PO bid x 12wk; **hypersecretory conditions:** 20mg PO q6h, max 800mg/d; **PRO GERD:** 10mg PO 10-15min before meals, max 20mg/d; DARF: CrCl (ml/min) <50: 50% dose or q36-48h

Nizatidine	EHL 1-2.8h, PRC B, Lact -
Axid *Cap 150mg, 300mg* **Generics** *Cap 150mg, 300mg*	**Active ulcers:** 300mg PO qhs or 150mg PO bid x 8wk; **ulcer (maint):** 150mg PO qhs; GERD: 150mg PO bid x 12wk; **heartburn PRO:** prn 75mg PO 1h ac, max 150mg/d; DARF: GFR (ml/min), 20-50: 150mg qd, <20: 150mg qod

Ranitidine

	EHL 2-2.5h, PRC B, Lact +

Novo-Ranidine *Tab 150mg, 300mg, Oral (sol) 168mg/10ml*
Nu-Ranit *Tab 150mg, 300mg*
Zantac *Tab 75mg, 150mg, 300mg, Syr 75mg/5ml, Inj 25mg/ml*
Generics *Tab 75mg, 150mg, 300mg*

Active ulcers: 150mg PO bid or 300mg qhs or 50mg IV/ IM q6-8h or 6.25mg/h as continuous IV inf, max 400mg/d;
ulcer (maint): 150mg PO qhs;
GERD: 150mg PO bid;
hypersecretory conditions: 150mg PO bid, max 6g/d;
Zollinger-Ellison syndrome: ini 100mg IV (bolus), then ini 0.5mg/kg/h continuous IV inf, prn incr by 0.5 mg/kg/h, max 4mg/kg/h or 9,000mg/24h;
esophagitis (erosive, active): 150mg PO qid; **esophagitis (erosive, maint):** 150mg PO bid; **DARF:** GFR (ml/min) <50: 150mg PO qd or 50mg IV q18-24h

5.1.2   Proton Pump Inhibitors

MA/EF: blockage of H^+/K^+-ATPase $\Rightarrow$ greatest suppression of acid production
AE: dizziness, headache, diarrhea, constipation, flatulence, exanthema, liver enz. ↑

Esomeprazole

	EHL 1.5h, PRC B, Lact ?

Nexium *Tab del. rel. 20mg, 40mg*

GERD: 20mg PO qd x 2-4wk;
Reflux esophagitis: 40mg PO qd x 4-8wk, maint 20mg PO qd

Lansoprazole

	EHL 0.9-1.5h, PRC B, Lact ?

PrevAcid *Cap del.rel. 15mg, 30mg*

Gastric, duodenal ulcers:
15mg PO ac qam x 2-4wk;
Erosive esophagitis (active):
30mg PO qam x 4-8wk;
erosive esophagitis (maint):
15mg PO ac qam;
Zollinger-Ellison syndrome:
60mg PO ac qam, >120mg/d div bid, max 90mg ac bid; **DARF:** not req,
Liver impairment: max 30mg/d

Omeprazole	EHL 0.5-1.5h, PRC C, Lact ?
Losec *Tab del. rel. 10mg, 20mg, 40mg* **Losec MUPS** *Tab del. rel. 10mg, 20mg* **Generics** *Cap 20mg, 40mg*	**GERD:** 20mg PO qd x 4-8-12wk; **active duodenal ulcers:** 20mg PO qd x 4-8wk; maint 20mg PO qd; **gastric ulcers:** 20mg PO ac qam x 4-8wk; **ulcer PRO:** 20mg PO/NG qd; **erosive esophagitis:** 20mg PO qd, maint 10mg PO qd; **hypersecretory conditions, Zollinger-Ellison syndrome:** 60mg PO qd, >80mg div prn, max 120mg PO tid; ini prn 60mg IV q8h; DARF: not req

Pantoprazole	EHL 1h, PRC B, Lact ?
Pantoloc *Tab ent.coat. 20mg, 40mg* **Panto IV** *Inj 40mg/vial*	**Duodenal/gastric ulcer:** 40mg PO/IV ac qam x 4-8wk, max 80mg/d; **GERD/reflux esophagitis:** 40mg PO/IV ac qam x 4-6wk, maint 20-40mg PO qd; **PRO NSAID:** 20mg PO qam; **Hypersecretion:** 80mg IV bid; **Acute upper GI bleed:** 80mg IV x1, then 8mg/h x 72h; DARF: max 40mg/d

Rabeprozole	EHL 0.85-2h, PRC B, Lact ?
Pariet *Tab 10mg, 20mg*	**GERD/reflux esophagitis:** 20mg PO qd x for 4-8 weeks; maint 10-20mg PO qd; **gastric/duodenal ulcer:** 20 mg PO qd x 4-6 weeks; **Hypersecretory conditions:** 60 mg PO qd

5.1.3   Helicobacter pylori Treatment

MA/EF (bismuth): antibacterial activity and protective effects on gastric mucosa
AE (bismuth): black coloration of tongue, teeth and feces; neurological and psychic DO
CI (bismuth): renal insufficiency, children <14

Amoxicillin + Clarithromycin + Lansoprazole PRC C , Lact ?

Hp-PAC *contains:* *Prevacid, Cap 30mg (lansoprazole),* *Amoxicillin, Cap 500mg,* *Biaxin, Tab 500mg (clarithromycin)* **Losec 1-2-3 A** *Cap 1000mg + 500mg + 20mg*	**Duodenal ulcers associated with H.p.:** Prevacid 1 Cap, Trimox 2 Cap, Biaxin 1 Tab PO bid x 10-14d **Duodenal ulcers associated with H.p.:** 2 bismuth Tab + 1 metronidazole Tab + 1 tetracycline Cap PO qid, at meals and hs x 2wk with H2 antagonist

Metronidazole + Clarithromycin + Lansoprazole PRC C , Lact ?

Losec 1-2-3 M *Cap 500mg + 250mg + 20mg*	**Duodenal ulcers associated with H.p.:** 400 mg PO bid x 4wk (ini + clarithromycin 500 mg PO tid x 2wk), DARF: GFR (ml/min) <25: not rec

5.1.4   Other Antiulcer Drugs

MA/EF (misoprostol): prostaglandin E_1 analog ⇒ prostaglandin-mediated inhibition of acid secretion, activation of bicarbonate and mucus secretion; **MA/EF** (sucralfate): forming of an adherent, protective protein complex at ulcer site; **AE** (misoprostol): diarrhea, dizziness, headache, metrorrhagia; **AE** (sucralfate): constipation, raise of aluminum level in renal insufficiency; **CI** (misoprostol): children, epilepsy, women of childbearing potential have to use adequate contraception, infectious intestinal illnesses
CI (sucralfate): hypersensitivity to sucralfate

Misoprostol	EHL rapid, metabol. 20-40min, PRC X, Lact -
Generics *Tab 0.1mg, 0.2mg*	**NSAID-ind. gastric ulcers (PRO), peptic ulcers (Tx):** 200 mcg PO qid; if not tolerated: 100 mcg PO qid; DARF: not req

Sucralfate	PRC B, Lact +
Novo-Sucralate *Tab 1g* Sulcrate *Tab 1g, Susp 1g/5ml* Generics *Tab 1g*	**Duodenal ulcers:** 1g PO qid (1h ac and hs) x 6-8wk; ulcer (maint): 1g PO bid; DARF: risk of aluminium accumulation in chronic RF

see Propantheline →86

5.2   Antacids

MA/EF: neutralization of stomach acid
AE (aluminium): constipation, ileus, phosphate deficiency;
AE (magnesium): diarrhea; **AE (calcium):** kidney stones, hypercalcemia, constipation
CI: hypersensitivity to antacids

Aluminium Hydroxide	PRC B, Lact ?
Amphojel *Tab 600mg, Sol (oral) 320mg/5ml*	**GERD, mild heartburn:** 500-1800mg PO tid-6 times/d between meals and hs; DARF: req in severe RF
Aluminium Hydroxide + Alginic acid	
Gaviscon Heartburn Relief *Susp (oral) 100mg+250mg/5ml*	**GERD, mild heartburn:** 10-20ml or 2-4 Tab PO qid, max 80ml or 16 tablets/d
Aluminium + Magnesium Hydroxide	PRC B, Lact ?
Diovol *Tab 184mg+100mg, Cap 200mg + 200mg, Susp (oral) 165mg+200mg/5ml, 494mg+300mg/5ml* **Gelusil** *Tab 153mg+200mg, 306mg+ 400mg, Susp (oral) 153mg+200mg/5ml* **Maalox** *Tab (chew) 600mg+300mg* **Mylanta DS Plain** *Susp (oral) 306mg+400mg/5ml*	**GERD, mild heartburn:** 10-20ml or 1-4 Tab PO qid; DARF: req in severe RF
Aluminium + Magnesium Hydroxide + Oxethazine	
Mucaine *Susp (oral) 300mg+100mg+10mg/5ml*	**GERD, mild heartburn:** 5-10ml PO qid
Aluminium + Magnesium Hydroxide + Simethicone	
Diovol Plus *Tab 184mg+100mg+25mg* **Maalox with Anti-Gas** *Susp(oral) 200mg+200mg+20mg/5ml, 400mg+400mg+40mg/5ml* **Mylanta Regular Strength** *Tab 153mg+200mg+20mg, Susp(oral) 153mg+200mg+20mg/5ml* **Mylanta DS** *Tab 306mg+400mg+30mg* **Mylanta Extra Strength** *Susp (oral) 497mg+350mg+30mg/5ml*	**GERD, mild heartburn:** 5-20ml or 2-4 Tab PO qid

ASA + Sodium Bicarbonate + Citric Acid	
Alka Seltzer *Tab 325mg + 1916mg + 1000mg*	**Heartburn**: adults and ch>12y: 2 tabs PO q4h PRN, max 8 tabs/d; age>60 max 4 tabs/d
Calcium Carbonate	PRC B, Lact ?
Maalox *Tab (chew) 600mg, 1000mg* **Tums** *Tab (chew) 500mg, 750mg, 1g*	**GERD, mild heartburn**: 0.5-1.5g PO prn, max 8g/d
Calcium Carbonate + Magnesium Carbonate + Sodium Alginate	
Maalox HRF *Susp (oral) 300mg+125mg+275mg/5ml*	**GERD, mild heartburn**: 5-10ml PO qid
Calcium Carbonate + Simethicone	PRC B, Lact ?
Maalox Quick Dissolve with Antigas *Tab (quick dissolve) 1000mg+60mg*	**GERD, mild heartburn**: 1-2 Tab PO qid
Magnesium Carbonate + Alginic acid	PRC B, Lact ?
Gaviscon Heartburn Relief (aluminium free) *Tab 40mg+200mg, 63mg+313mg*	**GERD, mild heartburn**: 2-4 Tab PO qid

5.3   Laxatives

MA/EF (bisacodyl, sodium sulfate): resorption and metabolism in liver ⇒ biliary excretion, effective in intestine as free diphenyl ⇒ antiresorptive, water binding;
MA/EF (lactulose): osmotic effect, fermented to acids through bacteria ⇒ peristaltic ↑;
MA/EF (polycarbophil): swelling effect;
MA/EF (senna): splitting of contained anthraglycosides through coli bacteria to anthrones/anthranols ⇒ antiresorptive and water binding effects
AE (laxatives): electrolyte loss (especially K^+), melanosis coli, albuminuria, hematuria
AE (polycarbophil): abdominal fullness, flatulence
CI (laxatives): ileus, gastroenteritis, acute surgical abdomen, appendicitis, intestinal obstruction, severe dehydration

Bisacodyl	PRC B, Lact ?
Dulcolax *Tab 5mg, Supp 5mg,10mg, Microenema 10mg/5ml* **Gentlax** *Tab 5mg* **Generics** *Tab 5mg, Supp 10mg*	**Constipation, colonic evacuation:** 10-15mg PO hs prn, 10mg PR prn, max 30mg/d; **CH** <2 y: 5mg PR prn, max 5mg/d; **CH** 2-12 y: 5-10mg PR prn, max 10mg/d

Bisacodyl + Magnesium Citrate	
Royvac *Kit: Tab 5mg, Supp 10mg (Bisacodyl) + Soln 17.46g/bottle (Mg Citrate)*	**Constipation, bowel evacuation:** Day before colonic procedure: 1 bottle oral Sol po at 12:30 pm, then 1 Supp PR at 10:00 PM
Castor Oil	PRC N, Lact ?
Generics *Liquid (oral) 100%*	**Constipation:** 15ml PO prn on empty stomach; colonic evacuation: 15-30ml PO prn on empty stomach; **CH** < 2 y: 1-2ml, max 5ml PO; **CH** 2-11 y: 5-15ml PO
Docusate Calcium	PRC C, Lact ?
Generics *Cap 240mg*	**Constipation:** 240mg PO prn
Docusate + Sennosides	
Senokot-S *Tab 50mg + 8.6mg*	**Constipation:** 2-4 Tab PO qhs, max 4 Tab bid
Docusate Sodium	PRC C, Lact ?
Colace *Liquid (oral) 10mg/ml, Cap 100mg, Syr 20mg/5ml* **Selax** *Cap 100mg, Syr 20mg/5ml* **Soflax** *Cap 100mg, 200mg* **Generics** *Cap 100mg, Liquid (oral)10mg/ml, Syr 4mg/ml, 50mg/ml*	**Constipation:** 50-400mg/d PO qd-qid; ch <3 y: 10-40mg/d PO prn, 3-6 y: 20-60mg/d PO prn, 6-12 y: 40-150mg/d PO prn, >12 y: 50-200mg/d PO prn
Lactulose	PRC B, Lact ?
Duphalac *Sol (oral) 10g/packet* **Laxilose** *Sol (oral) 667mg/ml* **Generics** *Sol (oral) 667mg/ml*	**Constipation:** 30-45ml PO qd-qid prn; infants: 2.5-10ml/d PO div tid-qid, **CH** adolescents: 40-90ml/d PO div tid-qid; **hepatic encephalopathy** (PRO/Tx): 30-45ml/dose PO q1h until effect, then 30-45ml PO tid-qid or 300ml PR with 700ml water, rep q4-6h prn
Magnesium Citrate	PRC B, Lact +
Citro-Mag *Sol (oral) 15g/bottle*	**Bowel evacuation:** 150-300ml PO qd; ch 6-12y: 0.5ml/kg PO q4-6h

Magnesium Hydroxide	PRC N, Lact +
Philipps' Milk of Magnesia *Tab (chew) 300mg, Liquid (oral) 80mg/ml* **Generics** *Tab (chew) 311mg, Liquid 375mg/5ml, 400mg/5ml, 800mg/5ml, 2400mg/10ml*	**Laxative:** 15-40 ml PO qd or 6-8 Tab PO/d prn; **CH** <2 y: 0.5 ml/kg PO qd, 2-5 y: 5-15 ml/d PO qd or 1-2 Tab PO/d prn, 6-11 y: 15-30 ml PO qd, 3-4 Tab PO/d prn; DARF: req in severe RF
Methylcellulose	PRC N, Lact ?
Entrocel *Sol (oral) 1.8%*	**Laxative:** 1 tablespoon in 8 oz cold water PO qd-tid; **CH** 6- 12 y: 50% of adult dose
Mineral Oil	PRC C, Lact ?
Fleet Enema Mineral Oil *Sol (rectal) 130ml/dose* **Lansoÿl** *Liq (oral) 75% mineral oil* **Lansoÿl sugar free** *Liq (oral) 75% mineral oil*	**Laxative:** 15-45ml PO or 120ml PR; ch 5-11 y: 5-15ml PO, 2-11 y: 30-60ml PR
Polyethylene Glycol with Electrolytes	PRC C, Lact ?
Colyte *Powder for Sol (oral) polyethylene glycol 240g/4L* **Klean-Prep** *Powder for Sol (oral) polyethylene glycol 236g/4L* **Peglyte** *Powder for Sol (oral) polyethylene glycol 238.18g/4L*	**Bowel preparation:** 1.5 l/h PO
Senna	EHL 4.0-12.1h, PRC C, Lact +
Senokot *Tab 8.6mg, Syr 1.7mg/ml, Gran 15mg/tsp., Supp 30mg* **X-prep** *Liq. 119mg/70ml, Powder 157.5mg/pouch* **Generics** *Tab 8.6mg, 12mg*	**Laxative or bowel preparation:** 1 tsp gran (15mg) in water or 10-15ml or 2 Tab (8.5mg) PO or 1 supp PR hs; max 4 tsp of gran or 30ml syrup or 8 Tab (34-50mg PO bid) or 2 supp/d; **CH** 6-12 y: 1 Tab or 1/2 tsp PO bid, 2-6 y: 1/2 Tab or 1/4 tsp PO qd
Sodium Phosphate	EHL 20h, PRC N, Lact ?
Fleet Enema *Enema 130ml/dose* **Fleet Phospho-Soda** *Sol (oral) monobasicsodium phosphate 2.4 g + dibasicsodium phosphate 0.9 g/5ml*	**Laxative:** 1 adult enema (118ml) PR prn or 20-45ml oral sol PO prn; **CH** 2-11 y: 1 pediatric enema (59ml) PR prn or 5-9 y: 5-10ml oral sol PO prn, 10-11 y: 10-20ml oral sol PO prn; DARF: contraind.

| **Nabilone** | EHL 2h, PRC C, Lact - |
| **Cesamet** *Cap 1mg* | **Nausea:** 1-2mg PO bid |

| **Perphenazine** | PRC C, Lact ? |
| **Trilafon** *Inj 5mg/ml*
 Generic *Tab 2mg, 4mg, 8mg, 16mg* | **Nausea:** 5-10mg IV |

| **Trifluoperazine** | |
| **Generic** *Tab 1mg, 2mg, 5mg, 10mg, 20mg* | **Nausea:** 2-5 mg PO |

| **Prochlorperazine** | EHL 6.8-9h, PRC C, Lact - |
| **Nu-Prochlor** *Tab 5mg, 10mg*
 Stemetil *Inj 5mg/ml, Liq 5mg/5ml, Supp 10mg, Tab 5mg, 10mg*
 Generics *Tab 5mg, 10mg* | **Nausea:** 5-10mg PO/IM tid/qid, max 40 mg/d or 25mg PR bid or 5-10mg IM q3-4h prn |

5.6   Anti-Inflammatory Drugs, Bowel

MA: influence on prostaglandin biosynthesis, inhibition of leukotriene synthesis
EF: locally anti-inflammatory; **AE:** headache, dizziness, nausea, agranulocytosis, pancytop., allerg. reactt., renal functi. impairment; **CI:** gastric/duodenal ulcer, intest. obstruct., hypersens. to salicylates, hemmorhagic diathesis, ch < 2y; **CI** (sulfasalazine): porphyria

| **Mesalamine/5-ASA** | EHL 0.6-1.4h, PRC B, Lact ? |
| **Asacol** *Tab ent. coat. 400mg*
 Mesasal *Tab 500mg*
 Novo-5-ASA *Tab 400mg*
 Pentasa *Tab del. rel. 500mg, Enema 1g, 4g, Supp 1g*
 Salofalk *Enema 2g, 4g, Supp 250mg, 500mg, 500mg, 1000mg* | **Ulcerative colitis:** 800-3200mg/d PO div, maint 1600mg/d PO div, max 4800mg/d or Tab del. rel. 500mg PO qid; Enema: 1-4g PR qhs; (Pentasa) Supp. 1g pr qhs, (Salofalk) 1g PO tid-qid, 500mg PR bid-tid or 1g PR qd; **Crohn's disease:** Tab ext. rel. 1g PO qid, maint 750mg PO qid, (Salofalk) 3g/d PO div |

| **Olsalazine** | EHL 0.9h, PRC C , Lact ? |
| **Dipentum** *Cap 250mg* | **Ulcerative colitis:** 500 mg PO qid, max 3g/d, maint 500mg po bid |

| **Sulfasalazine** | EHL 7.6h , PRC B , Lact ? |
| **Salazopyrin** *Tab 500mg, Tab ent. coat. 500mg*
 Generics *Tab 500mg, Tab ent. coat. 500mg* | **IBD:** 1-2g PO tid-qid, ch (25-35kg): 500mg PO tid, (35-50kg): 1g PO bid-tid; **PRO UC:** 1g PO bid-tid, ch (25-35kg): 500mg PO tid, (35-50kg): 500mg PO bid-tid |

5.7   GI Enzymes

MA/EF (pancrelipase): mixture of amylase, trypsin, and lipase
AE (pancrelipase): skin rash, hypersensitivity, nausea/diarrhea with large doses, hyperuricemia, hyperuricosuria
CI (pancreatic enzymes): hypersensitivity to pork protein

Lactase Enzyme   PRC N, Lact ?

Dairyaid Tab 3,000 FCC, Cap 4,500 FCC
Lactaid Tab (original strength) 3,000 FCC U of enzyme, Tab (extra strength) 4,500 FCC U of enzyme, Cap (ultra) 9,000 FCC U of enzyme, Cap (ultra, chew) 9,000 FCC U of enzyme, Gtt lactase
Lactrase Cap 250mg

Lactose intolerance: 3 Cap PO (original strength), 2 Cap PO (extra strength), 1 Cap PO (ultra), swallow Cap with first bite of dairy foods or 5-7 Gtt, max 15gtt PO/liter of milk

Pancrealipase (lipase+protease+amylase)   PRC C, Lact ?

Cotazym Cap 8000U+30000U+30000U
Cotazym 65B Cap 8000U+30000U + 30000U + 65mg conj. bile salts
Creon 5, Creon 10, Creon 20, Crean 25 Cap 5000U+18750U+16600U, 10000U+37500U+33200U, 20000U+75000U+66400U, 25000U+62500U+74000U
ECS 4, ECS 8, ECS 20 Cap 4000U +11000U +11000U, 8000U +30000U +30000U, 20000U+55000U+55000U
Pancrease Cap 4500U+25000U+20000U
Pancrease MT Cap 4000U +12000U +12000U, 10000U+30000U+30000U, 16000U+48000U+48000U
Ultrase Cap 4500U+25000U+20000U
Ultrase MT12, MT20 Cap 12000U +39000U+39000U, 20000U +65000U +65000U
Viokase Powder 16800U+70000U +70000U/ 1/4 tsp
Viokase-8,-16 Tab 8000U+30000U +30000U, 16000U+60000U+60000U

Pancreatic enzyme deficiency: 1-4 Tab/Cap PO with each meal, 1 Tab/Cap with snacks, (Creon): **CH** 6-12mo 2000 U lipase, 1-6y: 4000-8000 U lipase, 7-12y: 4000- 12000 U lipase (always with meals, feedings)

5.8   Gallstone Dissolving Drugs

MA/EF: inhibition of biliary cholesterol secretion and intestinal cholesterol resorption; inhibition of HMG-CoA-reductase ⇒ cholesterol synthesis ↓ ⇒ dissolving of cholesterol stones

AE: diarrhea, transaminases ↑

CI: infx of the gall bladder and ducts, common bile duct or cystic duct occlusion, disturbed contractility of the gall bladder, calcified gall stones

Ursodiol	PRC B, Lact ?
Urso *Tab 250mg, 500mg*	**Cholestatic liver disease, PBC:** 13-15mg/kg/d PO div bid-qid

5.9   Antispasmodics (Parasympatholytics)

MA/EF (dicyclomine): antimuscarinic ⇒ antispasmodic, smooth muscle relaxation

MA/EF (hyoscyamine): competitive inhibition of muscarinic acetylcholine receptors ⇒ antisecretory (exocrine glands, intestinal mucosa), smooth muscle relax, vagolytic effects

MA/EF (propantheline): anticholinergic, antispasmodic, bladder capacity ↑, urinary frequency ↓, gastric acid secretion ↓

AE (dicyclomine, hyoscyamine): urinary retention, constipation, blurred vision, dry mouth, tachycardia, dizziness, headache, nausea

AE (propantheline). urinary retention, constipation, blurred vision, dry mouth, tachycardia, dizziness, headache, sexual dysfunction

CI (dicyclomine, hyoscyamine): obstructive uropathy, GI obstruction, ulcerative colitis, glaucoma, children (<6m dicyclomine, <2 y hyoscyamine), reflux esophagitis, myasthenia gravis, megacolon

CI (hyoscine): myasthenia gravis, megacolon, glaucoma, obsructive prostatic hypertrophy

CI (hyoscyamine): hepatic, renal, or pulmonary insufficiency, intestinal atony in elderly or debilitated patients, myasthenia gravis, cardiospasm, unstable CVS status

CI (propantheline): hypersensivity to anticholinergic drugs, myasthenia gravis, narrow-angle glaucoma, obstructive GI disease, paralytic ileus, reflux esophagitis, ulcerative colitis, obstructive uropathy, unstable CVS status in acute hemorrhage

Dicyclomine	EHL 1.8h, PRC B, Lact ?
Bentylol *Tab 20mg, Tap 10mg, Syr 10mg/5ml, Inj 10mg/ml* **Formulex** *Cap 10mg* **Lomine** *Cap 10mg*	**Functional bowel syndrome:** ini 10-20mg PO tid-qid, max 160mg/d, 20mg IM qid (max 2d); **CH** 6 mo-2 y: 5- 10mg PO 15min ac tid-qid, max 40mg/d, 2-12 y: 10mg/d PO tid-qid

Hyoscine	EHL 2-3min, PRC C, Lact ?
Buscopan *Tab 10mg, Inj 20mg/ml*	**GI hypermotility, functional bowel syndr.:** 10-20mg/d, max 60mg/d, 10-20 IV/SC/IM, max 100mg/d

Hyoscyamine	EHL 3.5h, PRC C, Lact -
Levsin *Tab 0.125mg*	**GI hypermotility, functional bowel syndr.:** 0.125- 0.25mg PO/SL q4h or prn, max 1.5mg/d or 0.375-0.75mg PO q12h, max 1.5mg/d (ext. rel); **CH** 2-12 y: 0.0625- 0.125mg q4h prn or 0.375mg (ext. rel) PO q12h, max 0.75mg/24h, >12 y: adult dose

Propantheline	EHL (biphasic) 57.9min, 2.93h, PRC C, Lact ?
Pro-Banthine *Tab 7.5mg, 15mg*	**GI antispasmodic, peptic ulcer:** 15mg tid 30min ac, 30mg qhs; UT

5.10 Antiflatulents

MA/EF: altering surface tension of gas bubbles, antifoaming
AE: mild diarrhea, regurgitation

Simethicone	PRC B, Lact ?
Ovol *Drops 40mg/ml, Cap 180mg, Tab 80mg, 160mg* **Phazyme** *Softgel 95mg, 125mg, 180mg*	**GI discomfort due to gas:** 180mg PO pc or qhs, 80-160mg PO qid or 180mg PO bid, max 540mg/d; **CH** <12 y: 10-20mg PO tid

6.2   Ions, Minerals
6.2.1   Potassium

AE: N/V, belching, heartburn, flatulence, abdominal pain, diarrhea, mucosal ulcers, GI hemorrhage, ECG changes
CI: hyperkalemia, hyperchloremia, renal insufficiency, Addison's disease, acute dehydration, heat cramps

Potassium Chloride	PRC C, Lact ?
Apo-K *Tab (ext. rel)* 8mEq **K-10** *Liquid* 20mEq/15ml **K-Dur** *Tab (ext. rel)* 20mEq **K-Lor** *Powder* 20mEq/pkt **K-Lyte/Cl** *Powder* 25mEq/7.8g **Micro-K Extencaps, Micro-K-10 Extencaps** *Cap (ext.rel)* 8mEq, 10mEq **Roychol** *Liquid* 20mEq/15ml **Slow-K** *Tab (ext.rel)*, 8mEq	**Hypokalemia Tx:** 40-100mEq/d PO; 40-300mEq/d IV, max 40mEq/liter, max 15mEq/h; **hypokalemia PRO:** 20-40mEq/d PO qd- bid
Potassium Citrate	Lact +
K-Lyte *Tab (efferv)* 25mEq **Polycitra-K** *Crystals* 30mEq/pkt, *Sol (oral)* 10mEq/5ml	**Hypokalemia Tx:** 40-100mEq/d PO; 40-300mEq/d IV, max 40mEq/liter, max 15mEq/h; **hypokalemia** PRO: 20-40mEq/d PO qd- bid
Potassium Gluconate	PRC A
Generics *Tab* 550mg, 1000mg, *Liquid* 20mEq/15ml	**Hypokalemia Tx:** 40-100mEq/d PO; 40-300mEq/d IV, max 40mEq/liter, max 15mEq/h; **hypokalemia** PRO: 20-40mEq/d PO qd- bid

6.2.2   Calcium

AE (calcium IV): sensation of heat, fits of perspiration, BP ↓, N/V, arrhythmias
CI (calcium IV): hypercalcemia, nephrocalcinosis, digitalis intoxication, severe renal insuff.

Calcium Carbonate	PRC C, Lact +
Apo-Cal *Tab 250mg, 500mg* **Calcite 500** *Tab 1250mg (500mg Ca)* **Calcium 500** *Tab 1250mg (500mg Ca)* **Calcium Oyster Shell** *Tab 650mg (250mg Ca), 1250mg (500mg Ca)* **Caltrate 600** *Tab 1500mg (600mg Ca)* **Os-Cal** *Tab 1250mg (500mg Ca)* **Tums** *Tab (chew) 500mg, 750mg, 1000mg*	**Hypocalcemia:** 1-2g PO qd; **osteoporosis PRO:** 1-1.5g PO qd; **RDA:** 1200mg PO qd

Calcium Chloride	PRC C, Lact ?
Generics *Inj 10% (1.36 mEq/ml)*	**Hypocalcemia:** 500-1000mg IV q1-3d; **magnesium intoxication:** 500mg IV; **hyperkalemia:** dose must be titrated by ECG-changes

Calcium Citrate	PRC C, Lact ?
Generics *Tab 150mg, 300mg, 350mg*	**Dietary supplement:** 500-2000mg PO 2-4 times/day

Calcium Glucoheptonate	EHL n/a
Generics *Syr 100mg/5ml, 110mg/5ml, 125mg/ml*	**Dietary supplement:** 10 mL PO 1-3 times daily, **CH:** 2.5-5 mL PO tid.

Calcium Gluconate	PRC C, Lact ?
Generics *Inj 10% Sol (0.465mEq/ml)*	**Hypocalcemia:** 0.5-2g slowly IV; 500-1000mg PO bid-qid

6.2.3   Calcium Combinations

Calcium Carbonate + Cholecalciferol	
Os-Cal D *Tab 1250mg (500mg Ca) + 125 IU* **Viactiv** *Softchew 1250mg(500mgCa)+100IU*	**Dietary supplement:** 1-2 tab PO qd

Calcium Carbonate + Cholecalciferol + Magnesium	
Calcium + *Liq 1250mg (500mg Ca) + 200 IU + 200mg/2 tsp*	**Dietary supplement:** 1-2 tsp PO qd

Calcium Carbonate + Copper + Manganese + Magnesium + Vitamin D + Zinc

Caltrate Plus *Tab 1500mg (600mg Ca) + 1mg + 1.8mg + 50mg + 200 IU + 7.5mg*	**Dietary supplement:** 1-2 tab PO qd

Calcium Carbonate + Etidronate

Didrocal *Calcium Carbonate: Tab 1250mg (500mg Ca)* **Etidronate:** *Tab 400mg*	**Osteoporosis:** 90-d cycle, 400mg etidronate PO qd x 14d then 500mg calcium PO qd x 76d

Calcium Carbonate + Vitamin D

Calcite D–500 *Tab 1250mg (500mg Ca) + 125 IU* **Calcium 500 with Vitamin D** *Tab 1250mg (500mg Ca) + 125 IU* **Calcium D 500** *Tab 1250mg (500mg Ca) + 125 IU* **Caltrate Select** *Tab 1500mg + 400U* **Caltrate 600 + D** *Tab 1500mg (600mg Ca) + 125 IU*	**Dietary supplement:** 1-2 tab PO qd

Calcium Citrate + Cholecalciferol + Magnesium + Silicon

Active Calcium Plus *Tab 200mg + 100IU + 100mg + 2.25mg*	**Dietary supplement:** 2 tab PO bid

Calcium Glucoheptonate + Calcium Gluconate

Calcium Stanley *Liq 132 + 112 mg/ml* **ratio-Calcium** *Syr 172.1 + 58.7mg/ml*	**Dietary supplement:** 10 mL PO 1-3 times daily, ch: 2.5-5 mL PO tid

6.2.4   Magnesium

AE: sleepiness, diarrhea, CNS disturbances, arrhythmias, muscle weakness, respiratory depression, flushing, hypotension;
CI: restricted use in case of depressed renal function,
2 hrs preceding delivery, heart block; IV: AV block, myasthenia gravis

Magnesium Chloride   EHL n/a

Formule 454 *Liq 180mg/5mlFormule 575Liq 400mg/ml* **Magnonat** *Liq 200mg/ml* **Generics** *Tab 606.5mg*	**Hypomagnesemia:** 100-600mg/d elemental magnesium PO div

Magnesium Glucoheptonate	EHL n/a
ratio-Magnesium Sol (oral) 100mg (5mg Mg)/ml	**Hypomagnesemia:** 15-30ml PO 1-3x/d

Magnesium Gluconate	PRC A, Lact +
Maglucate *Tab 500mg (29.3mg Mg), Liquid 54mg Mg/5ml*	**Hypomagnesemia:** 100-600mg/d elemental magnesium PO div tid

Magnesium Oxide	PRC B, Lact ?
Generics *Tab 252mg, 420mg, 835mg, Powder 240mg/ml, 750mg/1.25ml*	**Hypomagnesemia:** 100-600mg/d elemental magnesium PO div tid

Magnesium Sulfate	PRC A, Lact +
Generics *Inj 500mg/ml*	**Ventricular arrhythmias:** 1-6g IV over several min, then 3-20mg/min IV for 5-48h; **preeclampsia, eclampsia:** 4g IV, simultaneously 4-5g IM each buttock; preterm labor: 4-6g IV over 20min, then 1-3g/h IV

6.2.5   Fluoride

AE: N/V, diarrhea
CI: areas where water fluoride content is greater than 0.7ppm

Fluoride	PRC no data currently available , Lact ?
Fluor-A-Day *Drops 1mg/ml, Lozen 1mg, Tab (chew) 0.25mg, 0.5mg, 1mg* **Fluotic** *Tab 20mg*	**Osteoporosis:** 25mg PO bid (in combination with calcium citrate 400mg bid)

6.2.6   Phosphorous

Potassium Phosphate	PRC no data, Lact no data
Generics *Inj 3mmol/ml*	**Severe hypophosphatemia (< 1mg/dl):** 1-3g PO/PR; **CH** 2-4mmol/kg/d PO; 25mmol IV over 24 hours

6.2.7 Iron

AE: N/V, diarrhea, constipation, dark-colored stools, when used intravenously: headaches, thrombophlebitis, allergic reactions, collapse; **CI:** hemochromatosis, hemolytic anemia, hemosiderosis, premature infants with vit. E deficiency

Ferrous Fumarate (33% elem. iron)	PRC C, Lact +
Palafer *Cap 300mg (100mg)*, *Susp 300mg/5ml (100mg)* **Palafer CF** *Cap 300mg (100mg)*	**Iron deficiency:** 2-3mg/kg/d elemental iron PO div bid- tid
Ferrous Gluconate (11.6% elem. iron)	PRC C, Lact +
Generics *Tab 300mg (35mg)*	**Iron deficiency:** 2-3mg/kg/d elemental iron PO div bid- tid
Ferrous Polysaccharide (100% elem. iron)	PRC C, Lact +
Triferexx *Cap 150mg*	**Iron deficiency:** 2-3mg/kg/d elemental iron PO div bid- tid
Ferrous Sulfate (20% elem. iron)	PRC C, Lact +
Fer-In-Sol *Drops 75mg/ml (15mg)*, *Syr 150mg/5ml (30mg)* **Ferodan Infant Drops** *Drops 75mg/ml (15mg)* **Ferodan** *Tab 300mg, Syr 150mg/5ml (30mg)* **Generics** *Tab 300mg (60mg)*	**Iron deficiency:** 2-3mg/kg/d elemental iron PO div bid- tid
Iron Dextran (100% elem. iron)	PRC C, Lact +
Dexiron *Inj 50mg/ml* **Infufer** *Inj 50mg/ml*	**Iron deficiency anemia:** total dose (ml) = 0.0442 x (desired Hb – observed Hb) x kg + [0.26 x kg] IV
Iron Sucrose (100% elem. iron)	EHL 6h, PRC C, Lact ?
Venofer *Inj 20mg/ml*	**Iron deficiency anemia in chronic hemodialysis:** 100mg IV 1-3x/wk up to 1g. rep prn

6.3   Drugs Affecting Electrolyte Imbalances

6.3.1   Biphosphonates

MA/EF: osteoclastic activity ↓ ⇒ osteal release of calcium ↓, bone degradation ↓
AE: allergic skin reactions, hypocalcemia, GI DO
AE (alendronate): abdominal pain, musculoskeletal pain, headache, diarrhea, constipation
AE (etidronate): loss of taste, osteomalacia, GI complaints, bone pain
AE (pamidronate): myelosuppression, HTN, thrombophlebitis, malaise, N/V
AE (risedronate): flu like syndrome, diarrhea, arthralgia, headache, abdominal pain, rash
CI: renal insufficiency, acute GI inflammation, children
CI (alendronate): hypersensitivity to alendronate products, esophageal abnormalities, inability to stand or sit upright for 30min, CrCl <35ml/min
CI (clodranate): Cr>440umol/L, severe inflammation of GI tract
CI (etidronate): hypersensitivity to etidronate products, osteomalacia
CI (pamidronate): hypersensitivity to biphosphonates
CI (risedronate): hypocalcemia, hypersensitivity to risedronate products

Alendronate	EHL up to 10y, PRC C, Lact ?
Fosamax *Tab 5mg, 10mg, 40mg, 70mg, Oral (sol) 70mg/75ml* **Generic** *Tab 5mg, 10mg*	**Postmenopausal osteoporosis PRO:** 5mg PO qd or 35mg qwk; **postmenopausal osteoporosis Tx:** 10mg PO qd or 70mg qwk; **osteoporosis Tx men:** 10mg PO qd; **steroid-induced osteoporosis PRO + Tx:** 5mg PO qd (men and pre-menopausal women) or 10mg PO qd (postmenopausal women not taking estrogen); **Paget's disease:** 40mg PO qd for 6mo; DARF: GFR (ml/ min) 35-60: 100%, <35: not rec

Clodronate	EHL 13h, PRC C, Lact ?
Ostac *Cap 400mg, Inj 30mg/ml*	**Hypercalcemia of malignancy, osteolytic bone lesions:** ini 300mg/d IV, maint 1600-2400mg PO qd or div bid, max 3200mg PO qd; DARF: dose should be reduced in severe renal failure

Hydrocortisone	EHL 8-12h, PRC C, Lact -	Glu	Min
Cortef *Tab 10mg, 20mg* **Cortenema** *Enema 100mg* **Cortifoam** *Foam 80mg/application* **Hycort** *Enema 100mg* **Solu-Cortef** *Inj 100mg/vial,* *250mg/vial, 500mg/vial, 1g/vial* **Generics** *Inj 100mg/vial, 250mg/vial,* *500mg/vial, 1g/vial*	**Adrenal insufficiency:** 5-30mg PO bid-qid; **inflamm. disease:** 10-320mg/d PO div tid-qid or 100-500mg IV/IM q12h; **IBD:** 80-100mg PR qd-bid x 2-3wk, then qod; **CH adrenal insufficiency:** 0.5-0.75mg/kg/d PO div tid; **CH inflamm. disease:** 2.5-10mg/ kg/d PO div tid-qid; DARF: not req	1	2
Methylprednisolone	EHL 18-36h, PRC C, Lact ?	5	0
Depo-Medrol *Inj (M.-acetate)* *20mg/ml, 40mg/ml, 80mg/ml* **Depo-Medrol with Lidocaine** *Inj 40mg (plus 10mg lidocaine)/ml* **Medrol** *Tab 4mg, 16mg* **Solu-Medrol** *Inj (M.-succinate)* *40mg/vial, 125mg/vial, 500mg/vial,* *1g/ vial* **Generics** *Inj 500mg/vial, 1g/vial*	**Inflamm. disease:** 10-250mg IV/IM q4h; 4-48mg PO/d; 4-80mg intraarticular (methylprednisolone acetate), may be repeated after 1-5wk **spinal cord injury:** ini 30mg/kg IV over 15min, then 45min. pause, then 5.4mg/kg/h IV for 23h; **lupus nephritis:** 1g IV qd for 3d; **Acute IBD:** 20mg IV q8h; **CH inflamm. disease:** 0.5- 1.7mg/kg/d PO/IV/IM div q6-12h; **CH spinal cord injury:** see adults; DARF: not req		
Prednisolone	EHL 18-36h, PRC C, Lact ?	4	1
Pediapred *Sol (oral) 5mg/5ml* **Generics** *Sol (oral) 5mg/5ml, Tab 5mg*	**Inflamm. disease:** 5-60mg PO/d; **CH** 0.1-2mg/kg/ d PO div qd-qid; DARF: not req		
Prednisone	EHL 18-36h, PRC C, Lact +	4	1
Winpred *Tab 1mg* **Generics** *Tab 1mg, 5mg, 50mg*	**Inflamm. disease:** 5-60mg/d PO qd or div bid-qid; **CH** 0.05-2mg/kg/d div qd-qid; DARF: not req		

Triamcinolone	EHL 18-36h, PRC C, Lact +	Glu	Min
Aristocort Inj 25mg/ml, 40mg/ml **Aristospan** Inj 20mg/ml **Kenalog** Inj (T.acetonide) 10mg/ml, 40mg/ml **Generics** Inj 10mg/ml, 40mg/ml	**Inflamm. disease:** 4-48mg/d PO div qd-qid; 2.5-15mg, max 40mg **Intraarticular RA/OA:** 2-20mg IA q3-4wk prn; DARF: not req	5	0

Glu: relative glucocorticoid potency, **Min:** relative mineralocorticoid potency

6.7 Oral Antidiabetics
6.7.1 Sulfonylureas – 1st Generation

MA/EF: blockage of ATP-dependent K^+ channels $\Rightarrow$ release of insulin from pancreatic β-cells ↑, sensitivity of peripheral tissues to insulin ↑
AE (sulfonylureas): N/V, hypoglycemia, cholestatic jaundice, pancytopenia
AE (chlorpropamide): hypoglycemia, N, allergic skin reactions
AE (tolbutamide): hypoglycemia, nausea, heartburn, allergic skin reactions
CI (sulfonylureas): type 1 DM, ketoacidosis, renal insufficiency, coma, severe infection, severe thyroid or liver disease, trauma or surgery

Chlorpropamide	EHL 36h, PRC C, Lact -
Novo-Propamide Tab 250mg **Generics** Tab 100mg, 250mg	**DM:** ini 250mg PO qd, maint 100-500mg, max 750mg PO qd; DARF: GFR (ml/min) >50: 50%, <50: not rec

Tolbutamide	EHL 4.5-6.5h, PRC C, Lact ?
Generics Tab 500mg	**DM:** ini 1g PO qd, maint 500mg-3g PO qd, max 3g/d

6.7.2 Sulfonylureas - 2nd Generation

MA/EF: see Sulfonylureas - 1st Generation →107 ; **AE** (glimepiride): hypoglycemia, N;
AE (glyburide): hypoglycemia, N, heartburn, allergic skin reactions; **CI:** as above

Gliclazide	EHL 10.4h, PRC ?, Lact ?
Diamicron Tab 80mg **Diamicron MR** Tab (modified release) 30mg **Generics** Tab 80mg	**DM:** ini 80mg PO bid, maint 80-320mg PO/d (div doses of > 160mg bid), max 320mg/d; (Modified release): ini 30mg PO qd, maint 30-120mg PO qd
Glimepiride	EHL 5h, PRC C, Lact -
Amaryl Tab 1mg, 2mg, 4mg	**DM:** ini 1-2mg PO qd, main. 1-4mg PO qd, max 8mg/d
Glyburide	EHL 5-10h, PRC C, Lact ?
DiaBeta Tab 2.5mg, 5mg **Euglucon** Tab 2.5mg, 5mg **Gen-Glybe** Tab 2.5mg, 5mg **Generics** Tab 2.5mg, 5mg	**DM:** ini 2.5-5mg PO qd, maint 2.5-20mg PO qd or div bid; max 20mg/d

6.7.3 Oral Antidiabetics - α-Glucosidase Inhibitors

MA (acarbose): inhibition of glucosidase ⇒ intestinal glucose resorption ↓
AE (acarbose): diarrhea, abdominal pain, flatulence ; **CI** (acarbose): hypersensitivity to
acarbose, DKA, inflammatory bowel diseases, colonic ulceration, partial obstruction

Acarbose	EHL 2h, PRC B, Lact ?
Prandase Tab 50mg, 100mg	**DM:** ini 50mg PO qd, incr to 50mg PO bid, then tid at 1-2wk increments, max 300mg/d

6.7.4 Oral Antidiabetics - Meglitinides

MA/EF: stimul. insulin secret. via inhib. (closing) of ATP-sensitive potassium
channels in beta cells (⇒ increases in beta-cell calcium influx)
AE: hypoglycemia
CI: diabetic ketoacidosis, type 1 DM, hypersensitivity to repaglinide products

Nateglinide	EHL 1.5h, PRC C, Lact ?
Starlix Tab 60mg, 120mg, 180mg	**DM:** ini 120mg PO tid, maint 60-180mg PO tid

Repaglinide	EHL < 1h, PRC C, Lact ?
GlucoNorm *Tab 0.5mg, 1mg, 2mg*	**DM:** ini 0.5-2mg PO tid within 30min before a meal; max 16mg/d

6.7.5 Oral Antidiabetics - Biguanides

MA: cellular glucose uptake ↑, non-oxidative glucose metabolism ↑;
AE: lactic acidosis, N/V/D, flatulence, anorexia, complete blood count changes;
CI: type 1 DM, ren./hep./respir./cardiac insuff., Cr >136 umol/l in men or >124 umol/l in women, CHF, sev.infect., hypersens. to metformin, metabolic acidosis, concomitant use of iiodin.contrast media, DKA, ethanol abusus

Metformin	EHL 1.5-6.2h, PRC B, Lact ?
Glucophage *Tab 500mg, 850mg* **Generics** *Tab 500mg, 850mg*	**DM:** ini 500mg PO qd-bid, maint 500mg PO tid-qid or 850mg PO bid-tid, max 2550mg/d; DARF: contraind. in RF

6.7.6 Oral Antidiabetics - Thiazolidinediones

MA/EF: binding to peroxisome proliferator activated (PPA)-receptor in insulin target tissue ⇒ insulin effectiveness↑ ⇒ cellular glucose uptake↑, hepatic gluconeogenesis↓
AE: edema, weight gain, anemia. Combination with metformin: anemia, hypo- and hyperglycemia, headache, diarrhea, stomachache, N, tiredness, edema. Combination with sulfonylureas: anemia, thrombopenia, hypo- and hyperglycemia, weight gain, edema
CI: acute heart failure, hepatic impairment, hypersensitivity to product ingredients

Pioglitazone	EHL 3-7h, PRC C, Lact ?
Actos *Tab 15mg, 30mg, 45mg*	**DM:** monotherapy or in combination with sulfonylureas, metformin, or insulin: ini 15-30mg PO qd, max 45mg/d; DARF: not req

Rosiglitazone	EHL 3-4h, PRC C, Lact -
Avandia *Tab 2mg, 4mg, 8mg*	**DM:** monotherapy or in combination with metformin or sulfonylureas: ini 4mg PO qd or 2mg bid, incr after 8- 12wk to max 8mg/d; DARF: not req

AE (Avandamet): diarrhea, anemia, upper resp. tract infx, headache, fatigue;
CI (Avandamet): renal disease, congestive heart failure, acute or chronic metabolic acidosis

Metformin + Rosiglitazone	PRC C, Lact -
Avandamet *Tab 500mg + 1mg, 500mg + 2mg, 500mg + 4mg*	**DM:** ini 500+1-2mg PO bid, max 2000+ 8mg/d; DARF: contraind. in RF

6.8   Insulins
6.8.1   Short-Acting Insulins

MA/EF: glucose resorption in muscle and fat cells↑ ⇒ anabolic metabolism↑ (glycogen-, lipid- and protein synthesis), catabolic metabolism↓ (glycogenolysis, lipolysis, proteolysis)
MA/EF: faster resorption because of amino acid changes ⇒ shorter inject-eat-interval
AE: hypoglycemia, transient injection site reaction, pain at injection site, lipodystrophy, allergic reactions
CI: current hypoglycemic episode, systemic allergic reaction to insulin (desensitize)

Insulin Aspart	EHL 81min, PRC no data, Lact ?
Novorapid *Inj 100 U/ml*	**DM:** individualized dosage SC 5-10min ac

Insulin Lispro	EHL 26-52min, PRC B, Lact ?
Humalog *Inj 100 U/ml*	**DM:** individualized dosage SC within 15min ac

Insulin Regular	EHL 5-15min (IV), PRC B, Lact +
Humulin R *Inj 100 U/ml* **Novolin ge Toronto** *Inj 100 U/ml* **Iletin II Pork regular** *Inj 100 U/ml*	**DM:** individualized dosage SC 30min ac; diabetic ketoacidosis: ini 0.1 U/kg IV bolus, then 0.1 U/kg/h, decrease when blood glucose falls to < 250mg/dl

6.8.2 Intermediate- and Long-Acting Insulins

MA, EF, AE, CI see short-acting insulins →110

Insulin Lente	PRC B, Lact ?
Humulin L *Inj 100 U/ml* **Iletin II Pork Lente** *Inj 100 U/ml* **Novolin ge Lente** *Inj 100 U/ml*	**DM:** individualized dosage
Insulin NPH	PRC B, Lact ?
Humulin N *Inj 100 U/ml* **Novolin ge NPH** *Inj 100 U/ml* **Iletin II Pork NPH** *Inj 100 U/ml*	**DM:** individualized dosage
Insulin Ultralente	PRC B, Lact ?
Humulin U *Inj 100 U/ml* **Novolin ge Ultralente** *Inj 100 U/ml*	**DM:** individualized dosage

6.8.3 Insulin Glargine

MA/EF (insulin glargine): genetically changed insulin molecule, badly soluble in physiological pH-span ⇒ slow resorption ⇒ longer action; **AE:** hypoglycemia, injection site pain, lipodystrophy, pruritus, rash, allergic reactions, hypersensitivity
CI: hypoglycemia, prior hypersensitivity to any component of insulin glargine formulation

Insulin Glargine	PRC C, Lact ?
Lantus *Inj 100 U/ml*	**DM:** individualized dosage SC qd hs

6.8.4 Biphasic Insulins

Insulin Lispro + Insulin Lispro-protamine	
Humalog Mix 25 *Inj 25 + 75 U/ml*	**DM:** individualized dosage SC within 15min ac
Insulin Regular + Insulin NPH	
Humulin 10/90, 20/80, 30/70, 40/60, 50/50 *Inj 10 + 90 U/ml, 20 + 80 U/ml, 30 + 70 U/ml, 40 + 60 U/ml, 50 + 50 U/ml* **Novolin ge 10/90, 20/80, 30/70, 40/60, 50/50** *Inj 10 + 90 U/ml, 20 + 80 U/ml, 30 + 70 U/ml, 40 + 60 U/ml, 50 + 50 U/ml*	**DM:** individualized dosage

6.12   Prolactin Inhibitors

MA: stimulation of hypophyseal dopamine receptors ⇒ inhibition of prolactin release
AE: N/V, GI disturbances, psychomotor- and extrapyramidal motor system DO,
hypotension, bradycardia, peripheral vascular perfusion disturbances
AE (bromocriptine): hypotension, periph. vasoconstriction, dyskinesias, fatigue, N/V
AE (cabergoline): dizziness, headache, weakness, fatigue, orthostatic hypotension
CI: limited use in psychiatric DO, gastroduodenal ulcers, serious CVS diseases
CI (bromocriptine): hypersensitivity to bromocriptine products, HTN disorders of
pregnancy, CAD, psychotic disorders
CI (cabergoline): hypersensitivity to ergot derivatives, uncontrolled HTN

Bromocriptine	EHL 50h, PRC C, Lact -
Parlodel *Tab 2.5mg, Cap 5mg* **Generics** *Tab 2.5mg, Cap 5mg*	**Hyperprolactinemia:** ini 1.25-2.5mg PO qhs, incr to 2.5mg PO bid in 2-3d, then incr to 2.5mg PO tid prn, max 20mg/d; **acromegaly:** ini 1.25-2.5mg PO qhs, incr to 10-20mg/d div qid over 2-4wks; **Parkinson's:** 1.25mg PO qhs, maint 2.5mg PO bib, incr 2.5mg/d q2-4wk, max 40mg/d; DARF: not req

Cabergoline	EHL 63-69h, PRC B, Lact ?
Dostinex *Tab 0.5mg*	**Hyperprolactinemia:** ini 0.25mg PO 2x/wk, incr by 0.25mg 2x/wk at 4wk intervals according to response, max 1mg 2x/wk

Quinagolide	EHL 17h, PRC C, Inhibits lactation
Norprolac *Tab 0.025mg, 0.05mg, 0.075mg, 0.15mg*	**Hyperprolactinemia:** ini 0.025mg PO qd x 3days, then 0.05mg PO qd x 3days, then 0.075mg PO qd, max 0.9mg/day

6.13 Anterior Pituitary Hormones

AE (somatropin): hyperglycemia, hypothyroidism, BP ↑, N/V, edema, retention of H_2O + natrium, developm. of antibodies; **AE** (somatrem): developm. of antibodies, periph. edema
CI (somatropin, somatrem): active malignancy, acute critical illness (post open heart or abdominal surgery; multiple accidental trauma; acute respiratory failure), closed epiphyses, hypersensitivity to growth hormone or product ingredients; **CI** (cosyntropin): Cushing's syndrome, active infection, pregnancy, lactation, CHF, PUD, acute psychosis

Clomiphene →289	
Cosyntropin	EHL no data, PRC C, Lact ?
Cortrosyn Inj 0.25mg/vial **Synachen Depot** Inj 1mg/amp	**Adrenal funct. screen. test:** 0.25mg IM/IV over 2min; **CH** <2y: 0.125mg IM/IV over 2min; >2y: see adults
Menotropins, FSH/LH, Follitropins, FSH, Chorionic Gonadotropins, hCG →288	
Somatrem	PRC C, Lact ?
Protropin Inj 5mg/vial, 10mg/vial	**Growth hormone deficiency:** individ. dos., upto 0.3mg/kg/wk SC/IM admin qd in div dos.
Somatropin (Growth Hormone)	EHL 18min, PRC C, Lact ?
Humatrope Inj 5mg/vial; 6, 12mg/vial, **Nutropin** Inj 5mg/vial, 10mg/vial, **Saizen** Inj 1.33mg/vial, 3.33mg/vial, 5mg/vial **Serostim** Inj 5mg/vial, 6mg/vial	**GH deficiency:** ini 0.006mg/kg/d SC, max 0.0125mg/kg/d

6.14 Posterior Pituitary Hormones

MA (desmopressin): renal H_2O resorpt. ↑, vasoconstr.; **AE** (desmopressin): flushing, headache, nausea; **CI** (desmopressin): hypersens. to desmopressin prod., CH< 3mo, Type IIB v.Willebrand

Desmopressin	EHL 75.5min, PRC B, Lact ?
DDAVP Tab 0.1, 0.2mg, Spray (nasal) 0.01mg/Spray, Inj 0.004mg/ml **DDAVP Rhinyle Nasal Sol.** Spray 0.25mg/bot **Minirin** Tab 0.1mg **Octostim** Spray (nasal) 0.15mg/Spray, Inj 0.015mg/ml **Generics** Spray (nasal) 0.01mg/Spray	**Central diabetes insipidus:** 10-40mcg (0.1-0.4ml) intranasally qd or div bid-tid; 0.1-1.2mg/d PO qd or div bid-tid; 2-4mcg/d SC/IV div bid; **CH central diabetes insipidus:** 3mo - 12y: 5-30mcg (0.05-0.3 ml) intranasally qd or div bid; 0.05mg PO bid; **hemophilia A;** enuresis

7.   Infections

7.1   Organism – Antibiotic

Organisms (rows):

- Streptococci A, B, C, G
- Strept. viridans group
- Strept. pneumoniae
- Enterococcus
- Staph. aureus (MSSA)
- Staph. aureus (MRSA)
- Corynebact. diphtheriae
- Gonococcus (Neiss.gon.)
- Meningococc. (Neiss.men.)
- Haemophilus influenza
- Escherichia coli
- Klebsiella
- Salmonella
- Shigella
- Proteus mirabilis
- Proteus vulgaris
- Enterobacter
- Serratia
- Pseudomonas aeruginosa
- Borrelia
- Legionella
- Actinomyces
- Clostridium (exc. Cl.dif.)
- Bacteroides fragilis
- Treponema
- Chlamydia
- Mycoplasma
- Rickettsia

Penicillin G, Penicillin V, Dicloxacillin, Ampicillin, Mezlocillin, Ampic.+sulbact, Cefadroxil, Cefazolin, Cefotaxime, Imipenem, Doxycyline, Clindamycin, Clarithromycin, Tobramycin, Ciprofloxacin, Moxifloxacin, Co-trimoxazole, Metronidazole, Vancomycin, Linezolid

Legend:

- effective
- low effectiveness
- not recommended
- ■ first choice
- ■ alternative

from Antibiotics pocketcard 2005; Hof, Börm Bruckmeier Publishing

7.2 Penicillins

7.2.1 Penicillins - 1st Generation (Benzylpenicillins, Penicillinase-Sensitive)

S: Pneumo-, Strepto-, Meningo-, Staphylococcus, Actinomyces, Leptospira, C. diphtheria, Treponema, Borrelia, Past. multocida, Fusobacteria, Peptococcus, Clostridia
R: Enteric bacteria, Pseudomonas, B. fragilis, E. faecium, Nocardia, Mycoplasma, Chlamydia, beta-lactamase producing bacteria, Salmonella, V. cholerae
AE: allergic skin reactions, Lyell-syndrome, anaphylaxis, vasculitis, myoclonia, seizures, oral dryness, N/V, diarrhea, Herxheimer- reaction, complete blood count changes, hemolytic anemia, interstitial nephritis, superinfection by multiresistant bacteria or yeasts
CI: hypersensitivity to prod ingredients, penicillins (Pen G procaine: additional sulfites), hx of anaphylaxis, accelerated or serum sickness reaction to previous penicillin administration

Benzylpenicilloyl Polylysine	PRC C, Lact ?
Pre-Pen *Inj. 0.0006 M/amp*	**Penicillin sensitivity detection:** scratch test or 0.01-0.02ml intradermally

Penicillin G	EHL 20-50min, PRC B, Lact +
Crystapen *Inj 1,000,000 U/vial, 5,000,000 U/vial, 10,000,000 U/vial* **Penicillin G Potassium** *Inj 1,000,000 U/vial, 5,000,000 U/vial, 10,000,000 U/vial* **Penicillin G Sodium** *Inj 1,000,000 U/vial, 5,000,000 U/vial, 10,000,000 U/vial*	**Streptococcal, pneumococcal, meningococcal infx:** 1-5 mio U/d IV div q4-6h; **streptococcal or staphylococcal endocarditis:** 12-18 mio U/d IV div q4h; **enterococcal endocarditis:** 18-30 mio U/d continuous IV inf or div q4h with aminoglycoside; **meningococcal meningitis:** 20-40 mio U/d IV div q2-4h; **CH** <12y: 25,000-400,000 U/kg/d IV div q4-6h, neonates: see Prod Info

Penicillin G Benzathine	EHL 20-50min
Penicillin G *Inj 600,000 U/ml*	**Group A streptococcal upper respiratory infx:** 1.2 mio U IM x 1; **CH** 25,000-50,000 U/kg IM x 1, max 1.2 mio U; **PRO of rheumatic fever:** 1.2 mio U IM q mo; **CH** 25,000-50,000 U/kg IM q3-4wks, max 1.2 mio U/dose; **early syphilis:** 2.4 mio U IM x 1; **CH early/congenital syphilis:** 50.000 U/kg IM x 1, max 2.4 mio U; **late syphilis:** 2.4 mio U IM qwk x 3 wk; **CH** 50.000 U/kg IM qwk x 3wk, max 2.4 mio U

Penicillin G Procaine	EHL 20-30min
Generics Inj 300,000 U/vial, 1,500,000 U/vial	**Anthrax (postexposure PRO, inhal):** 1.2 mio U IM q12h, **CH** 25,000U/kg IM q12h, max 1.2 mio U/dose, **cutaneous**: 600,000-1.2 mio U/d IM; **Streptococcal, staphylococcal infx:** 0.6-1.0 mio U IM qd for 7-10d **neurosyphilis:** 2.4 mio U IM qd + probenecid 500mg PO q6h for 10-14d; **CH** 300.000 U IM qd; **congenital syphilis:** 50.000 U/kg IM qd for 10d; DARF: GFR (ml/min): 10-30: q8-12h, <10: q12-18h

Penicillin V	EHL 30-40min, PRC B, Lact +
Apo-Pen VK Sol (oral) 125mg/5ml, 300mg/5ml, Tab 300mg **Novo-Pen-VK** Sol (oral) 300mg/5ml, Tab 300mg **Nu-Pen-VK** Tab 300mg **Pen-Vee** Sol (oral) 180mg/5ml, 300mg/5ml, Tab 300mg **PVF K** Tab 300mg **Generics** Tab 300mg	**Infection:** 125-500mg PO q6-8h; **CH** <12y: 25mg/mg/kg/d PO div q6-8h, max 3g/d; **PRO of recurrent rheumatic fever/pneumococcal infections:** 250mg PO bid; **CH** <5y: 125mg PO bid; ≥5y: 250mg PO bid; DARF: CrCl (ml/min): 10-15: q8-12h, <10: q 12-16h

7.2.2 Penicillins - 2nd Generation (Penicillinase-Resistant)

S/R: highly effective against beta-lactamase producing S. aureus; otherwise very narrow spectrum + lower activity against all other gram-positive bacteria than penicillin G
AE/CI: see benzylpenicillins →119
AE (cloxacillin): fever, rash, N/V, diarrhea, hepatotoxicity; **CI:** hypersensitivity to product ingredients/penicillins

Cloxacillin	EHL 0.5-1h, PRC B, Lact ?
Apo-Cloxi Cap 250mg, 500mg, Sol (Oral) 125mg/5ml **Novo-Cloxin** Cap 250mg, 500mg, Sol (Oral) 125mg/5ml **Nu-Cloxi** Cap 250mg, 500mg, Sol (Oral) 125mg/5ml **Cloxacillin sodium** Inj 500mg/vial, 1000mg/vial, 2000mg/vial	**Staphylococcal infx:** 250-500mg PO q6h; 250-250mg IV/IM q4-6h, severes: upto 2g IV/IM q4h **CH** 50-100mg/kg/d PO/IV/IM div q6h, max 4g/d; severe infections: 150-200mg/kg/d IV/IM div q6h, max 12g/d; DARF: not req

7.2.3 Penicillins - 3rd Generation (Aminopenicillins)

S: compared to penicillin G additional action against Enterococcus, H. influenza, E. coli, Listeria, P. mirabilis, Salmonella, Shigella
R: B. fragilis, Pseudomonas, E. faecium, Nocardia, Mycoplasma, Chlamydia, beta-lactamase producing bacteria, Klebsiella, Yersinia
AE/CI: see benzylpenicillins →119 ; **CI:** history of allergy to penicillins

Amoxicillin

EHL 1-2h, PRC B, Lact +

Apo-Amoxi *Cap 250mg, 500mg, Sol (oral) 125mg/5ml, 250mg/5ml*
Lin-Amox *Cap 250mg, 500mg, Sol (oral) 125mg/5ml, 250mg/5ml*
Novamoxin *Cap 250mg, 500mg, Sol (oral) 125mg/5ml, 250mg/5ml, Tab (chew) 125mg, 250mg*
Nu-Amoxi *Cap 250mg, 500mg, Sol (oral) 125mg/5ml, 250mg/5ml*
Generics *Cap 250mg, 500mg, Sol (oral) 125mg/5ml, 250mg/5ml*

Respiratory tract, ENT, genitourinary tract, skin, infx: 250-500mg PO q8h or 500-875mg PO q12h, max 2-3g/d; **CH** <20kg: 20-40mg/kg/d PO div q8h; **endocarditis PRO:** 2g PO 1h before the procedure; **CH** 50mg/kg PO 1h before the procedure, max 2g; **DARF:** GFR (ml/ min) 10-50: q8-12h, <10: q12-24h

Ampicillin

EHL 1-1.8 h and 15-20 h, PRC B, Lact +

Apo-Ampi *Cap 250mg, 500mg, Susp (oral) 125mg/5ml, 250mg/5ml*
Nu-Ampi *Cap 250mg, 500mg, Susp (oral) 125mg/5ml, 250mg/5ml*
Generics *Cap 250mg, 500mg, Susp (oral) 125mg/5ml, 50mg/5ml Inj 250mg/vial, 500mg/vial, 1g/vial, 2g/vial*

Respirat. tract, GI infx, UTI: 250-500mg PO/IV/IM q6h; **CH** <40kg 25-50mg/kg/d IV/IM div q6h; <20kg 50-100mg/kg/d PO div q6-8h; **meningitis or septicemia:** 8-14g/d IV div q3-4h; **CH** <40kg 100-200mg/kg/d IV/IM div q3-4h; **endocarditis PRO:** 2g IM/IV 30min before procedure; **CH** 50mg/kg IV/IM 30min before procedure; **endocard. Tx:** 12g/d IV contin. or div q4h; **DARF:** GFR (ml/min)>50: q6h, 10-50:q6-12h, <10: q12-24h

Pivampicillin

EHL 1h, PRC B, Lact ?

Pondocillin *Sol (oral) 175mg/5ml, Tab 500mg*

Respirat. tract, ENT, gyne, urinary tract infect.: 500mg PO bid, 15-30ml (525-1050mg) PO bid; **CH** 7-10y 10ml (350mg) PO bid, 4-6y 7.5ml (262.5mg) PO bid, 1-3y 5ml (175mg)PObid, max 500mg PO bid; **gonoc. urethr.:** 1.5g single dose with 1g probenecid

7.2.4　Penicillins - 4th Generation (Extended Spectrum, Antipseudomonal)

S/R: similar to aminopenicillins, but highly effective against Ps. aeroginosa
AE/CI: see benzylpenicillins →119
AE (piperacillin): fever, headache, rash **CI:** hypersensitivity to piperacillin

Piperacillin	EHL 3.33h, PRC B, Lact +
Generics *Inj 2g/vial, 3g/vial, 4g/vial*	**Sepsis, nosocomial pneumonia, intra-abdominal, urinary tract, skin and soft tissue infx:** 2-3g IM q6-12h; 3-4g IV q4-6h, max 24g/d; CH 200-300mg/kg/d div q4-6h; DARF: GFR (ml/min): 10-50: q6-8h, <10: q8h

7.2.5　Penicillin + β-Lactamase Inhibitor

AE (amoxicillin + clavulanate): headache, rash, N/V, diarrhea
AE (piperacillin + tazobactam): rash, diarrhea, headache, N/V
AE (ticarcillin + clavulanate): hypersensitivity reactions, seizures, pseudomembranous colitis, thrombophlebitis
CI (amoxicillin + clavulanate, piperacillin + tazobactam): hypersensitivity to penicillins + product ingredients, (amoxicillin + clavulanate): suspected or confirmed mononucleosis

Amoxicillin + Clavulanate	PRC B, Lact +
Apo-Amoxi-Clav *Tab 250mg + 125mg, 500mg + 125mg, 875mg + 125mg, S usp (oral) 125mg + 31.25mg/5ml, 250mg + 62.5mg/5ml* **Clavulin** *Tab 250mg + 125mg, 500mg + 125mg, 875mg + 125mg, Susp (oral) 125mg/5ml + 31.25mg/ 5ml, 200mg/5ml + 28.5mg/5ml, 250mg/5ml + 62.5mg/ 5ml, 400mg/5ml + 57mg/5ml* **Novo-Clavamoxin** *Tab 875mg + 125mg* **Ratio-Aclavulanate** *Tab 250mg + 125mg, 500mg + 125mg, 875mg + 125mg, Susp (oral) 125mg + 31.25mg/5ml, 250mg + 62.5mg/5ml*	**UTI, respiratory tract, skin infx, sinusitis, otitis media:** 500-875 + 125mg PO q12h or 250-500 +125mg PO q8h; **CH** (amoxicillin component) 25-45mg/kg/d PO div q12h or 20-40mg/kg/d PO div q8h; DARF: GFR (ml/min): 10-30: 250-500 + 125mg q12h; <10: 250-500 + 125mg PO q24h

Piperacillin + Tazobactam	PRC B, Lact +
Tazocin *Inj 2g/vial + 0.25g/vial, 3g/vial + 0.375g/vial, 4g/vial + 0.5g/vial*	**Intra-abdominal, skin infx, community-acquired pneumonia, febrile neutropenia:** 3 + 0.375g IV q6h; DARF: GFR (ml/min): 20-40: 2 + 0.25g IV q6h; <20: 2 + 0.25g IV q8h

Ticarcillin + Clavulanate	PRC B, Lact +
Timentin *Inj 3g/vial + 0.1g/vial, 30g/vial + 1g/vial*	**Systemic infx, UTI:** 3 + 0.1g IV q4-6h; **CH** 300mg/kg/d ticarcillin component IV div q6h; DARF: ini 3.1g, then GFR (ml/min): 30-60: 2g IV q4h; 10-30: 2g IV q8h; <10: 2g IV q12h; <10 with hepatic dysfunction: 2g IV q24h

7.3 Cephalosporins

7.3.1 Cephalosporins - 1st Generation

S: act as penicillin G substitutes, but resistant to staphylococcal penicillinase; also activity against Proteus mirabilis, E. coli + Klebsiella pneumoniae; cefazolin-group: Staphylo-, Strepto-, Pneumococcus, N. meningitis, E. coli, Klebsiella, Prot. mirabilis, H. influenza
R (cefazolin-group): Enterococcus, Pseudomonas, Acinetobact., Listeria, Chlamydia, Mycoplasma, gram-neg. ß-lactamase- producing bacteria
AE (cephalosporins): allergic skin reactions, Lyell-syndrome, anaphylaxis, N/V, diarrhea, transaminases↑, cholestasis, interstitial pneumonia, complete blood count changes, hemolytic anemia, creatinine↑, interstitial nephritis, superinfection by bacteria or yeasts
CI (cephalosporins): hypersensitivity to cephalosporins

Cefazolin	EHL 1.5-2.5h, PRC B, Lact +
Generics *Inj 500mg/vial, 1g/vial, 10g/vial*	**Pneumonia:** 500mg IV/IM q12h, **mild infx from gram pos. cocci:** 250-500mg IV/IM q8h, **uncomplicated UTI:** 1g IV/IM q12h **mod-severe infections:** 500mg-1g IV/IM q6-8h, **surgical PRO:** 1g IM/IV 30-60min preop, 0.5-1g during surgery >2h, 0.5-1g q6-8h for 24h postop; **CH** 25-50mg/kg/d IM/IV div q6-12h; 100mg/kg/d for severe infx; DARF: GFR (ml/min): >55: 100%, 35-54: 100% at least q8h, 11-34: 50% q12h, 0-10: 50% q18-24h

7.3.2   Cephalosporins - 1st Generation - Oral Cephalosporins

S: similar spectrum to cefazolin-group, highly effective against gram-positive bacteria, low effectiveness against gram-negative bacteria
R: Pseudomonas, Enterococcus, Prot. vulgaris, Morganella, Citrobacter, Serratia, enteric bacteria, Acinetobact., B. fragilis, Listeria, Chlamydia, Mycoplasma
AE/CI: see Cephalosporins - 1st Generation →123

Cefadroxil	EHL 1.2-1.7h , PRC B, Lact +
Duricef Cap 500mg **Generics** Cap 500mg	**UTI:** 1-2g/d PO qd or div bid; **skin and soft tissue infx, pharyngitis, tonsillitis:** 1g/d PO qd or div bid for 10d; **CH** 30mg/kg/d PO div bid; DARF: ini 1g, then: GFR (ml/min): 26-50: 0.5g q12h; 10-25: 0.5g q24h; 0-10: 0.5g q36h

Cephalexin	EHL 0.9h, PRC B, Lact +
Apo-Cephalex Tab 250mg, 500mg **Novo-Lexin** Cap 250mg, 500mg, Susp (oral) 125mg/5ml, 250mg/5ml, Tab 250mg, 500mg **Nu-Cephalex** Tab 250mg, 500mg	**Pneumonia, skin infx, UTI:** 250-500mg PO q6h, max 4g/ d; **CH** 25-50mg/kg/d PO div q6h, max 4g/d; **acute osteomyelitis:** (after IV therapy) 500mg-1g PO q6h, **CH** 100-150mg/kg/d div q6h; DARF: GFR (ml/min) >50: 100%, <50: 250-500mg q12h

7.3.3   Cephalosporins - 2nd Generation

S (cephalosporins - 2nd generation): greater activity against three additional gram-negative organisms, H. influenzae, some Enterbacter aerogenes and some Neisseria species, whereas activity against gram-positive organisms is weaker; cefuroxim group: see Cephalosporins - 1st Generation →123, higher effectiveness against E. coli, Klebsiella, Prot. mirabilis, H. influenza, ß- lactamase producing bacteria; cephamycins/cefoxitin group (S/R): highly effective against ß-lactamase-producing anaerobic bacteria (for example Bacteroides)
R (cefuroxime-group): Enterococcus, Pseudomonas, Acinetobact., Listeria, Chlamydia, Mycoplasma
AE/CI: see Cephalosporins - 1st Generation →123

Cefotetan	EHL 2.8-4.6h, PRC B, Lact +
Cefotan Inj 1g/vial, 2g/vial	**UTI, skin, lower respiratory, abdominal infx:** 500mg-3g IM/IV q12h; DARF: GFR (ml/min) 10-30: q24h, <10: q48h

Cefoxitin	EHL 0.8-1h, PRC B, Lact +
Generics *Inj 1g/vial, 2g/vial, 10g/vial*	**Pneumonia, genitourinary and gynecologic infx, sepsis, intra-abdominal, skin, bone and joint infx:** 1-2g IV q6-8h, **CH** 80-160mg/kg/d IV div q4-6h, max 12g/d; DARF: ini: 1-2g IV, then GFR (ml/min) 30-50: 1-2g IV q8- 12h 10-29: 1-2g IV q12-24h, 5-9: 0.5-1g IV q12-24h, <5: 0.5g IV q24-48h
Cefuroxime-Sodium	EHL no data, PRC B, Lact +
Zinacef *Inj 750mg/vial, 1.5g/vial, 7.5g/vial* **Generics** *Inj 750mg/vial, 1.5g/vial, 7.5g/vial*	**uncomplicated infections/UTI/soft tissue/ pneumonia:** 750mg IV/IM q8h; **CH** 30-100mg/kg/d div tid-qid; **Bone + joint infx, severe infection, gram neg. pneumonia:** 1.5g IV/IM q8h; **CH** 70-150mg/kg/d IV div q8h; **meningitis:** 3gIV q8h; **CH** 200-240mg/kg/d IV div tid-qid; **gonorrhea:** 1.5g IM as single dose together with 1g Probenecid PO; **CH** ; DARF: GFR (ml/min): >20: 750-1500mg q8h; 10-20: 750mg q12h; <20: 750mg q24h

7.3.4 Cephalosporins - 2nd Generation - Oralcephalosporins

S/R (oral cephalosporins 2nd generation): see cefuroxime-group →124
AE/CI: see Cephalosporins - 1st Generation →123

Cefaclor	EHL 30-60min, PRC B, Lact +
Ceclor *Cap 250mg, 500mg, Susp (oral) 125mg/5ml, 250mg/5ml, 375mg/5ml* **Generics** *Cap 250mg, 500mg, Susp (oral) 125mg/5ml, 250mg/5ml, 375mg/5ml*	**Respiratory tract infx, otitis media, UTI, skin infx, bone and joint infx:** 250-500mg PO tid; **CH** 20-40mg/kg/d PO div q8-12h, max 2g/d; DARF: GFR (ml/min): <50: 50%
Cefprozil	EHL 1-2h, PRC B, Lact +
Cefzil *Tab 250mg, 500mg, Susp (oral) 125mg/5ml, 250mg/5ml*	**Pharyngitis, tonsillitis, UTI:** 500mg PO qd; **sinusitis:** 250-500mg PO bid; **skin infx:** 250mg PO bid or 500mg PO qd; **CH** 6mo-12y: 7.5-15mg/kg PO q12h; DARF: GFR (ml/min) <30: 50%

Cefuroxime-Axetil	EHL 1.1-1.3h , PRC B, Lact +
Ceftin *Tab 250mg, 500mg,* *Susp (oral) 125mg/5ml, 250mg/5ml* **Generics** *Tab 250mg, 500mg*	**Early lyme disease:** 500mg PO bid for 20d; **bronchitis, tonsillitis, pharyngitis,** **sinusitis, skin infx:** 250mg PO bid; **pneumonia:** 500mg PO bid; **gonorrhea:** 1g PO x 1; **UTI:** 125-250mg PO bid for 7-10d; **CH** >3mo: 10-15mg/kg PO bid, max 1g/d

7.3.5 Cephalosporins - 3rd Generation

S (cephalosporins - 3rd generation): inferior to first generation cephalosporins against gram-positive cocci, but enhanced activity against gram-negative bacilli (see 2nd generation cephalosporins →124 plus most other enteric organisms) and Serratia marcescens. (ceftriaxone or cefotaxime: agents of choice in Tx of meningitis; ceftazidime: activity against Ps. aeruginosa); cefotaxime sodium-group: higher bactericidal effect against gram-negative germs (i.e. Klebsiella, H. influenza)
R: cefotaxime sodium-group: Enterococcus, Legionella, Chlamydia, Mycoplasma, Listeria, Clostridium diff.;
AE/CI: see Cephalosporins - 1st Generation →123

Cefotaxime	EHL 0.8-1.4h, PRC B, Lact +
Claforan *Inj 500mg/vial, 1g/vial, 2g/vial*	**Pneumonia, UTI, gynecologic, skin,** **intra-abdom., bone, joint, CNS infx,** **uncomplicated:** 1g IM/IV q12h; **moderate/severe:** 1-2g IM/IV q8h; **severe:** 2g IV q6-8h. **life-threatening:** 2g IV q4h, max 12g/d; **neonates** 1-4 wk: 50mg/kg IV q8h, **CH** 1mo-12y: 50-180mg/kg/d IM/IV div q4-6h; DARF: GFR (ml/min): <20: 50%

Ceftazidime	EHL 1.6-2h, PRC B, Lact +
Fortaz *Inj 1g/vial, 2g/vial, 6g/vial* **Generics** *Inj 1g/vial, 2g/vial, 6g/vial*	**unompl. UTI:** 250mg IM/IV q12h; **skin infx, uncomplicated pneumonia:** 500mg IM/IV q8h; **complicated UTI:** 500mg IM/IV q8-12h; **bone inx:** 2g IV q12h; **life-threatening infx:** 2g IV q8h; **CH** 1-2m 12.5-25mg/kg IV q12h; 2m-12y 10-33mg/kg IV q8h; **cystic fibrosis with pseudomonas infx:** 50-75mg/kg IV q8h; DARF: GFR (ml/min): 31-50: 1g IV q12h, 16-30: 1g IV q24h; 6-15: 500mg IV q24h, <5: 500mg IV q48h

Ceftizoxime	EHL 1.1-2.3h, PRC B, Lact +
Cefizox *Inj 1g/vial, 2g/vial*	**uncomplicated UTI:** 500mg IM/IV q12h; **Pneumonia, sepsis, intra-abdom., skin, bone/joint, UTI:** 1-2g IM/IV q8-12h, **life-threatening infx:** 3-4g IV q8h, **CH** >6mo: 50mg/kg IV q6-8h; DARF: ini 0.5-1g IV/IM, GFR (ml/min): 50-79: 0.5-1.5g q8h; 5-49: 250mg-1g q12h; 0-4: 250-500mg q24h

Ceftriaxone	EHL 5-9h, PRC B, Lact +
Rocephin *Inj 250mg/vial, 1g/vial, 2g/vial, 10g/vial*	**UTI, respir. tract, intra-abdom. infx, sepsis, endocarditis, meningitis, lyme disease:** 1-2g IM/IV q24h or div q12h, max 4g/d; **gonorrhea:** 250mg IM x 1; **CH** 50-75mg/kg/d IM/IV div q12- 24h, max 2g/d; **CH meningitis:** 100mg/kg/d div q12h, max 4g/d; DARF: not req

7.3.6 Cephalosporins – 3rd Generation – Oralcephalosporins

S/R (oral cephalosporins 3rd gen.): more effective and broader spectrum then 2nd gen. cephalosporins against gram-neg. bacteria; less effective against gram-positive bacteria
AE/CI: see Cephalosporins – 1st Generation →123

Cefixime	EHL 3-4h, PRC B, Lact ?
Suprax *Tab 400mg, Susp (oral) 100mg/5ml*	**Respiratory tract infx, UTI, pharyngitis, tonsillitis:** 400mg PO qd; **gonorrhea:** 400mg PO as single dose; **CH** >6mo: 8mg/kg/d qd or div bid;DARF: GFR (ml/min): >60: 100%, 21-60: 75%, <20: 50%

7.3.7 Cephalosporins – 4th Generation

S: wide antibacterial spectrum, Strepto- and Staphylococci (only methicillin susceptible ones); also aerobic gram-negatives like Enterobacter, E. coli, Klebsiella pneumoniae, Proteus mirabilis and Ps. aeruginosa
see Cephalosporins – 1st Generation →123

Cefepime	EHL 2h, PRC B, Lact ?
Maxipime *Inj 1g/vial, 2g/vial*	**uncompl or complicated UTI, skin infx, mild-mod. pneumonia:** 0.5-1g IM/IV q12h; **intra-abdominal, severe pneumonia:** 2g IV q12h; **febrile neutropenia:** 2g IV q8h; **CH** 2mo-12y: 50mg/kg IV q12h; DARF: GFR (ml/ min): <11: 0.25-1g q24h, 11-29: 0.5-2g q24h

7.4 Carbapenems

S: almost all gram-positive and gram-negative bacteria
R: Mycoplasma, Chlamydia, Legionella, Ps. cepacia, Xanthonomas maltophilia, E. faecium
AE: N/V, diarrhea, liver enz.m, allergic reactions, complete blood count changes, CNS DO
CI: hypersensitivity to product ingredients, penicillins, cephalosporins, and other beta lactams

Imipenem–Cilastatin	EHL 1h, PRC C, Lact ?
Primaxin *Inj 250mg/vial, 500mg/vial*	**mild infx:** 250mg IV q6h; **moderate:** 500mg IV q8h; **severe:** 500mg q6h; **life threatening:** 1g IV q6-8h; max 4g/d; **CH** >3mo: 15-25mg/kg IV q6h; DARF: GFR (ml/min) 31-70 max 2g q6h, 21-30 max 1.5g q8h, 0-20 max 1g q12h

Meropenem	EHL 1h, PRC B, Lact ?
Merrem *Inj 500mg/vial, 1g/vial*	**complicated UTI, skin infx, gyne infx, PID, comm. aquired pneumonia:** 500mg IV q8h; **nosocomial pneumonia, intra-abdominal infx, septicemia:** 1g IV q8h; **meningitis:** 2g IV q8h; **CH** 3-12y: 20-40mg/kg tid; DARF: GFR (ml/min) 26-50: 0.5-2g q12h; 10-25: 50% q12h; <10: 50% q24h

7.5   Glycopeptides

S: aerobic and anaerobic gram-positive bacteria, methicillin resistant S. aureus (MRSA)
R: all gram-negative Bacteria, Mycoplasma, Chlamydia
AE: allergic reactions, thrombophlebitis, ototoxicity, nephrotoxicity, complete blood count changes, red man/neck syndrome, N/ V; **CI:** hypersensitivity to product ingredients

Vancomycin	EHL 4-6h, PRC C, Lact + serum-lev. (mcg/ml): peak 30-40; trough 5-10
Vancocin *Cap 125mg, 250mg, Inj 500mg/vial, 1g/vial, 10g/vial* **Generics** *Inj 500mg/vial, 1g/vial*	**MRSA infx, other staphylococcal or streptococcal infx, endocarditis:** 500mg IV q6h or 1g IV q12h or 30mg/kg/d IV div q12; **CH** >1mo: 40mg/kg/d IV div q6h; **clostridium difficile diarrhea:** 125-500mg PO q6-8h for 7-10d; **CH** 40mg/kg/d PO div tid-qid; DARF: GFR (ml/min) >50: 500mg IV q12h, 10-50: 500mg IV q24-48h, <10: 500mg IV q48-96h

Clarithromycin	EHL 3-7h, PRC C, Lact ?
Biaxin *Tab 250mg, 500mg, Susp (oral) 125mg/5ml, 250mg/5ml* **Biaxin XL** *Tab ext. release 500mg*	**upper/lower respiratiry infx, exacerbation of chronic bronchitis:** 250-500mg PO bid or 1g ext rel. PO qd for 7d; **pharyngitis/tonsilitis:** 250mg PO bid for 10d; **pneumonia, sinusitis:** 500mg PO bid or 1g ext. rel. PO qd for 14d; **uncomplicated skin infx:** 250mg PO bid; **PRO/Tx of mycobacterium avium complex:** 500mg PO bid in combination with **antimyco-bacterial drugs; h. pylori triple Tx:** 500mg PO bid with omeprazole 20mg bid and amoxicillin 1g bid for 10d; **CH** >6mo: 7.5mg/kg PO bid; DARF: GFR (ml/min) <30: 50%

Erythromycin Base	EHL no data, PRC B
Apo-Erythro Base *Tab 250mg* **Apo-Erythro E-C** *Cap 250mg, 333mg* **Erybid** *Tab ext. rel. 500mg* **Eryc** *Cap ext.rel. 250mg, 333mg* **PCE** *Tab 333mg*	**Respiratory, campylobacter jejuni, chlamydia, mycoplasma pneumoniae infx, nongonococcal urethritis, legionnaire's disease:** 250mg PO q6h or 333mg PO q8h or 500mg bid, max 4g/d; **CH** 7.5-25mg/kg PO q6h or 15-25mg PO q12h; DARF: GFR (ml/min): <10: 50-75%, max 2g/d

Erythromycin Estolate	EHL no data, PRC B, Lact +
Generics *Cap 250mg*	250mg PO q6h or 333mg PO q8h or 500mg bid, max 4g/d; **CH** 7.5-25mg/kg PO q6h or 15-25mg PO q12h DARF: GFR (ml/min): <10: 50-75%, max 2g/d

Erythromycin Ethylsuccinate	EHL no data, PRC B, Lact +
Apo-Erythro-ES *Tab 600mg* **E.E.S.** *Tab 600mg, Gran (oral) 200mg/5ml, Susp (oral) 200mg/5ml, 400mg/5ml* **Novo-Rythro ethylsuccinate** *Susp (oral) 200mg/5ml, 400mg/5ml*	400mg PO q6h, max 4g/d; **CH** 12-40mg/kg PO q6h; DARF: GFR (ml/min): <10: 50-75%, max 2g/d

Erythromycin Ethylsuccinate + Sulfisoxazole PRC C, Lact ?	
Pediazole *Susp (oral) 200 + 600mg/5ml*	**CH >2m otitis media:** 50mg/kg/d erythromycin + 150mg/kg/d sulfisoxazole div tid-qid for 10d

Erythromycin Lactobionate	EHL no data, PRC B, Lact +
Generics *Inj 500mg/vial, 1g/vial*	**Infx:** 250-500mg IV q6h, or 15-20mg/kg/d IV div q6h, max 4g/d, **CH** 20-40mg/kg/d div q6h, max 4g/d; DARF: GFR (ml/min): <10: 50-75%, max. 2g/d

Erythromycin Stearate	EHL no data, PRC B, Lact +
Apo-Erythro-S *Tab 250mg* **Generics** *Tab 250mg*	**Infx:** 250-500mg PO q6-12h

7.8 Aminoglycosides

S: enteric bacteria, Pseudomonas, Staphylococcus, Serratia, Yersinia, Pasteurella, Brucella
R: Enterococcus, Anaerobic bacteria, Streptococcus, Pneumococcus
AE: nephrotoxicity, ototoxicity, neurotoxicity, neuromuscular blockage, paresthesia, renal damage, complete blood count changes, allergic reactions, N/V/D, dizziness
CI: hypersensitivity to product ingredients **CI** (paromomycin) intestinal obsruction

Amikacin	EHL no data, PRC D, Lact + serum-lev. (mcg/ml): peak: 30; trough: 5-10
Amikin *Inj 250mg/ml*	**Gram-negative infx:** 15mg/kg/d IV/IM bid, max 1.5g/d, max 15g total course; **neonates:** ini 10mg/kg, then 7.5mg/kg IM/IV q12h; DARF: GFR (ml/min) >50: 60-90% q12h, 10-50: 30-70% q12-18h, <10: 20-30% q24-48h

Gentamicin	EHL 2h, PRC C, Lact ? serum-level (mcg/ml): peak 5-10; trough <2
Garamycin *Inj 10mg/ml, 40mg/ml* **Generics** *Inj 0.8mg/ml, 1mg/ml, 1.2mg/ml, 1.6mg/ml, 10mg/ml, 40mg/ml*	**Gram-negative infx:** 3-6mg/kg/d IV/IM div tid, **neonates:** 2.5-3mg/kg IM/IV q12h, **CH** 5-6mg/kg/d IM/IV div q8h; DARF: GFR (ml/min) 35-70: q12h, 24-34: q18h,16-23: q24; 10-15: q36h; 5-9: q48h

Paromomycin	PRC ?, Lact ?
Humatin Cap 250mg	**Intestinal amebiasis:** 25-35mg/kg/d div tid for 5-10days

Streptomycin	EHL 2.5h, PRC D, Lact +
Generics Inj 1g/vial	**Streptococcal endocarditis:** 1g IM/IV bid for 1wk, then 0.5g bid for 1wk; **TB:** 15mg/kg IM qd, max 1g/d, can reduce to 25mg/kg IM 2-3x/wk; **tularemia:** 1-2g/d div doses for 7-14d orafebrile for 5-7d; **plague:** 2-4g/d div doese until afebrile for 3days; **CH TB:** 20-40mg/kg IM qd, max 1g/d; DARF: GFR (ml/min) >50: 7.5mg/kg q24h, 10-50: 7.5mg/kg q24-72h, <10: 7.5mg/kg q72-96h

Tobramycin	EHL 2h, PRC D, Lact + serum-level (mcg/ml): peak 5-10; trough <2.
TOBI Sol (inhal) 300mg/amp **Generics** Inj 10mg/ml, 40mg/ml	**Infx:** 3-5mg/kg/d IV/IM div tid; **cystic fibrosis/chronic P. aeruginosa:** 300mg inhal nedulizer bid for 28d, then 28d off, **neonates:** 4mg/kg/d IV div bid; **CH** 6-7.5mg/kg/d IV/IM div tid-qid; ; DARF: GFR (ml/min): ini 1mg/kg IM/IV, >50: 60-90% q8-12h; 10-50:30-70% q12h-24,<10:20-30% q24- 48h

7.9 Lincosamides

S: Pneumo-, Staphylo-, Streptococcus, C. diphtheria, anaerobics, B. fragilis, Cl. perfringens
R: Enteric bacteria, P. aeruginosa, Entero-, Gono-, Meningococcus, H. influenza, Mycoplasma, Listeria; **AE:** N/V, diarrhea, pseudomembranous enterokolitis, allergic skin reactions, LFT↑, erythema exsudativum, thrombophlebitis (when used iv)
CI: caution with Myasthenia gravis, hypersensitivity to product ingredients, newborn
CI: (lincomycin) monilial infection

Clindamycin	EHL 1.5-5h, PRC B, Lact ?
Dalacin C *Cap 150mg, 300mg, Sol (oral) 75mg/5ml, Inj 150mg/ml* **Generics** *Cap 150mg, 300mg*	**Anaerobic and other infx:** 1.2-1.8g/d IV/IM div bid-qid, max 4.8g/d or 150-450mg PO qid; **CH** > 1m 20-40mg/kg/d IV div q6-8h or 8-20mg/kg/d PO div tid-qid; DARF: not req, reduce dose with hep. impairment

Lincomycin	PRC A, Lact ?
Lincocin *Inj 300mg/ml*	**Gram positive infection:** 600mg IM q12-24h, 600mg IV q8-12h, **CH** 10mg/kg IM q12-24h, 10-20mg/kg/d IV div q8-12h

7.10 Chloramphenicol

S: wide range of gram-positive and gram-negative organisms (note: because of its toxicity limited clinical use)
AE: N/V, irreversible aplastic anemia, rash, myelosuppression, gray baby syndrom
CI: hypersensitivity to chloramphenicol products

Chloramphenicol	EHL 1.6-3.3h, PRC C, Lact -
Generic *Inj 1g/vial*	**Infx:** 50mg/kg/d IV div q6h, max 100mg/kg/d; **CH** >4wk 50mg/kg/d IV div q6h, upto 100mg/kg/d IV div q6h, DARF: not req

7.11 Quinolones
7.11.1 Nonfluorinated Quinolone

S: only enteric bacteria; **AE:** allergic skin reactions, photosensitivity, muscle weakness, muscle pain, tachycardia, BP↓,headache, malaise, visual DO, cholestasis, hepatitis, N/V; **CI:** children < 3m, hypersensitivity to nalidixic acid

Nalidixic Acid	EHL 60-90min, PRC B, Lact ?
NegGram *Cap 500mg*	**UTI:** 1g PO qid for 7-14d; **CH** 55-60mg/kg/d PO div qid; DARF: avoid if GFR <50ml/min

7.11.2 Fluoroquinolones 1st Group

Group I: indicated almost exclusively for UTI; **S:** enteric bacteria, Campylobacter, Salmonella, Shigella, Gonococcus; **R:** Anaerobic bacteria, Chlamydia, Mycoplasma, E. faecium, Ureaplasma; **AE** (quinolones): allergic skin reactions, phototoxicity, muscle weakness, muscle pain, tachycardia, BP↓, CNS disturbances, cholestasis, hepatitis, cristalluria; **AE** (norfloxacin): dizziness, nausea, headache, abdominal cramping; **CI** (norfloxacin): hypersensitivity to norfloxacin or other fluoroquinolones

Norfloxacin	EHL 2-4h, PRC C, Lact ?
Apo-Norflox Tab 400mg **Generics** Tab 400mg	**Simple UTI:** 400mg PO bid for 3d; **complicated UTI:** 400mg PO bid for 10-21d; **traveler's diarrhea:** 400mg PO bid for 3d; **gonorrhea:** 800mg PO as single dose; **DARF:** GFR (ml/min) <30: 400mg PO qd

7.11.3 Fluoroquinolones - 2nd Group

S: high activity vs. gram-negatives like enterobacteria + H. influenzae, different activity vs. pseudomonas, low activity vs. Staphylo-, Pneumo-, Enterococcus, Mycoplasma, Chlamydia
AE/CI (quinolones): see Fluoroquinolones - 1st Group →135; **AE** (ciprofloxacin): dizziness, headache, diarrhea; **AE** (ofloxacin): nausea, insomnia, headache, dizziness, diarrhea; **CI** (ciproflox., oflox.): hypersensitivity to product ingredients/quinolones

Ciprofloxacin	EHL 3-6h, PRC C, Lact -
Apo-Ciproflox Tab 100mg, 250mg, 500mg, 750mg **Cipro** Tab 250mg, 500mg, 750mg, Susp (oral) 500mg/5ml, Inj 2mg/ml, 10mg/ml **Cipro XL** Tab ext. rel. 500mg, 1000mg **Generics** Tab 250mg, 500mg, 750mg	**Simple UTI:** 250mg PO bid for 3d or ext. rel. 500mg PO qd x 3d; **UTI, bone and joint infx:** 250-500mg PO bid or 400-1200mg IV/d div bid-tid; **chronic bacterial prostatitis:** 500mg PO bid for 28d; **traveler's diarrhea:** 500mg PO bid for 5-7d; **typhoid fever:** 500mg PO bid for 10d; DARF: GFR (ml/min) 30-50: 250-500mg PO q12h; 5-29: 250-500mg PO q18h or 200-400mg IV q18-24h

Ofloxacin	EHL 5-7.5h, PRC C, Lact -
Apo-Oflox Tab 200mg, 300mg, 400mg **Floxin** Tab 300mg, 400mg	**Infx:** 300-400mg PO bid for 7-14d; **prostatitis:** 300-400mg PO bid for 6wk; DARF: GFR (ml/min): 20-50: 100% q24h, <20: 50% q24h

7.11.4 Fluoroquinolones – 3rd Group

S: additional activity Staphylo-, Pneumo-, Streptococcus, Chlamydia, Mycoplasma
AE, CI (quinolones): see Fluoroquinolones – 1st Group →135
AE (levofloxacin): N/V, diarrhea, headache
CI (levofloxacin): hypersensitivity to levofloxacin products/quinolones

Levofloxacin	EHL 6-8h, PRC C, Lact -
Levaquin *Tab 250mg, 500mg, Inj 5mg/ml, 25mg/ml*	**Infx:** 250-500mg PO/IV qd for 3-14d; **Complicated skin infx.:** 500mg PO/IV bid for 10-14d; DARF: ini 250- 500mg PO/IV, then GFR (ml/min): 20-49: 250mg q24h; 10-19: 250mg q48h; <10, dialysis: 250mg q48h

7.11.5 Fluoroquinolones – 4th Group

S: additional activity against anaerobic bacteria
AE, CI (quinolones): see Fluoroquinolones – 1st Group →135
AE (gatifloxacin, moxifloxacin): nausea, diarrhea, headache, dizziness
AE (trovafloxacin): dizziness, headache, N/V/D, liver disease including liver failure
CI (gatifloxacin, moxifloxacin): hypersensitivity to product ingredients/quinolones

Gatifloxacin	EHL 7-14h, PRC C
Tequin *Tab 200mg, 400mg, Inj 10mg/ml*	**Infx:** 400mg IV/PO qd for 5-14d; DARF: ini 400mg PO then GFR (ml/min): <40: 200mg qd

Moxifloxacin	EHL 9-16h, PRC C
Avelox *Tab 400mg, Inj 400mg/250ml*	**Infx:** 400mg PO qd for 5-10d; DARF: not req

7.12 Urinary Tract Antiseptics

AE (methenamine): N/V, diarrhea, cramping; **AE (nitrofurantoin):** pulmonary hypersensitivity, hemolytic anemia, peripheral neuropathy, N/V/D
CI (methenamine): severe dehydration, renal or hepatic insufficiency, use of sulfonamides, hypersensitivity to methenamine**CI (nitrofurantoin):** anuria, CrCl <60ml/min, pregnant patients (38-42wk gestation), neonates, hypersensitivity to nitrofurantoin

Methenamine Hippurate	EHL 4.3h, PRC C, Lact +
Hiprex *Tab 1g*	**Tx/PRO of recurrent or chronic UTI:** 1g PO bid; **CH** 6- 12y: 25-50mg/kg/d div bid; **DARF:** GFR (ml/min): >50: 100%; <50: not rated

Methenamine Mandelate	EHL 4.3h, PRC C, Lact +
Mandelamine *Tab 500mg*	**Tx/PRO of recurrent or chronic UTI:** 1g PO qid; **CH** 6- 12y: 50-75mg/kg/d div qid; **DARF:** GFR (ml/min): >50: 100%; <50: not rated

Nitrofurantoin	EHL 20min-1h, PRC B, Lact
Macrobid *Cap 100mg* **Macrodantin** *Cap 50mg, 100mg* **Novo-Furantoin** *Cap 50mg, 100mg* **Generics** *Cap 50mg, 100mg*	**UTI:** 50-100mg PO qid for 7d or at least 3d after sterile urine; **CH** >1mo: 5-7mg/kg/d PO div qid for 7d or at least 3d after sterile urine; **DARF:** GFR (ml/min): >50: 100%; <50: not rated

7.13 Folate Antagonists
7.13.1 Sulfonamides

S (sulfonamids, including co-trimoxazole): active against selected enterobacteria, chlamydia, Pneumocystis, nocardia
AE (sulfonamids): N/V, allergic reactions, erythema exudativum multiforme, photosensitivity, renal damage, complete blood count changes; **AE (sulfadiazine):** crystalluria, RF; **AE (sulfamethoxazole):** crystalluria, blood dyscrasias
AE (sulfisoxazole): N/V, diarrhea, blood dyscrasias
CI: hypersensitivity to sulfonamides, previous erythema exudativum, severe hepatic + renal dysfunction, newborns, infants < 2mo, patients receiving methenamine

Sulfamethoxazole	EHL 10h, PRC C, Lact ?
Generics *Tab 500mg*	**UTI:** ini 2g, then 1g PO bid-tid; **CH** > 2mo: ini 50-60mg/kg, then 25-30mg/kg PO bid, max 75mg/kg/d

Sulfisoxazole	EHL 7h, PRC C, Lact ?
Sulfizole *Tab 500mg* **Generics** *Tab 500mg*	**UTI:** ini 2-4g, then 4-8g/d PO div q4-6h; **CH** >2mo: ini 75mg/kg, then 150mg/kg/d PO div q4-6h; DARF: GFR (ml/min): >50: q6h; 10-49: q8-12h; <10: q12-24h

7.13.2 Trimethoprim

AE: rash, pruritus, effects of folate deficiency (megaloblastic anemia, leukopenia, granulozytopenia)
CI: hypersensitivity to trimethoprim products, megaloblastic anemia (folate deficiency)

Trimethoprim	EHL 5-17h, PRC C, Lact +
Generics *Tab 100mg, 200mg*	**Uncomplicated UTI:** 100mg PO q12h or 200mg PO q24h; DARF: GFR (ml/min): 15-30: 50mg PO q12h; <15: not rated

7.13.3 Co-trimoxazole

S: almost all aerobic bacteria, Pneumocystis carinii; **R:** P. aeruginosa, Treponema, Clostridium, Leptospiria, Rickettsia, Chlamydia psittaci, Mycoplasma
AE: exanthema, photodermatosis, Lyell-Syndrome, complete blood count changes, hemolytic anemia, N/V, rash, urticaria
CI: hypersensitivity to sulfonamides or trimethoprim, glucose-6-phosphat-dehydrogenase deficiency, severe complete blood count change, severe renal insufficiency, infants < 2mo

Sulfamethoxazole + Trimethoprim (Co-trimoxazole)	PRC C, Lact ?
Apo-Sulfatrim *Tab 100+20mg, 400+80mg, 800+160mg, Susp 200+40mg/5ml* **Novo-Trimel** *Tab 400+80mg, 800+160mg Susp 200+40mg/5ml* **Nu-Cotrimox** *Tab 400+80mg, 800+160mg Susp 200+40mg/5ml* **Protrin** *Tab 400+80mg, 800+160mg* **Septra** *Inj 400+80mg/5ml* **Trisulfa** *Tab 400+80mg*	**UTI:** 800mg + 160mg PO q12h for 3-7d; **exacerbation of chronic bronchitis:** 800mg + 160mg PO q12h for 14d; **travelers' diarrhea:** 800mg + 160mg PO q12h for 5d; **pneumocystis Tx:** 15-20 (TMP) + 75-100 (SMZ) mg/kg/ d IV div q6-8h or PO div q6h for 14-21d; **pneumocystis PRO:** 800mg + 160mg PO qd; **CH** 40- 100mg/kg + 8-20mg/kg PO/IV/; DARF: GFR (ml/min): > 30: 100%; 15-30: 50%, <30: not rated

7.14 Nitroimidazoles

S: obligate anaerobic bacteria (i.e. Bacteroides, Clostridium), Campylobacter, H. pylori, Gardnerella vaginalis, Trichomonas vaginalis, Giardia lamblia, Entamoeba histolytica
R: all aerobic and facultative anaerobic bacteria, Actinomyces, Propionibacteria
AE: GI disturbances, bitter/metallic taste, CNS-disturbances, seizures, allergic skin reactions, alcohol intolerance; **CI:** hypersensitivity to metronidazole

Metronidazole	EHL 6-11h, PRC B, Lact ?
Flagyl *Cap 500mg* **Florazole ER** *Tab ext. release 750mg* **Generics** *Tab 250mg* *Inj 5mg/ml*	**Anaerobic bacterial infx:** 500mg PO/IV q8h or 1.5g IV q24h; **Bacterial vaginosis:** 500mg PO bid x 7d; **Trichomoniasis:** 2g PO x 1 or 250mg PO bid x 10d; **Amebiasis:** 750mg PO q8h x 5-7d; **Giardiasis:** 250mg PO bid x 5-7d; **pseudomembranous colitis:** 500mg PO tid; **CH anaerobic bacterial infx:** ini 15mg/kg IV, then 7.5mg/kg IV bid or 30mg/kg/d PO div qid; DARF: GFR (ml/min) >10: 100%, <10: 50%

7.15 Streptogramines

S: all gram-positive cocci, incl. MRSA, E. faecium, penicillin-G-resistent Pneumococcus, Mor. catarrhalis, Legionella, Mycoplasma pneumoniae, Chlamydia, Prevotella, Fusobacteria, Peptostreptococcus, Clostridia; **R:** H. influenza, E. faecalis, B. fragilis
AE: vein irritation, pruritus, erythema and burning on the face and upper body, N/V, arthralgia, myalgia, transaminases ↑, bilirubin ↑, alkaline phosphatase ↑
CI: severe hepatic insufficiency, combination with drugs that prolong QT interval, hypersensitivity to dalfopristin/quinupristin/ streptogramins

Dalfopristin + Quinupristin	PRC B, Lact ?
Synercid *Inj 350mg/vial + 150mg/vial*	**Vancomycin-resistant E. faecium infx:** 7.5mg/kg IV q8h; **complicated staphyl. skin infx:** 7.5mg/kg IV q12h; DARF: not req

7.16 Other Antimicrobials

AE (fosfomycin): diarrhea, headache, N/V; **AE (linezolid):** diarrhea, headache, nausea
CI (fosfomycin, linezolid): hypersensitivity to product ingredients

Fosfomycin	EHL 5.7 (+/- 2.8)h, PRC B, Lact ?
Monurol *Susp 3g/pkt*	**UTI:** 3g PO as single dose

Linezolid	EHL 5h, PRC N, Lact ?
Zyvoxam *Tab 600mg, Inj 2mg/ml*	**MRSA, vancomycin-resistant E. faecium infx:** 600mg IV/PO q12h for 14-28 d; **complicated skin infx, pneumonia:** 600mg IV/PO q12h for 10-14d; **uncompl. skin infx:** 400mg PO q12h for 10-14d; **DARF:** not req

7.17 Antimycobacterials
7.17.1 Antituberculosis Drugs – Single Ingredient Drugs

S (ethambutol): M. tuberculosis, M. kansasii, M. avium-intracellulare
S (isoniazid): M. tuberculosis, M. kansasii
S (pyrazinamide): M. tuberculosis
S (rifampicin): M. tuberculosis, gram-positive cocci, Legionella, Chlamydia, M. lepra, Meningococcus, Gonococcus, H. influenza, Bacteroides
S (streptomycin): M.tuberculosis, Brucella, Yersinia pestis, Francisella tularensis
AE (ethambutol): optic neuritis, transaminases ↑, allergic reactions;
AE (isoniazid): peripheral neuropathy, transaminases ↑, hepatotoxicity, acne, leukopenia, microhematuria;
AE (pyrazinamide): hyperuricemia, vomiting, transaminases ↑, liver toxicity, disturbances of hematopoiesis, mild nausea + anorexia, arthralgia;
AE (rifampicin): transaminases ↑, cholestasis, red discoloration of the urine, neutropenia, thrombopenia, RF
AE (streptomycin): nephrotoxicity, neurotoxicity, hypersensitivity, ototoxicity
CI (ethambutol): optic neuritis, hypersensitivity to ethambutol products
CI (isoniazid): acute liver disease, previous isoniazid-associated hepatitis
CI (pyrazinamide): severe hepatic dysfunction, hypersensitivity to pyrazinamide products, acute gout
CI (rifampicin): severe hepatic dysfunction
CI (streptomycin): severe renal insufficiency, inner ear damage, hypersensitivity to streptomycin/aminoglycosides

Ethambutol	EHL 2.5-4h, PRC B, Lact +
Etibi *Tab 100mg, 400mg*	**TB:** 15-25mg/kg PO qd **mycobacterium avium complex:** 15-25mg/kg PO qd, **CH** see adults; **DARF:** GFR (ml/min) 10-50: q24-36h, <10: q48h

Isoniazid	EHL 0.7-4h, PRC C, Lact +
Isotamine *Tab 300mg* *Syr 50mg/5ml* **Generics** *Tab 50mg, 100mg, 300mg,* *Syr 50mg/5ml*	**TB Tx:** 5-10mg/kg PO/IM qd, max 300mg/d PO or 15mg/kg, max 900mg 2x/wk; **CH** 10-20mg/kg/d PO, max 300mg; **TB PRO:** 300mg PO qd, **CH** 10-15mg/kg/d PO, max 300mg; DARF: GFR (ml/min) >10: 100%, <10: 50%
Pyrazinamide	EHL 9-23h, PRC C, Lact ?
Tebrazid *Tab 500mg*	**TB Tx:** 15-30mg/kg PO qd, max 2g/d or 50-70mg/dose, max 4g/dose 2x/wk; **CH** see adults; DARF: endstage RF: 12-20mg/kg/d
Rifampin	EHL 3h, PRC C, Lact +
Rifadin *Cap 150mg, 300mg* **Rofact** *Cap 150mg, 300mg*	**TB:** 10mg/kg PO qd, max 600mg/d, **meningococcal PRO:** 600mg PO bid for 2d, **CH** 10-20mg/kg PO/IV qd, max 600mg/d; **CH meningococcal PRO:** 10mg/kg PO bid for 2d
Streptomycin	EHL 2.5h, PRC D, Lact +
Generics *Inj 1g/vial*	**TB:** 15mg/kg IM qd, max 1g/d or 25-30mg/kg IM max 1.5g/d biw-tiw; **CH** TB: 20-40mg/kg IM qd, max 1g/d; DARF: GFR (ml/min) >50: 100% q24h, 10-50: 100% q24-72h, <10: 100% q72-96h

7.17.2 Antituberculosis Drugs - Combinations

Isoniazid + Pyrazinamide + Rifampin	
Rifater *Tab 50mg + 300mg + 120mg*	**TB:** > 55kg: 6 Tab PO qd; 45-54kg: 5 Tab PO qd, < 44kg: 4 Tab PO qd

7.17.3 Other Antimycobacterials

S (dapsone): M. tuberculosis, M. leprae, Pneumocystis carinii
S (rifabutin): M. tuberculosis, M. marinum, M. kansasii, M. leprae, M. avium-intracellulare, gram-positive cocci, Legionella, Chlamydia, Gonococcus
AE (dapsone): dose-related hemolysis, methemoglobinemia, peripheral neuropathy, N/V
AE (rifabutin): red-orange discoloration of urine, N/V, liver enzymesl, jaundice, anemia, leukopenia, eosinophilia, neutropenia, thrombopenia, fever, skin discoloration, reversible uveitis, rash
CI (dapsone): hypersensitivity to dapsone products
CI (rifabutin): hypersensitivity to other rifamycins

Dapsone	EHL 10-50h, PRC C, Lact -
Generics *Tab 100mg*	**Leprosy:** 50-100mg PO qd with other anti-leprosy drugs; **CH** 1-2mg/kg/d PO, max 100mg/d; **pneumocystis PRO:** 100mg PO qd; **pneumocystis Tx:** 100mg PO qd; **CH** 2mg/kg/d PO, max 100mg/d

Rifabutin	EHL 45h, PRC B, Lact ?
Mycobutin *Cap 150mg*	**Mycobacterium avium PRO:** 300mg PO qd or 150mg PO bid; **mycobacterium avium Tx:** 300mg PO qd in combination with a macrolide

7.18 Antivirals
7.18.1 Anti-CMV Drugs

MA/Ind (ganciclovir, valgancicl.): nucleoside analogue, inhibition of DNA synthesis of CMV
AE (ganciclovir): neutropenia, thrombopenia, fever, headache, nausea
AE (valganciclovir): diarrhea, neutropenia, thrombocytopenia, anemia, fever, headache, nausea, abdominal pain, insomnia, peripheral neuropathy
CI (ganciclovir): severe leuko- or thrombopenia, children and adolescents < 18
CI (valganciclovir): hypersensitivity to valganciclovir or ganciclovir

Ganciclovir	EHL 2.5-5h, PRC C, Lact ?
Cytovene *Cap 250mg, 500mg, Inj 500mg/vial*	**CMV retinitis:** 5 mg/kg IV bid for 14-21 d, then 5mg/kg IV qd or 1g PO tid; **CMV PRO in AIDS:** 1g PO tid; DARF: see Prod Info

Valganciclovir	EHL 4h, PRC C, Lact -
Valcyte *Tab 450mg*	**CMV retinitis:** ini 900mg PO bid for 21d, then 900mg qd; DARF: GFR (ml/min): >60: 100%; 40-59: ini 450mg bid, then 450mg qd; 25-39: ini 450mg qd, then 450mg qod; 10-24: ini 450mg qod, then 450mg biw

7.18.2 Anti-Herpetic Drugs

MA/Ind (acyclovir): inhibition of the viral DNA-polymerase; herpes simplex, varicella zoster
MA/Ind (famciclovir): inhibition of the DNA-Polymerase; herpes genitalis, varicella zoster
MA/Ind (valacyclovir): better resorption than acyclovir, varicella zoster infx
AE (acyclovir): renal dysfunction, exanthema, complete blood count changes, N/V headache, rash, phlebitis; **AE (famciclovir):** headache, dizziness, diarrhea;
AE (valacyclovir): headache, N/V
CI (famciclovir): hypersensitivity to famciclovir or penciclovir; **CI (acyclovir):** hypersensitivity to acyclovir; **CI (valacyclovir):** hypersensitivity to valacyclovir or acyclovir

Acyclovir	EHL 3h, PRC B, Lact ?
Zovirax *Tab 200mg, 400mg, 800mg, Susp 200mg/5ml* **Generics** *Tab 200mg, 400mg, 800mg, Inj 500mg/vial*	**CMV infx:** 500mg/square meter IV q8h; **herpes simplex encephalitis:** 10mg/kg IV q8h for 10d; **mucocutaneous herpes:** 5-10mg/kg IV q8h for 5-7d; **varicella zoster in immunocompromised patients:** 10-12mg/kg IV q8h for 7-14d; **varicella zoster in immunocompetent patients:** 5mg/kg IV q8h for 5-7d or 800mg PO q4h for7-10d; **ini herpes genitalis:** 200mg PO 5 x/d for 7-10d; **recurrent herpes genitalis:** 400mg PO bid for up to 12 mo; **chickenpox:** 800mg PO qid for 5d; DARF: GFR (ml/ min): >50: 100% q8h (IV), 25-50: 100% q12h (IV), 10-25: 100% q24h (IV), 0-10: 50% q24h (IV)

Famciclovir	EHL 2-2.3h, PRC B, Lact ?
Famvir *Tab 125mg, 250mg, 500mg*	**Herpes simplex in AIDS:** 500mg PO bid for 7d; **recurrent genital herpes:** 125mg PO bid for 5d; **herpes PRO:** 250 mg PO bid; **herpes zoster:** 500mg PO q8h for 7d; DARF: see Prod Info

Valacyclovir	EHL 2.5-3.6h, PRC B, Lact -
Valtrex *Tab 500mg*	**Herpes zoster:** 1g PO tid for 7 d; **ini. genital herpes:** 1g PO bid for 10 d; **recurrent genital herpes:** 500mg PO bid for 5d; **herpes PRO:** 500-1000 mg PO qd; DARF: see Prod Info

7.18.3 Anti-Influenza Drugs

MA/Ind (amantadine): prevents uncoating and maturation of influenza viruses
MA/Ind (zanamivir): inhibition of the viral neuraminidase, inhibition of the release of newly built influenza A + B viruses; **AE** (amantadine): nausea, dizziness, insomnia;
AE (oseltamivir): N/V, bronchitis, insomnia, vertigo; **AE** (zanamivir): respiratory symptoms, thrombotic thrombocytopenic purpura, hemolytic uremic syndrome
CI (amantadine, oseltamivir, zanamivir): hypersensitivity to product ingredients

Amantadine	EHL 10-14h, PRC C, Lact -
Endantadine *Cap 100mg* **Symmetrel** *Cap 100mg, Syr 50mg/5ml* **Generics** *Cap 100mg*	**Influenza A:** 100mg PO bid; **CH** 1-9 yr or <40kg: 5mg/kg/ d PO, max. 150mg/d div bid, 10 yr and older: 100mg PO bid; **Parkinsonism**; DARF: ini 200mg, then GFR (ml/ min) 30-50: 100mg qd, 15-29: 100mg qod, <15: 200mg q7d,

Oseltamivir	EHL 1-3h, PRC C, Lact ?
Tamiflu *Cap 75mg, Susp (oral) 12mg/ml*	**Influenza A, B Tx:** 75mg PO bid for 5d; **Influenza A, B PRO:** 75mg PO qd; DARF: GFR (ml/min) <30: 75mg qd

Zanamivir	EHL 1.6-5.1h, PRC B, Lact ?
Relenza *Cap (inhal) 5mg*	**Influenza A, B Tx:** 2 inhal bid for 5d; **CH** >7 yr: see adults; DARF: not req

7.18.4 Interferons

MA/EF: antiviral, growth inhibiting and immune regulatory effects
AE: fever, sweating, chills, tiredness, joint and soft-tissue pains, complete blood count changes, cardiac arrhythmias, depression, tremors, convulsions, paresthesia, GI disturbances, hair loss, exanthema, pruritus; **AE** (interferon alfacon-1): flu like symptoms, depression, N/V, granulocytopenia; **AE** (interferon alfa-2b + Ribavirin): anemia, insomnia, irritability, depression, headache, nausea
CI: coronary diseases, CNS DO, severe hepatic dysfunction, RF, severe bone marrow damage
CI (interferon alfacon-1): hypersensitivity to alfa interferons/E. coli derived products
CI (interferon alfa-2b + Ribavirin): hypersensitivity to ribavirin or alfa interferon, autoimmune hepatitis

Interferon alfa 2a	EHL 3.7-8.5 h
Roferon A Inj 3, 9, 18 million U/vial	**Chronic hepatitis C:** 3 mio U 3x/wk SC/IM
Interferon alfa 2b	EHL 2-3 h
Intron A Inj 3,10,18, 30, 60 million U/vial	**Chronic hepatitis B:** 5 mio U qd or 10 mio U 3x/wk SC/ IM for 16 wk; **chronic hepatitis C:** 3 mio U SC/IM 3x/wk upto 18months
Interferon alfacon-1	EHL 0.5-7h, PRC C, Lact ?
Infergen Inj 0.03mg/ml	**Chronic hepatitis C:** 9mcg SC 3x/wk for 24 wk; 15mcg SC 3x/wk for 24 wk for relapse or no response-9mcg dose
Interferon beta 1a	EHL 69h, PRC C, Lact ?
Avonex Inj 33mcg/vial **Rebif** Syr 22mcg/0.5ml, 44mcg/0.5ml Inj 11mcg/vial, 44mcg/vial	**Relapsing form of multiple sclerosis:** (Avonex): 30mcg IM qwk; (Rebif): 22-44mcg SC tiw
Interferon beta 1b	PRC C , Lact ?
Betaseron Inj 0.3mg/vial	**Relapsing form of multiple sclerosis:** ini 0.25mg sc qod
Peginterferon alfa 2a	EHL 60h, PRC C, Lact ?
Pegasys Syr 180mcg/0.5ml, Inj 180mcg/ml	**Chronic hepatitis C:** 180mcg SC qwk

Peginterferon alfa-2a + Ribavirin	
Pegasys RBV *Syr 180mcg/0.5ml, Inj 180mcg/ml, Cap 200mg*	**Chronic hepatitis C:** ini 1.5 mcg/kg SC qweek of Peginterferon alfa-2b and Ribavirin 800-1200mg PO/d div bid

Peginterferon alfa 2b	EHL 40h, PRC C, Lact ?
Unitron PEG *Inj 74mcg/vial, 118.4mcg/vial, 177.6mcg/vial, 222mcg/vial*	**Chronic hepatitis C:** 1mcg/kg/wk SC;

Peginterferon alfa-2b + Ribavirin	PRC X, Lact ?
Pegetron *Inj 74mcg/vial, 118.4mcg/vial, 177.6mcg/vial, 222mcg/vial, + Cap 200mg*	**Chronic hepatitis C:** ini 1.5 mcg/kg SC qweek of Peginterferon alfa-2b and Ribavirin 800-1200mg PO/d div bid

7.18.5 Anti-Respiratory-Syncytial-Virus Drugs

MA/Ind (ribavirin): guanosine analogue, inhibition of the RNA polymerase of HCV
AE (palivizumab): rash, rhinitis, upper respiratory tract infx; **AE** (ribavirin): rash, respiratory dysfunction, conjunctivitis; **CI** (ribavirin): hypersensitivity to ribavirin products
CI (palivizumab): hypersensitivity to palivizumab products

Palivizumab	EHL 20d (age<24m), 18d (adults), PRC C
Synagis *Inj 50mg/vial, 100mg/vial*	**Prevention of severe respiratory syncytial virus infx:** 15mg/kg IM

Ribavirin	EHL Inhal 9.5h, IV/PO 24-36h, PRC X, Lact ?
Virazole *Sol (inhal) 6g/vial*	**Severe respiratory syncytial virus infx:** aerosol 12h/d for 3d; **CH** see adults

7.18.6 Anti-HIV Drugs: Nucleoside Reverse Transcriptase Inhibitors

MA/Ind (nucleoside analogues): blockage of the transformation of RNA into DNA through chemically altered nucleosides in HIV-infx
AE (abacavir): N/V, fatigue, fever, headache, diarrhea, loss of appetite, lactic acidosis/severe hepatomegaly with steatosis, hypersensitivity reactions (some fatal)
AE (didanosine, stavudine): polyneuropathy, pancreatitis, diarrhea, exanthema
AE (lamivudine): headache, N/V, pancreatitis, lactic acidosis/hepatomegaly, fatigue
AE (zalcitabine): polyneuropathy, dermatitis, mucositis, pancreatitis, granulocytopenia, anemia; **AE** (zidovudine): anemia, leukopenia, myopathy, nausea, headache
CI (abacavir): severe hepatic dysfunction, hypersensitivity to abacavir products
CI (didanosine): acute pancreatitis, combination with rifampicin, hypersensitivity to product ingredients; **CI** (lamivudine): hypersensitivity; **CI** (stavudine): hypersensitivity to product ingredients; **CI** (zalcitabine): polyneuropathy, pancreatitis, hypersensitivity to product ingredients; **CI** (zidovudine): leukopenia<750/μl, Hb<7.5g/dl, hypersensitivity

Abacavir (ABC)	EHL 1-2h, PRC C, Lact -
Ziagen Tab 300mg, Sol (oral) 20mg/ml	**HIV infx:** 300mg PO bid in combination with other antiretroviral drugs; **CH** 3 mo - 16 yr: 8mg/kg PO bid, max. 300mg PO bid; DARF: not req

Abacavir + Lamivudine + Zidovudine	PRC C, Lact +
Trizivir Tab 300 + 150 + 300mg	**HIV inx:** 1 tab PO bid; DARF: not recommended if CrCL <50

Didanosine (ddI)	EHL 1.3-1.5h, PRC B, Lact ?
Videx Tab (chew) 25mg, 50mg, 100mg, 150mg, Sol (oral) 4g/240ml, Tab ent. coated 125mg, 200mg, 250mg, 400mg	**HIV infx:** >60kg: 400mg PO qd or 200mg PO bid as Tab or 250mg PO bid buffered powder; <60kg: 250mg PO qd or 125mg PO bid as Tab or 167mg PO bid buffered powder in combination with other antiretroviral drugs; **CH** 120mg/square meter PO bid; DARF: see Prod Info

Lamivudine (3TC)	EHL 3-7h, PRC C Lact ?
3TC *Tab 150mg,* *Sol (oral) 10mg/ml* **Heptovir** *Tab 100mg,* *Sol (oral) 5mg/ml*	**HIV infx:** 150mg PO bid in combination with other antiretroviral drugs; **chronic hepatitis B:** 100mg PO qd, **CH** 3 mo -16 yr, **HIV infx:** 4mg/kg, max. 150mg PO bid DARF: HIV-Tx GFR (ml/min): >50: 150mg bid, 30-49: 150mg qd, 15-29:ini. 150mg, then 100mg qd, 5-14: ini. 150mg, then 50mg qd, <5: ini. 50mg, then 25mg qd
Lamivudine + Zidovudine	PRC C, Lact ?
Combivir *Tab 150 + 300mg*	**HIV infx:** 1 Tab PO bid; DARF: not rec in RF
Stavudine (d4T)	EHL 0.9-1.6h, PRC C, Lact ?
Zerit *Cap 15mg, 20mg, 30mg, 40mg*	**HIV infx:** >60kg: 40mg PO bid <60kg: 30mg PO bid; **CH** <30kg: 1mg/kg PO bid, >30kg: see adults; DARF: GFR (ml/min) >50: 100% q12h, 26-50: 50% q12h, 10-25: 50% q24h
Tenofovir	PRC B Lact +
Viread *Tab 300mg*	**HIV infx:** 300mg PO qd
Zalcitabine (ddC)	EHL 1-3h, PRC C Lact ?
Hivid *Tab 0.375mg, 0.75mg*	**HIV infx:** 0.75mg PO tid in combination with other antiretroviral drugs; **CH** 0.015-0.04mg/kg PO qid; DARF: GFR (ml/min): 10-40: 100% q12h, <10: 100% q24h
Zidovudine (AZT, ZDV)	EHL 1h, PRC C, Lact ?
Retrovir *Cap 100mg, Syr 50mg/5ml, Inj* *10mg/ml* **Generics** *Cap 100mg*	**HIV infx:** 600 mg/d PO div bid or tid; 1mg/kg IV over 1h 5-6x/d in combination with other antiretroviral drugs; **PRO of** **maternal-fetal HIV transmission:** mother (>14 wk of pregnancy): 100mg PO 5x/d until start of labor, during labor, 2mg/kg IV over 1h, then 1mg/kg/h until delivery; newborn: 2mg/kg PO q6h within 12h of birth for 6 wk, **CH** 3 mo - 12 yr: 180mg/square meter q6h, max. 200mg q6h

Abacavir + Lamivudine + Zidovudine	PRC C, Lact -
Trizivir *Tab 300 + 150 + 300mg*	**HIV infx:** 1 Tab PO bid; DARF: GFR (ml/min) <50: not rec

7.18.7 Anti-HIV Drugs: Non-Nucleoside Reverse Transcriptase Inhibitors

MA/Ind (efavirenz, nevirapine): direct binding on the reverse transcriptase ⇒ blockage of DNA-polymerase of HIV-1; **AE** (delavirdine): N/V, rash, headache, fatigue
AE (efavirenz): dizziness, drowsiness, impaired concentration, sleeplessness, exanthema, liver enzymesm; **AE** (nevirapine): rash, nausea, diarrhea, fever, headache, liver enzymesm, hypersensitivity to product ingredients
CI (delavirdine): hypersensitivity to delavirdine products, concomitant use with rifampin or rifabutin
CI (efavirenz): combination with astemizole, cisapride, midazolam, triazolam, fexofenadine, ergotamine derivatives; children < 3 yr, hypersensitivity to product ingredients
CI (nevirapine): hypersensitivity to nevirapine products

Delavirdine (DLV)	EHL 2-11h, PRC C, Lact ?
Rescriptor *Tab 100mg*	**HIV infx:** 400mg PO tid combined with other antiretroviral; **CH** >16yr: see adults

Efavirenz (EFV)	EHL 52-76 h (1 dose), 40-55 h (x dose), Lact -
Sustiva *Cap 50mg, 100mg, 200mg, 600mg*	**HIV infx:** 600mg PO qd combined with other antiretroviral drugs; **CH** >3 yr: 10-15kg: 200mg PO qd, 15- 20kg: 250mg PO qd, 20-25kg: 300mg PO qd, 25-32.5kg: 350mg PO qd, 33-40kg: 400mg PO qd, >40kg: 600mg qd

Nevirapine (NVP)	EHL 22-84h, PRC C, Lact ?
Viramune *Tab 200mg*	**HIV infx:** 200mg PO qd for 14d, then 200mg PO bid combined with other antiretroviral drugs; **CH** 2 mo - 8 yr: 4mg/kg PO qd for 14d, then 7mg/kg bid, >8 yr: 4 mg/kg PO qd x 2 wk, then 4 mg/kg bid, max. 400mg/d; **PRO of maternal-fetal HIV transmission:** mother 200mg PO as single dose at onset of labor; neonate 2mg/kg PO within 3d of birth

7.18.8 Anti-HIV Drugs: Protease Inhibitors

MA/Ind: specific inhibition of HIV protease ⇒ protein production ↓ (i.e. rev. transcriptase)
AE (amprenavir): N/V, diarrhea, rash, paresthesia;
AE (indinavir, ritonavir): nausea, headache, diarrhea, tiredness, exanthema;
AE (nelfinavir, saquinavir): diarrhea, nausea, exanthema
CI (amprenavir): concomitant interacting drugs, hypersensitivity to amprenavir products, children < 4yr, hepatic or RF, under metronidazole Tx;
CI (indinavir): hypersensitivity to indinavir products;
CI (nelfinavir): combination w/rifampicin, fexofenadine;
CI (ritonavir): severe hepatic insufficiency;
CI (saquinavir): combination w/rifampicin

Amprenavir (APV)	EHL 7-10h, PRC C, Lact -
Agenerase Cap 50, 150mg, Sol (oral) 15mg/ml	**HIV-1 infx:** 1200mg PO bid in combination with ohther antiretroviral drugs; **CH** 4-16yr, <50kg: Cap: 20mg/kg PO bid, max. 2400mg/d, Sol: 22.5mg/kg bid
Atazanavir	EHL 7h, PRC B, Lact ?
Reyataz Cap 150mg, 200mg	**HIV-1 infx:** 300-400mg PO qd
Indinavir (IDV)	EHL 1.5-2h, PRC C, Lact -
Crixivan Cap 200mg, 400mg	**HIV infx:** 800mg PO tid in combination with other antiretroviral drugs; DARF: not req
Nelfinavir (NFV)	EHL 3.5-5h, PRC B, Lact ?
Viracept Tab 250mg, 625mg Susp 50mg/scoopful	**HIV infx:** 750mg PO tid or 1250mg PO bid in combination with other antiretroviral drugs; **CH** 2-13 yr: 20-30 mg/kg tid
Ritonavir (RTV)	EHL 3-3.5h, PRC B, Lact ?
Norvir Cap 100mg, Sol (oral) 80mg/ml	**HIV infx:** ini. 300mg PO bid, incr. at 2-3d intervals by 100mg bid to 600mg bid in combination with other antiretroviral drugs; **CH** ini 250mg/m2 PO bid, incr. at 2-3d intervals by 50mg/m2/dose to 400 mg/m^2 PO bid, max. 600mg PO bid
Ritonavir + lopinavir	
Kaletra Cap 33.3mg + 133.3mg, Sol 20 + 80mg	**HIV infx:** ini 100 + 400mg PO bid

Mefloquine	EHL 13-30 d, PRC C, Lact ?
Lariam *Tab 250mg*	**Malaria PRO:** 250mg PO 1x/wk from 1wk before exposure to 4 wk after **malaria Tx:** 1250mg PO single dose; **CH malaria PRO:** 1x/wk, 15-19kg: ¼ Tab PO, 20- 30kg: ½ Tab PO, 31-45kg: ¾ Tab PO, >45kg: 1 Tab PO; **malaria Tx** <45 kg: 15mg/kg PO, then 10 mg/kg given 6- 8h after first dose
Primaquine Phosphate	EHL 4-7h, PRC C, Lact ?
Primaquine *Tab 15mg*	**PRO of p. vivax and p. ovale relapse:** 15mg PO qd for 14d; **CH** 0.3mg/kg PO for 14d
Quinidine Gluconate	EHL no data, PRC ? Lact ?
Generics *Inj 80mg/ml, Tab ext.rel. 324mg*	**Severe p. falcip. malaria:** ini. 10 mg/kg IV over 1-2h, then 0.02 mg/kg/min for 72 h or until parasitemia <1%, or PO meds tolerated
Quinine Sulfate	EHL no data, PRC X, Lact ?
Quinine-odan *Cap 200mg, 300mg* Generics *Cap 200mg, 300mg*	**Malaria Tx:** 650mg PO tid for 3-7 d with doxycycline or pyrimethamine/sulfadoxine

7.21.2 Antimalarials - Combinations

AE (a. + p.): fever, headache, myalgia
CI (a. + p.): hypersensitivity to atovaquone, hypersensitivity to proguanil

Atovaquone + Proquanil	PRC C, Lact ?
Malarone *Tab 250 + 100mg*	**Malaria PRO:** 1 Tab PO qd from 2d before to 7d after exposure; **malaria Tx:** 4 Tab PO qd for 3d; **CH malaria PRO:** from 2d before to 7d after exposure, 11-20kg: 1 ped Tab PO qd, 21-30kg: 2 ped Tab PO qd, 31-40kg: 3 ped Tab PO qd, >40kg: 1 adult Tab PO qd; **malaria Tx:** for 3 d, 11-20kg: 1 adult Tab PO qd, 21-30kg: 2 adult Tab PO qd, 31-40kg: 3 adult Tab PO qd, >40kg: 4 adult Tab PO qd

8. Immunology

8.1 Vaccines

8.1.1 Combinations

AE (Diphtheria + Tetanus + Acellular Pertussis vaccine): injection site reaction, fever, irritability, drowsiness
CI (Diphtheria + Tetanus + Acellular Pertussis vaccine): hypersensitivity to the vaccine or thimerosal, adults and children > 7y, active infection, febrile illness, history encephalopathy secondary to DPT vaccine

Diphtheria + Tetanus + Acellular Pertussis Vaccine (DTaP)	EHL no data, PRC C, Lact -
Adacel *Inj 0.5ml single dose*	**Diphtheria, tetanus, pertussis immunization:** 0.5ml IM for age 11-54 years

Diphtheria + Tetanus + Poliomyelitis Vaccine (DT Polio)	
Generics *0.5ml single dose*	**Diphtheria, tetanus, poliomyelitis immunization:** 0.5ml IM at 2, 4, 6 and 18mo of age; booster dose at 4-6y

Diphtheria + Tetanus + acellular Pertussis + Poliomyelitis Vaccine (DTaP Polio)	
Quadracel *0.5ml single dose*	**Diphtheria, tetanus, acellular pertussis, poliomyelitis:** 0.5ml IM at 2, 4, 6 and 18mo of age; booster dose at 4-6y

Diphtheria + Tetanus + acellular Pertussis + Poliomyelitis Vaccine + Haemophilus b	
Pentacel *Inj 0.5ml single dose*	**Diphtheria, tetanus, acellular pertussis, poliomyelitis, haemophilus b:** 0.5ml IM at 2, 4, 6 and 18mo of age

Diphtheria + Tetanus Toxoid (Td)	EHL no data
Generics *Inj 2LF U + 5 LF U/0.5ml*	**Tetanus, diphtheria immunization:** >7y: 0.5ml IM, rep after 4-8wk and after 6-12mo; 0.5ml booster dose q10y

Measles + Mumps + Rubella Vaccine (MMR)	
	Measles, mumps, rubella immunization: 0.5ml IM at 12mo and 18mo or 4-6 years of age

8.1.2 Toxoids (Bacteria)

AE (tetanus toxoid): injection site pain, fever
CI (tetanus toxoid): hypersensitivity to tetanus tox. products, infx, poliomyelitis outbreak

Tetanus Toxoid	EHL no data, PRC C, Lact ?
Generics *Inj 5 LF U/0.5ml*	**Tetanus immunization:** 0.5ml IM, rep after 4-8wk and after 6-12mo; give 0.5ml booster dose q10y; **CH** <1y: 0.5ml IM, rep after 4 and 8wk and after 6-12mo; > 1y: see adults

Vi Polysaccharide Typhoid + Inactivated Hepatitis A	
ViVaxim *Inj 1ml*	**Typhoid and Hepatitis A immunization:** 1ml IM

8.1.3 Polysaccharid-Vaccines (Bacteria)

AE (pneumococcal vaccine): injection site pain, anaphylaxis;
AE (meningococcal vaccine): see Prod Info;
CI (pneumococcal vaccine): hypersensitivity to pneumococcal vaccine products, Hodgkin's disease within 10d of or during Tx;
CI (meningococcal vaccine): any acute illness, sensitivity to thimerosal or any other component of the vaccine

Haemophilus B Vaccine	PRC X
Act-HIB *Inj 10mcg purified polysaccharide/0.5ml* PedvaxHIB *Inj 7.5mcg purified polysaccharide/0.5ml*	**Haemophilus B:** 0.5ml IM at 2, 4, 6 and 18mo of age

Meningococcal Polysaccharide Vaccine	EHL no data, PRC C
Menjugate *Inj 0.5ml Group C-CRM197 conjugate vaccine* Meningitec *nj 0.5ml Group C-CRM197 conjugate vaccine* NeisVac-C *Inj 0.5ml Group C-TT conjugate vaccine* Generics *Inj 50mcg of "isolated product" from each of Groups A, C, Y and W-135/0.5ml*	**Meningococcal infx PRO:** 0.5ml IM; **CH** 3-18mo: 0.5ml SC, rep after 3mo; > 2y: see adults

Pneumococcal Vaccine	EHL no data
Pneumo 23 *Inj 25mcg of each of the 23 polysaccharide types/0.5ml* **Pneumovax 23** *Inj 25mcg of each of the 23 polysaccharide types/0.5ml* Prevnar *Inj 25mcg of each of the 23 polysaccharide types/0.5ml*	**Pneumococcal infx PRO:** 0.5ml IM/SC

Salmonella TyphiVi Vaccine	PRC C, Lact ?
Typherix *Inj 25mcg polysaccharide/0.5ml* **Typhim Vi** *Inj 25mcg polysaccharide/0.5ml*	**Salmonella Typhi immunization:** 0.5ml IM

8.1.4 Inactivated Vaccines (Bacteria)

AE (cholera vaccine): fever, malaise, headache
CI (cholera vaccine): illness, hypersensitivity to cholera vaccine

Cholera Vaccine	EHL no data, PRC C, Lact ?
Mutacol Berna *Sol (oral) 2-10 X 108 CFU viable V. Cholerae + 20-100X108 CFU non-viable V. Cholerae/package*	**Cholera immunization:** 1 packet PO

8.1.5 Live Attenuated Vaccines (Bacteria)

AE: flu-like syndrome, hematuria, urinary frequency, dysuria
CI: positive tuberculin tests, burns, AIDS, immunocompromised status, fever unknown origin, UTI (intravesical BCG), hypersensitivity to BCG vaccine

BCG Vaccine	EHL no data
BCG Vaccine *Inj 50mg/vial*	**Different BCG vaccine products are available for TB immunization;** route of immunization and dose depends on product; see Prod Info; TB immunization: 0.2-0.3ml percutanous; **CH** >1mo: see adults, **CH** <1mo: 50%

8.1.6　Inactivated Vaccines (Viruses)

AE (hepatitis A vaccine): fever, injection site pain/soreness, headache
AE (hepatitis B vaccine): fever, injection site soreness/erythema
AE (influenza vaccine): fever, pain, redness at injection site, malaise
AE (japanese encephalitis vaccine): fever, headache, injection site pain
AE (poliovirus vaccine): fever, injection site reaction, fussiness and crying in children
AE (rabies vaccine): dizziness, malaise, injection site reaction, myalgias, nausea
CI (hepatitis A vaccine): hypersensitivity to hepatitis A vaccine
CI (hepatitis B vaccine): hypersensitivity to hepatitis B vaccine/yeast
CI (influenza vaccine): allergy to chicken feathers/dander/eggs, hypersensitivity to vaccine/thimerosol, active acute respiratory disease/infections
CI (japanese encephalitis vaccine): hypersensitivity to japanese encephalitis vaccine
CI (poliovirus vaccine): hypersensitivity to streptomycin, neomycin, polymixin B, hypersensitivity to polio vaccine products
CI (rabies vaccine): hypersensitivity to rabies vaccine products, fever

Hepatitis A Vaccine	EHL no data, PRC C, Lact ?
Avaxim *Inj 160U/0.5ml* **Avaxim-Pediatric** *Inj 80U/0.5ml* **Havrix** *Inj 720U/ml, 1440U/ml* **Vaqta** *Inj 25U/0.5ml, 50U/ml*	**Hep. A immunization:** Avaxim, Epaxal Berna: 0.5ml IM, rep after 6- 12mo Havrix: 1440 U IM, rep after 6- 12mo; Vaqta: 50 U IM, rep after 6mo; **CH** 2-17y: Havrix: 720 U IM, rep after 6-12mo; Vaqta: 25 U IM, rep after 6-18mo

Hepatitis B Vaccine	EHL no data, PRC C, Lact ?
Engerix-B *Inj 10mcg/0.5ml (pediatric), Inj 20mcg/ml, 200mcg/10ml (adult)* **Recombivax HB** *Inj 10mcg/ml, 40mcg/ml*	**Hep. B immunization:** Engerix-B: 20mcg IM, rep after 1 + 6mo **Recombivax HB:** 10mcg IM, rep after1 + 6mo; **CH Engerix-B:** 10mcg IM within 7d of birth, rep after 1 + 6mo; **Recombivax HB:** 5mcg IM within 7d of birth, rep after 1 + 6mo

Hepatitis A + B Vaccine	PRC C, Lact ?
Twinrix *Inj 360U + 10mcg/0.5ml (Junior), 720U + 20mcg/ml (adult)*	**Hep. A+B immunization:** 720 + 20mcg IM, rep after 1 + 6mo

Influenza Vaccine	EHL no data, PRC C, Lact +
Fluviral S/F *Inj 45mcg/0.5ml* **Fluzone** *Inj 45mcg/0.5ml* **Vaxigrip** *Inj 45mcg/0.5ml*	**Influenza virus PRO:** 0.5ml IM once yearly; **CH** 6-35mo: 0.25ml IM, rep after 4wk; 3-8y: 0.5ml IM, rep after 4wk; 9- 12y: see adults

Japanese Encephalitis Vaccine	EHL no data
JE-Vax *Inj single dose vial*	**Japanese encephalitis immunization:** 1ml SC on d 0, 7, 30; 1ml booster dose may be given after 2y; **CH** 1-3y: 0.5ml SC on d 0, 7, 30; > 3y: see adults

Poliovirus Vaccine	EHL no data
Inactivated Poliomyelitis Vaccine (IPV) *Inj 40 D antigen U of Type1 + 8 D antigen U of Type2 + 32 D antigen U of Type 3 poliovirus/0.5ml*	**poliomyelitis immunization:** IPOL: 0.5ml SC, rep after 1 and 6-12mo

Rabies Vaccine 9	EHL no data, PRC C, Lact ?
Imovax Rabies *Inj: 1ml is equal to or greater than 2.5 U of rabies antigen*	**Rabies immunization, pre exposure:** 1ml IM on d 0, 7, 21 or 28; **post exposure:** 1ml IM on d 0, 3, 7, 14, 28, 90 with a concommitant dose of 20 U/kg rabies IG on d 0; **CH** see adults

8.1.7 Live Attenuated Vaccines (Viruses)

AE (varicella vaccine): fever, N/V, injection site pain/swelling
AE (yellow fever vaccine): fever, malaise, headache
CI (varicella vaccine): hypersensitivity to varicella vaccine products, blood dyscrasias, immunodeficiency, active TB
CI (yellow fever vaccine): hypersensitivity to yellow virus vaccine products/eggs, child younger than 4mo of age, blood transfusion or IG therapy within 8wk

Varicella Vaccine	EHL no data, PRC C, Lact ?
Varivax *Inj 1350 PFU (plaque forming U) of Oka/Merck varicella virus/0.5ml*	**Varicella immunization:** 0.5ml SC, rep after 4-8wk; **CH** > 12y: see adults; 1-12y: 0.5ml SC as single dose

Yellow Fever Vaccine	EHL no data, PRC C, Lact +
YF-Vax *5.04 Log 10 Plaque Forming Units (PFU)/0.5ml*	**Yellow fever immunization:** 0.5ml SC as single dose; **CH** > 9mo: see adults

8.1.8   Other Vaccines

AE (lyme disease vaccine): injection site reaction, flu like symptoms
AE (plague vaccine): see Prod Info
AE (typhoid vaccine): fever, rash, N/V, myalgia, diarrhea
CI (lyme disease vaccine): hypersensitivity to vaccine or its components)
CI (plague vaccine): see Prod Info
CI (typhoid vaccine): hypersensitivity to typhoid vaccine products, immunodeficiency, persistent diarrhea, GI illness

Lyme Disease Vaccine	EHL no data, PRC C, Lact ?
LYMErix Inj 30mcg/0.5ml	**Lyme disease immunization:** 30mcg IM, rep after 1 and 12mo; **CH** >15y: see adults

Typhoid Vaccine	EHL no data
Vivotif Berna Cap 2-10 X 109 colony-forming U of viable S. typhi Ty21a / 5-60 X 109 bact. cells of non-viable S. typhi Ty21a	**Typhoid fever immunization:** **Typhim Vi:** 0.5ml IM as single dose; **Typhoid Vaccine USP:** 0.5ml SC,rep after 4wk; **CH** >10y: see adults; **CH** <10y: 0.25ml SC, rep after 4wk; Vivotif Berna: 1 Cap PO 1h ac on d 1, 3, 5, 7; **CH** >6y: see adults

8.2   Immunoglobulins

AE (hepatitis B IG): rash, pain at injection site, joint pain
AE (IG): flushing of face, hypotension, tachycardia, chest tightness, rash
AE (rabies IG human): fever, pain at injection site, hypersensitivity reaction
AE (tetanus IG): fever, redness, pain at injection site, myalgia
AE (varicella-zoster IG): injection site reaction
CI (hepatitis B IG): hypersensitivity to IG products
CI (IG): hypersensitivity to IG, blood products, IgA deficiency
CI (rabies IG human): hypersensitivity to rabies IG/thimerosal
CI (tetanus IG): hypersensitivity to tetanus IG products, patients with IgA deficiency
CI (varicella-zoster IG): IgA deficiency, hypersensitivity to IG products/neomycin, immunodeficiency, blood dyscrasias, fever/ respiratory, illness/active TB

Anti-Thymocyte Globulin	EHL 5.7d, PRC C, Lact ?
Atgam Inj 50mg/ml	**Immunosuppression:** 7-30mg/kg IV qd, duration is dependent on indication for immunosuppresion

Black Widow Spider Antivenin	PRC C, Lact ?
Antivenin (Latrodectus Mactans) *Inj 6000 U/vial*	**Black widow spider bite:** 1 vial IM/IV
Botulism Antitoxin	EHL n/a,
Botulism Antitoxin *Inj 5000 U/vial (type E)*	**Botulism toxin poisoning:** 1 vial IV (1:10 dilution) or IM
Diphtheria Antitoxin	PRC D, Lact ?
Diphtheria Antitoxin *Inj 20000 U/vial*	**Diphtheria:** 10000-150000 U IV (1:10 dilution) or IM
Hepatitis B Immune Globulin	EHL 17.5d/25d, PRC C, Lact ?
Bayhep B *Inj 0.5ml syringe, 1ml vial, 5ml vial*	**Post-exposure PRO:** 0.06ml/kg IM, repeat in 1mo for persons, who are not given hepatitis B vaccine. Initiate hepatitis B vaccine series PRO of infants born to HbsAG (+) mothers: 0.5ml IM within 12h of birth. Initiate hepatitis B vaccine series
Immune Globulin	EHL 3-5wk, PRC C, Lact no data
Baygam *Inj (IM form) 2ml, 5ml, 10ml single dose vials* **Gamimune N** *Inj (5%) 0.5g, 1g, 2.5g, 5g, 12.5g, 25g size vials* *Inj (10%) 1g, 2.5g, 5g, 10g, 20g size vials* **Gammagard S/D** *Inj 0.5g, 1g, 2.5g, 5g, 10g size vials* **Iveegam Immuno** *Inj 5g/vial*	**Hep. A post-exposure PRO (i.e. household or institutional contacts):** 0.02ml/kg IM; hep. A pre-exposure PRO: < 3mo length of stay = 0.02ml/kg IM;> 3mo length of stay = 0.06ml/kg IM and rep. q4-6mo; measles: 0.2-0.25ml/kg IM within 6d of exposure, max 15ml; **CH** pediatric HIV: 400mg/kg IV inf q28d; measles: 0.2-0.25ml/kg IM within 6d of exposure, max 15ml
Rabies Immune Globulin	EHL 21d, PRC C, Lact ?
Bayrab *Inj 300 U/vial, 1500 U/vial* **Imogam Rabies Pasteurized** *Inj 150 U/ml*	**Post-exposure PRO:** 20IU/kg (0.133ml/kg), infiltrated in the area around the wound and the rest given IM

Tetanus Immune Globulin	EHL 3-5wk, PRC B/C, Lact no data
Baytet Inj 250U/vial, 250U/single dose syringe **Tetanus Immune Globulin** Inj 250U/vial	**Tetanus PRO:** 250U IM at time of injury; higher doses in severe injuries, severely contaminated wounds, or wounds >24h old, see Prod Info ; **tetanus Tx:** dose adjusted to severitiy of infx/clinical situation; usually TIG 3000-6000 U IM; **CH** >7y: see adults; **CH** <7y: 4 U/kg IM
Varicella-Zoster Immune Globulin	EHL 3wk, PRC C, Lact ?
Varicella-Zoster Immune Globulin Inj 100 U/ml	**Passive immunization to varicella: IM (gluteal):** ≤10kg: 125U at one site; 10.1-20kg: 250U at a single site, 20.1-30kg: 375U with no > 2.5ml at a single site, 30.1-40kg: 500 U with no > 2.5ml at a single site, > 40kg: 625U with no > 2.5ml at a single site; spezialized dosing for post-exposure PRO in immundeficient patients

8.3   Immunosuppressives

AE (cyclosporine): renal damage, hepatic DO, cardiotoxic, tremors, hirsutism, gingival hypertrophy, edema; **MA** (anakinra): recombinant interleukin-1 receptor antagonist **AE** (daclizumab): N/V, headache, dizziness, tremor; **AE** (mycophenolate mofetil): myelosuppression, HTN, tremor, diarrhea, N/V; **AE** (sirolimus): thrombocyto-, leukopenia, hyperlipidemia, headache, periph. edema; **AE** (anakinra): neutropenia, infections, headache, injection site reactions; **AE** (tacrolimus): HTN, N/V, diarrhea, headache/tremor, infx; **CI** (cyclosporine): renal dysfunction, uncontrollable HTN, uncontrollable infx, tumors, severe hepatic diseases; **CI** (daclizumab, sirolimus, tacrolimus): hypersens. to product; **CI** (anakinra): hypersensitivity to E. coli-derived products; **CI** (mycophenolate mofetil): hypersens. to mycophenolate mofetil/mycophenolic acid, hypersens. to IV formulation

Anakinra	EHL 4-6h, PRC B, Lact ?
Kineret Inj 150mg/ml	**Rheumadoid arthritis:** 100mg sc qd; DARF: CrCl<30 decrease by 70-75%

Basiliximab	EHL 7.2 +/- 3.2d, PRC B, Lact ?
Simulect *Inj 20mg/vial*	**Renal transplant:** 20mg IV 2h prior to transpl., rep after 4d; **CH** 2-15y: 12mg/square meter 2h prior to transpl., rep after 4d
Cyclosporine	EHL 19h, PRC C, Lact -
Neoral *Cap 10mg, 25mg, 50mg, 100mg, Sol (oral) 100mg/ml* **Sandimmune** *Inj 50mg/ml* **Generics** *Cap 100mg*	**Organ transplant:** ini 15mg/kg/d PO for 7-14d, then decrease 5%/wk, maint 5-10mg/kg/d; IV: 1/3 of PO dose; **rheum. arthritis:** ini 2.5mg/kg/d PO div bid, incr prn after 8-12wk by 0.5-0.75mg/kg/d, max 4mg/kg/d
Daclizumab	EHL 44-360h, PRC C, Lact ?
Zenapax *Inj 25mg/5ml*	**Renal transplant:** 1mg/kg IV 24h prior to transpl., rep q14d for a total of 5 doses
Muromonab-CD3	
Orthoclone OKT 3 *Inj 1mg/ml*	**Acute allograft rejection:** 5mg IV qd for 10-14d
Mycophenolate Mofetil	EHL 16-18h, PRC C, Lact ?
Cellcept *Tab 500mg, Cap 250mg, Susp 200mg/ml, Inj 500mg/vial*	**Renal transplant:** 1g IV/PO bid; **heart transplant:** 1.5g IV/PO bid; **liver transplant:** 1.5g PO bid; 1g IV bid
Sirolimus	EHL 57-63h, PRC C, Lact ?
Rapamune *Sol (oral) 1mg/ml*	**Renal transplant:** ini 6mg for 1d, maint 2mg PO qd; DARF: not req
Tacrolimus	EHL 8.7-11.3h, PRC C, Lact -
Prograf *Cap 1mg, 5mg, Inj 5mg/ml*	**Liver/renal transplant:** ini 0.03-0.05mg/kg/d IV contin. inf, maint 0.1-0.2mg/kg PO div bid

8.4   Recommended Childhood Immunization Schedule

Vaccine	Months Birth	2	4	6	Years 12	18	4–6	14–18
Diphtherie, tetanus, pertussis (acell.) [1]		DTap	DTap	DTap		DTap	DTap	
Inactivated poliovirus		IPV	IPV	IPV [5]		IPV	IPV	
Haemophilus influenza type b [2]		Hib	Hib	Hib		Hib		
Measles, mumps and rubella					MMR	MMR [5] or MMR [6]		
Tetanus [3] and diphterica toxoid [10]								Td
Hepatitis B (3 doses) [4]	Infancy or preadolescence (9–13 years)							
Varicella					V [7]			
Pneumococcal conjugate		PC [8]	PC	PC	PC			
Meningococcal conjugate		MC [9]	MC	MC	or			MC [9]

6th Edition 2002 Canadian Immunization Guide

1. DTaP (diphtheria, tetanus, acellular or component pertussis) vaccine is the preferred vaccine for all doses in the vaccin. series, including completion of the series in children who have received > 1 dose of DPT (whole cell) vaccine.
2. Hib schedule shown is for PRP-T or HbOC vaccine. If PRP-OMP is used, give at 2, 4 and 12 months of age.
3. Td (tetanus and diphtheria toxoid), a combined adsorbed "adult type" preparation for use in people > 7 years of age, contains less diphtheria toxoid than preparat. given to younger childr. and is less likely to cause react. in older people.
4. Hepatitis B vaccine can be routinely given to infants or preadolescents, depending on the provincial/territorial policy; three doses at 0, 1 and 6 month intervals are preferred. The second dose should be administered at least 1 month after the first dose, and the third at least 2 months after the second dose. A two-dose schedule for adolescents is also possible (see 6th Edition 2002 Canadian Immunization Guide).
5. This dose is not needed routinely, but can be included for convenience.
6. A second dose of MMR is recommended, at least 1 month after the first dose for the purpose of better measles protection. For convenience, options include giving it with the next scheduled vaccination at 18 months of age or with school entry (4-6 years) vaccinations (depending on the provincial/territorial policy), or at any intervening age that is practicable. The need for a 2nd dose of mumps and rubella vaccine is not estab. but may benefit (given for conven. as MMR). The 2nd dose of MMR should be given at the same visit as DTaP IPV (+ Hib) to ensure high uptake rates.
7. Children aged 12 months to 12 years should receive one dose of varicella vaccine. Individuals > 13 years of age should receive two doses at least 28 days apart.
8. Recommended schedule, number of doses and subsequent use of 23 valent polysaccharide pneumococcal vaccine depend on the age of the child when vaccination is begun (see 6th Edition 2002 Canadian Immunization Guide).
9. Recomm. schedule and numb. of doses of meningoc. vaccine depends on the age of the child (see 6th Edition 2002).
10. dTap adult formulation with reduced diphtheria toxoid and pertussis component

9. Antirheumatics, Analgesics

9.1 Antirheumatics

9.1.1 Gold

MA: inhibition of leukocyte migration into synovial membrane
EF: influence on rheumatoid process
AE: hair loss, dermatitis, stomatitis, pancytopenia, renal damage
AE (auranofin): rash, abdominal cramps, N/V, pruritus, proteinuria, diarrhea, anemia
AE (aurothioglucose): stomatitis, proteinuria, blood dyscrasias, pruritus/dermatitis
AE (gold sodium thiomalate): pruritus/rash, mucous membrane reactions, nephrotic syndrome, hematologic toxicity
CI: renal insufficiency, complete blood count changes, hepatic damage
CI (auranofin): hypersensitivity to gold salts, severe colitis, pulmonary fibrosis, exfoliative dermatitis, bone marrow aplasia, hematological DO
CI (aurothioglucose): SLE, untreat. CHF/DM, blood DO, severe HTN, urticaria, eczema, colitis
CI (gold sodium thiomalate): toxicity to gold/heavy metals, SLE, severe debilitation

Auranofin	EHL 15-31d, PRC C, Lact ?
Ridaura *Cap 3mg*	**Rheumatoid arthritis:** 3mg PO bid or 6mg PO qd; max 9mg/d; **CH** 0.1-0.15mg/kg/d PO; max 0.2mg/kg/d

Gold Sodium Thiomalate	EHL 5d, PRC C, Lact ?
Myochrysine *Inj 10mg/ml, 25mg/ml, 50mg/ml*	**Rheumatoid arthritis:** 1st wk: 10mg IM, 2nd wk: 25mg, then 25-50mg/wk until cumulative dose of 0.8-1g; maint 25-50mg q other wk for 2-20wk; **CH** test dose 10mg IM, then 1mg/kg/wk until cumulative dose of 0.8-1g; max 50mg/dose maint 1mg/kg q2-4wk; DARF: GFR (ml/min) >50: 100%, <50: not rec

9.1.2   Hydroxychloroquin

AE: agranulocytosis, ocular toxicity, skin/mucosal pigmentation, N/V;
CI: retinal or visual field changes from prior use, hypersens. to hydroxychloroquine, long-term use in children

Hydroxychloroquine Sulfate	EHL 40d, PRC C, Lact ?
Plaquenil *Tab 200mg*	**Rheumatoid arthritis:** 400-600mg PO qd maint.: 200- 400mg PO qd; LE: 400mg PO qd-bid maint 200-400mg PO qd; **CH** 3-5mg/kg/d PO, max 400mg/d or max 7mg/kg/ d

9.1.3   Sulfasalazine

MA: prostaglandin synthesis ↓ ⇒ influence on rheumatoid process
AE: headache, N/V, GI distress, reversible oligospermia
CI: hypersensitivity to sulfasalazine/sulfa drugs/salicylates

Sulfasalazine	EHL 7.6h, PRC B, Lact ?
Salazopyrin *Tab 500mg* **Salazopyrin En-Tabs** *Tab ent. coat. 500mg* **Generics** *Tab 500mg, Tab ent. coat. 500mg*	**Rheumatoid arthritis:** ini 500mg PO qd-bid; maint 1g bid; **CH** ini 10mg/kg/d PO; maint 30-50mg/kg/d div bid, max 2g/d

9.1.4   Immunosuppressants

MA (methotrexate): immunosuppressive, synthesis of cytokines ↓
EF: influence on rheumatoid process
AE (azathioprine): leukopenia/thrombocytopenia, N/V, pancreatitis, GI hypersensitivity
AE (methotrexate): exanthema, hair loss, GI ulcers, N/V, hematopoietic DO, lung fibrosis
CI (azathioprine): hypersensitivity to azathioprine, history of taking alkylating agents
CI (methotrexate): acute infx, severe bone marrow depression, hepatic DO, GI ulcers, RF

Azathioprine	EHL 3h, PRC D, Lact -
Imuran *Tab 50mg, Inj 100mg/20ml* **Generics** *Tab 50mg*	**Rheumatoid arthritis:** ini 1mg/kg/d PO, maint 1-2.5mg/ kg/d; DARF: GFR (ml/min) >50: 100%, 10-50: 75%, <10: 50%

Methotrexate	EHL no data, PRC X, Lact -
Generics *Tab 2.5mg, 10mg* *Inj 10mg/ml, 25mg/ml*	**Rheumatoid arthritis:** 7.5-15mg/wk PO/IM; DARF: GFR (ml/min) >50: 100%, 10-50: 50%

9.1.5 New Disease-Modifiying Anti-Rheumatic Drugs

MA (anakinra): recombinant interleukin-1 receptor antagonist
MA (etanercept): genetically engineered fusion protein composed of TNF receptors
⇒ binds 2 molecules of TNF and prevents them from binding to cellular receptors
MA (leflunomide): inhibition of dihydroorotate dehydrogenase ⇒ inhibition of pyrimidine synthesis ⇒ lymphocyte proliferation ↓
EF: influence on rheumatoid process
AE (anakinra): neutropenia, infections, headache, injection site reactions;
AE (etanercept): injection site reaction, headache, rhinitis;
AE (leflunomide): diarrhea, HTN, transaminases ↑, exanthema, hair loss, bone marrow depression, susceptibility to infx ↑
CI (anakinra): hypersensitivity to E. coli-derived products
CI (etanercept): hypersensitivity to etanercept products
CI (leflunomide): severe immunodeficiencies, restricted hematopoiesis, severe infections, hepatic dysfunction, moderate and severe RF, children and adolescents < 18

Anakinra	EHL 4-6h, PRC B, Lact ?
Kineret *Inj 150mg/vial*	**Rheumatoid arthritis**: 100mg SC qd
Etanercept	EHL 90-300h, PRC B, Lact ?
Enbrel *Inj 25mg/vial*	**Rheumatoid arthritis**: 25mg SC 2x/wk; **CH** 4-17y: 0.4mg/ kg SC 2x/wk; max 25mg/dose; DARF: not req
Leflunomide	EHL 4-28d, PRC X, Lact -
Arava *Tab 10mg, 20mg, 100mg*	**Rheumatoid arthritis**: 100mg PO qd for 3d; maint 10- 20mg PO qd; DARF: not req

9.2 Nonsteroidal Anti-Inflammatory Drugs

9.2.1 NSAID - Salicylates

MA/EF: inhibition of cyclooxygenase ⇒ synthesis of prostaglandins ↓ ⇒ analgesic, antiinflammatory, antipyretic; inhibition of blood platelet aggregation (aspirin)
Note: salicylate-containing products are not recommended for use in children and teenagers with chicken pox, influenza or flu symptoms
AE: allergic skin reactions, dizziness, nausea, tinnitus, GI ulcerations, bronchospasm, hematopoietic DO, renal dysfunctions, abscess formation after IM administration
AE (aspirin): pancytopenia, acid-base balance DO, bleeding time ↑
AE (diflunisal): GI distress, rash
CI (acid NSAIDs): GI ulcerations, hematopoietic DO
CI (aspirin): restricted use in children and adolescents with febrile diseases (danger of Reye's syndrome)
CI (diflunisal): hypersensitivity to diflunisal, asthma, allergic reactions to ASA or other anti-inflammatories

Aspirin (Acetylsalicylic Acid)	EHL 4.7-9h, PRC D, Lact ?
Asaphen *Tab 80mg* **Asaphen E.C.** *Ent. coated tab 80mg* **Aspirin** *Tab 80mg, 325mg, 500mg, 650mg, Coated Tab 81mg* **Entrophen** *Cap 325mg, 650mg, Tab 325mg, 500mg, 650mg* **MSD Enteric Coated ASA** *Tab 325mg, 650mg* **Novasen** *Ent. coated tab 325mg, 650mg* **Generics** *Tab 325*	**Pain,fever:** 325-650mg PO/PR q4h prn, max 3.9g/d; **rheumatoid arthritis:** 3.2-6g/d in div doses; **rheumatic fever:** 1g q3-6h; **CH 2-14y: fever:** 10-15mg/kg PO q4h, max 60-80mg/kg/d; DARF GFR < 10ml/h: not rated

Diflunisal	EHL 8-12h, PRC C, Lact ?
Generics *Tab 250mg, 500mg*	**Pain:** ini 1g PO, maint 250-500mg q8-12h; **rheumatoid arthritis, osteoarthritis:** 500mg-1g PO div bid, max 1.5g/d; DARF: GFR (ml/min) > 50: 100%, <50: 50%

9.2.2 NSAID - Propionic Acid Derivatives

MA/EF: see NSAID, Aspirin + other salicylates →172 ; **AE** (flurbiprofen): headache, GI distress, ocular burning/ stinging, rash, ulcers; **AE** (ibuprofen): nausea, heartburn, ulcers, rash; **AE** (ketoprofen): malaise, dizziness, GI distress, rash, tinnitus; **AE** (ketorolac): GI distress, ulcers, headache/dizziness; **AE** (naproxen): GI upset, headache, edema, dizziness; **AE** (oxaprozin): GI distress, rash **CI** (ibuprofen, ketoprofen, naproxen): hypersensitivity to product ingredients, asthma, allergic reactions to ASA, other anti-inflammatories; **CI** (flurbiprofen): hypersensitivity to flurbiprofen products, asthma, allergic reaction to ASA/other anti-inflammatories, ocular epithelial herpes simplex keratitis; **CI** (ketorolac, oxaprozin): hypersensitivity to product ingredients, allergy to ASA or other inflammatories, syndr. of nasal polyps and angioedema

Flurbiprofen	EHL 5.7h, PRC B, Lact ?
Ansaid *Tab 50mg, 100mg* **Froben** *Tab 50mg, 100mg* **Froben SR** *Cap sust rel 200mg* **Novo-Flurprofen** *Tab 50mg, 100mg* **Generics** *Tab 50mg, 100mg*	**Rheumatoid arthritis, osteoarthritis:** 200-300mg/d PO div bid-qid

Ibuprofen	EHL 1.8-2.0h, PRC D, Lact +
Advil *Tab 200mg, Cap 200mg, Susp 100mg/5ml* **Novo-Profen** *Tab 200mg, 300mg, 400mg, 600mg* **Generics** *Tab 200mg, 300mg, 400mg, 600mg*	**Rheumatoid arthritis, osteoarthritis:** 1200-3200mg/d PO div tid-qid; **pain, dysmenorrhea:** 400mg PO q4-6h; **CH juv. rheum. arthritis:** 30-50mg/kg/d PO div tid- qid, max 2.4g/d; **CH fever, pain:** 5-10mg/kg PO q6-8h prn, max 40mg/kg/d; DARF: not req

Ketoprofen	EHL 2-4h, PRC B, Lact ?
Apo-Keto *Cap 50mg* **Apo-Keto-E** *Ent coat Tab 50mg, 100mg* **Apo-Keto SR** *Ent coat Tab Sust Rel 200mg* **Novo-Keto** *Supp 100mg* **Novo-Keto-EC** *Ent Coat Tab 50mg, 100mg* **Oruvail** *Cap ext.rel. 150mg, 200mg* **Rhodis** *Cap 50mg, Supp 100mg* **Rhodis-EC** *Ent Coat Tab 50mg, 100mg* **Rhodis SR** *Sust Rel Tab 200mg* **Rhovail** *Cap 150mg, 200mg* **Generics** *Cap 50mg, Ent Coat Tab 50, 100mg*	**Rheumatoid arthritis, osteoarthritis:** 100-300mg/d PO div tid-qid; pain, **dysmenorrhea:** 25-50mg PO q6-8h **CH juv. rheumatoid arthritis:** 25-50mg bid; DARF: see Prod Info

Ketorolac	EHL 5.3h, PRC C, Lact ?
Toradol *Tab 10mg, Inj 10mg/ml, 30mg/ml* **Generics** *Tab 10mg, Inj 30mg/ml*	**Pain:** ini 30-60mg IM or 15-30mg IV or 15-30mg IV/IM q6h; max IV/IM, 120mg/d; 10mg PO q4-6h prn; max PO 40mg/d; DARF: see Prod Info

Naproxen	EHL 12-15h
Anaprox *Tab 275mg, 550mg* **Apo-Napro-Na** *Tab 275mg, 550mg* **Naprosyn** *Supp 500mg, Susp 125mg/5m, Tab 500mg, Ent coat tab 250mg, 375mg, 500mg, Sust rel tab 750mg* **Novo-Naprox** *Tab 125mg, 250mg, 275mg, 375mg, 500mg, 550mg, Novo-Naprox SR Sust rel tab 750mg* **Novo-Naprox-EC** *Ent. coated Tab 250mg, 375mg, 500mg* **Nu-Naprox** *Tab 125mg, 250mg, 375mg, 500mg* **Generics** *Tab 125mg, 250mg, 375mg, 500mg, Sust rel tab 750mg, Supp 500mg*	**Rheumatoid arthritis, osteoarthritis, ankylosing spondylitis:** 250-500mg PO bid; **pain, dysmenorrhea:** ini 500mg, maint 250mg q6-8h prn; **CH** (rheumatoid arthritis): 10mg/kg/d div bid; DARF: not req

Oxaprozin	EHL 24-69h, PRC C, Lact ?
Daypro *Tab 600mg* **Generics** *Tab 600mg*	**Rheumatoid arthritis, osteoarthritis:** 1200mg PO qd, max 1800mg/d; DARF: severe renal impairment: 600mg PO qd

Tiaprofenic Acid	EHL 1.7h, PRC C, Lact ?
Surgam *Tab 300mg* **Surgam SR** *Cap sust rel 300mg* **Generics** *Tab 200mg, 300mg*	**Rheumatoid arthritis, osteoarthritis:** 300-600mg PO daily in div doses, max 600mg/d

9.2.3   NSAID - Acetic Acid Derivatives

MA/EF: see NSAID, Aspirin + other salicylates →172
AE (diclofenac): nausea/diarrhea, constipation, headache, burning/stinging, ulcers;
AE (diclofenac): abdominal pain, nausea, diarrhea; **AE** (etodolac): GI distress, malaise, dizziness; **AE** (indomethacin): headache, GI distress; **AE** (nabumetone): headache/dizziness, edema, GI distress; **AE** (sulindac): headache, dizziness, rash/pruritus, GI distress, edema;
AE (tolmetin): edema, dizziness, GI distress, BP ↑
CI (diclofenac): hypersensitivity to diclofenac or misoprostol, asthma or allergic reactions with aspirin or NSAIDS
CI (diclofenac, etodolac, nabumetone, sulindac): hypersensitivity to product ingredients, allergic reactions to ASA or other anti-inflammatories, asthma
CI (indomethacin, in addition): history of recent rectal bleeding or proctitis

Diclofenac	EHL 2h, PRC B, Lact ?
Apo-Diclo *Tab 25mg, 50mg,* *Tab ext.rel. 75mg, 100mg* **Novo-Difenac-K** *Tab 50mg* **Nu-Diclo** *Tab 25mg, 50mg* **Nu-Diclo SR** *Tab ext.rel. 75mg, 100mg* **Voltaren** *Tab 25mg, 50mg, Supp 50mg, 100mg* **Voltaren-SR** *Tab ext.rel. 75mg, 100mg* **Generics** *Tab 25mg, 50mg, Tab ext.rel. 75mg, 100mg, Supp 50mg, 100mg*	**Osteoarthritis, rheumatoid arthritis:** 50mg PO bid-tid or 75mg bid or 100mg qd; **ankylosing spondylitis:** 25mg PO qid **pain, dysmenorrhea:** 50mg PO tid

Diclofenac + Misoprostol	
Arthrotec *Tab ext. rel. 50mg + 200mcg, 75mg + 200mcg*	**Osteoarthritis:** 50mg/200mcg PO bid-tid or 75mg/ 200mcg bid; **rheumatoid arthritis:** 50mg/200mcg PO bid-qid or 75mg/200mcg bid ; DARF: GFR < 30ml/min: contraind.

Etodolac	EHL 6-7h, PRC C, Lact ?
Ultradol *Cap 200mg, 300mg* **Generics** *Cap 200mg, 300mg*	**Pain:** 200-400mg PO q6-8h; max 1000 mg/d; max in patients weighing < 60kg is 20mg/kg/d; **rheumatoid arthritis, osteoarthritis:** ini 400-500mg PO bid or 300mg bid-tid; maint 400-1000mg/d

Indomethacin	EHL 4.5h, PRC D, Lact +
Indotec *Cap 25mg, 50mg,* *Supp 50mg, 100mg* **Novo-Methacin** *Cap 25mg, 50mg,* *Supp 50mg, 100mg* **Nu-Indo** *Cap 25mg, 50mg* **Rhodacine** *Supp 50mg, 100mg* **Generics** *Cap 25mg, 50mg*	**Rheumatoid arthritis, osteoarthritis:** 25mg PO bid-tid, max 200mg/d **bursitis, tendinitis:** 75-150mg/d PO/PR div tid-qid; DARF: not req

Ketorolac	EHL 5.3h, PRC C, Lact ?
Toradol *Tab 10mg, Inj 10mg/ml, 30mg/ml* **Generics** *Tab 10mg, Inj 30mg/ml*	**Pain:** ini 30-60mg IM or 15-30mg IV or 15-30mg IV/IM q6h; max IV/IM 120mg/d; 10mg PO q4-6h prn; max PO 40mg/d; DARF: see Prod Info

Nabumetone	EHL unknown, PRC C, Lact ?
Relafen *Tab 500mg, 750mg* **Generics** *Tab 500mg*	**Rheumatoid arthritis, osteoarthritis:** 500mg PO bid, maint 1-2g/d; DARF not req

Sulindac	EHL 7.8h, PRC D, Lact -
Apo-Sulin *Tab 150mg, 200mg* **Novo-Sundac** *Tab 150mg, 200mg* **Generics** *Tab 150mg, 200mg*	**Rheumatoid arthritis, osteoarthritis,** **ankylosing spondylitis:** 150mg PO bid **bursitis, tendinitis, gout:** 200mg PO bid; max 400mg/d; **CH** limited data, 4mg/kg/d PO div bid has been used; DARF: not req

9.2.4 NSAID - Cyclooxygenase-2-Inhibitors

MA/EF (celecoxib, rofecoxib, valdecoxib): high selectivity for cyclooxygenase-2; inhibition of cyclooxygenase ⇒ synthesis of prostaglandins ↓
AE (celecoxib): dyspepsia, abdominal pain, GI effects
AE (valdecoxib): dyspepsia, headache, abdominal pain, nausea, diarrhea, edema
CI (celecoxib): hypersensitivity to celecoxib products, hypersensitivity to ASA or other anti-inflammatory drugs, hypersensitivity to sulfonamides
CI (valdecoxib): hypersensitivity to valdecoxib, allergic or asthma reaction to ASA/NSAIDs

Celecoxib	EHL 11h , PRC C, Lact ?
Celebrex *Cap 100mg, 200mg*	**Osteoarthritis:** 100mg PO bid or 200mg qd; **rheumatoid arthritis:** 100-200mg PO bid

Valdecoxib	EHL 8-11h, PRC C, Lact ?
Bextra *Tab 10mg, 20mg*	**Osteoarthritis:** 10mg PO qd; **dysmenorrhea:** 20mg PO bid; DARF: not rec in advanced RF

9.2.5 Other NSAIDs

MA/EF: see NSAID, Aspirin + other salicylates →172
AE (meloxicam): dyspepsia, flatulence, abdominal pain, diarrhea
AE (piroxicam) GI distress, rash, dizziness, ulcers, edema
CI (meloxicam): hypersensitiviy to meloxicam, allergic reactions to aspirin/NSAIDS
CI (piroxicam): hypersensitivity to piroxicam products, asthma, allergic reactions to ASA or other anti-inflammatories

Floctafenine	EHL 8h, PRC C, Lact -
Idarac *Tab 200mg, 400mg* **Generics** *Tab 200mg, 400mg*	**Pain:** 200-400mg PO q6-8 h PRN, max 1 200 mg/d
Mefenamic Acid	EHL 3-4h, PRC D, Lact -
Generics *Cap 250mg*	**Muscular aches, pain, primary dysmenorrhea, headache, dental pain:** ini 500mg PO then 250mg PO q6h PRN
Meloxicam	EHL 15-20h, PRC N, Lact ?
Mobicox *Tab 7.5mg, 15mg* **Generics** *Tab 7.5mg, 15mg*	**Osteoarthritis:** 7.5mg PO qd, max 15mg/d; DARF: see Prod Info
Piroxicam	EHL 50h, PRC C, Lact +
Novo-Pirocam *Cap 10mg, 20mg* **Nu-Pirox** *Cap 10mg, 20mg* **Generics** *Cap 10mg, 20mg*	**Rheumatoid arthritis, osteoarthritis:** 20mg PO qd or div bid; DARF: not req
Tenoxicam	EHL 60-75h, PRC D, Lact ?
Generics *Tab 20mg*	**Rheumatoid arthritis, osteoarthritis, ankylosing spondylitis, acute gouty arthritis, dysmenorrhoea:** 20mg PO qd

9.3　Other Non-Opiod Analgesics

9.3.1　Aniline Derivatives

MA: inhibition of cyclooxygenase ⇒ synthesis of prostaglandins ↓
EF: anti-inflammatory, analgesic, only mildly antiphlogistic
AE: allergic skin reactions, headache, bronchospasm, renal damage (tubular and papillary necrosis, interstitial nephritis), hepatic damage
CI: restricted use in presence of hepatic DO, Meulengracht's syndrome, renal DO

Acetaminophen (Paracetamol)	EHL no data, PRC B, Lact +
Abenol Supp 120mg, 325mg, 650mg **Atasol** Cap 325mg, 500mg, Drops 80mg/ml, Tab 325mg, 500mg **Novo-Gesic** Tab 325mg, 500mg **Pediatrix** Drops 80mg/ml, Sol (oral) 160mg/5ml **Tempra** Drops 80mg/ml, Syr 80mg/5ml, 160mg/5ml, Tab (chew) 80mg, 160mg, Tab (quick dissolve) 160mg **Tylenol** Cap 325mg, 500mg, 650mg, Soft chews 80mg, Elixir 160mg/5ml, Susp (oral) 160mg/5ml, Gelcaps 500mg, Drops 80mg/ml, Tab (chew) 160mg, Tab 325mg, 500mg **Generics** Cap 325mg, 500mg, Tab 325mg, 500mg	**Pain, fever:** 325-1000mg PO/PR q4-6h, max 4g/d; **CH** 10- 15mg/kg/dose PO/PR q4-6h, max 5 doses/d; DARF: GFR (ml/min) >50: q4h, 10-50: q6h, <10: q8h

9.3.2　Non-Opioid Analgesic Combinations

Acetaminophen + Methocarbamol	PRC D, Lact ?
Methoxacet Extra Strength Tab 500 + 400mg	**Acute painful musculoskeletal conditions:** 2 Tab PO qid

Aspirin + Butalbital + Caffeine	PRC D, Lact ?
Fiorinal Tab 330 + 50 + 40mg, Cap 330 + 50 + 40mg **ratio-Tecnal** Tab 330 + 50 + 40mg, Cap 330 + 50 + 40mg **Trianal** Tab 330 + 50 + 40mg, Cap 330 + 50 + 40mg	**Tension headache:** 1-2 Tab/Cap PO q4h

Aspirin + Caffeine	PRC D, Lact ?
Alka Seltzer Morning Relief *Tab 500mg + 65mg*	**Headache** : adults and ch>12y: 2 tabs PO q6h PRN, max 8 tabs/d; age>60 max 4 tabs/d
Aspirin + Caffeine + Orphenadrine	PRC D, Lact ?
Norgesic *Tab 385 + 30 + 25mg* **Norgesic forte** *Tab 770 + 60 + 50mg*	**Musculoskeletal pain:** 1-2 Tab PO tid-qid; forte: 1/2-1 Tab PO tid-qid
Aspirin + Methocarbamol	PRC D, Lact ?
Methoxisal *Cap 325 + 400mg, 500 + 400mg* **Robaxisal** *Cap 325 + 400mg* *Tab 325 + 400mg* **Robaxisal Extra Strength** *Cap 500 + 400mg*	**Acute painful musculoskeletal conditions:** 2 Tab PO qid

9.4 Opioids
9.4.1 Opioid Agonists

MA/EF: stimulation of central opiate receptors ⇒ analgesic, sedative, respiratory depression, antitussive, emetic and antiemetic (see AE);
AE: respiratory depression, sedation, bradycardia, hypotensive circulation DO, pruritus, bronchospasm, transpiration, spasms of pancreatic and bile ducts, constipation, seizures, miosis, tolerance development, urinary retention;
CI: restricted use for children < 1, addiction to opiates, pancreatitis, respiratory DO; Note: all are PRC D if used for prolonged periods or in high doses at term

Codeine	EHL 2.5-3.5h, PRC C, Lact + Equivalent dose compared to morphine 10mg IM (IM/oral): 120 / 200
Linctus codeine *Liq (oral) 0.2%* **Generics** *Tab 15mg, 30mg, 50mg, 100mg, 150mg, 200mg, Inj 30mg/ml, 60mg/ml, Liq (oral) 143mg/30ml*	**Pain:** 15-60mg PO/IM/SC q4-6h; **cough:** 10-20mg PO/ SC q4-6h prn; **CH pain:** > 2y: 0.5-1mg/kg/dose PO/SC/IM q4-6h, **cough:** 2-6y: 1mg/kg/d PO div qid, max 30mg/ 24h; 6-12y: 5-10mg PO q4-6h prn; max 60mg/24h; DARF: GFR (ml/min) > 50: 100%, 10-50: 75%, <10: 50%

10.1.4   Ketamine

EF: analgesic, hypnotic without considerable respiratory depression
AE: BP ↑, tachycardia, intracranial pressure ↑, hypersalivation, unpleasant/vivid dreams, muscle hyperactivity, N/V
CI: severe HTN, pre-eclampsia, intracranial pressure ↑ without adequate artificial respiration, hypersensitivity to ketamine products, conditions where HTN is hazardous

Ketamine	EHL 2-3h, PRC D, Lact -
Ketalar *Inj* 10mg/ml, 50mg/ml	**Anesthesia:** 1-2mg/kg IV; 5-10mg/kg IM; maint. 0.1-0.5mg/min IV; **sedation, analgesia:** 0.2- 0.75mg/kg IV, maint 5-20mcg/kg/min, **CH anesthesia:** 1- 2mg/kg IV; 5-10mg/kg IM; maint 0.01-0.03mg/kg/min IV; **CH sedation, analgesia:** 0.2-1mg/kg IV maint 5-20mcg/ kg/min

10.1.5   Propofol

MA/EF: hypnotic for induction and maintenance of anesthesia, no analgesia
AE: BP ↑, respiratory depression, bradycardia, seizures, adrenal suppression, apnea, injection site pain, cardiac arrest
CI: decompensated cardiac insufficiency, ch < 3y, hypersensitivity to propofol products

Propofol	EHL 40-200min, PRC B, Lact ?
Diprivan *Inj* 10mg/ml **Generics** *Inj* 10mg/ml	**Anesthesia induction:** 1-2.5mg/kg IV, maint 100- 200mcg/kg/min IV; **ICU sedation:** 5-50mcg/kg/min; **CH > 3y: anesthesia induction:** 2.5-3.5mg/kg IV, maint 125-300mcg/kg/min; **sedation:** 1-2mg/kg IV, maint 75- 100mcg/kg/min; DARF: not req

10.2 Neuromuscular Blockers
10.2.1 Depolarising Muscle Relaxants

MA/EF: permanent depolarization of the motor endplate, prevention of the immediate repolarization;
AE: allerg. skin react., fasciculations, muscle pain, coronary dysrythmias, bradycardia, hyperkalemia, malignant hyperthermia, IOP ↑;
CI: impossibility of artificial respir.n, anamnestic malign.t hyperthermia, susceptibility to hyperkalemia ↑, acute phase of major trauma/major burns, hypersensit. to succinylcholine

Succinylcholine	EHL < 1min, PRC C, Lact ?
Quelicin *Inj 20mg/ml, 100mg/ml* **Generics** *Inj 20mg/ml*	**General anesthesia:** ini 0.6mg/kg IV, maint 0.5-10mg/ min; **CH general anesthesia:** ini 1-2mg/kg IV; DARF: not req

10.2.2 Non-Depolarising Muscle Relaxants

MA/EF: competitive displacement of acetylcholine at the nicotinergic receptors of the motor endplate ⇒ prevention of depolarization
AE: bronchospasm, tachycardia, urticaria, hypotension
AE (cisatracurium): bradycardia, flushing;
AE (mivacurium): flushing;
AE (pancuronium): HTN, salivation;
AE (rocuronium): severe pain on injection, HTN;
AE (vecuronium): brady-/tachycardia, allergic reactions, hypotension
CI: impossibility of artificial respiration; caution with myasthenia gravis and Eaton-Lambert-Syndrome
CI (cisatracurium, mivacurium): hypersensitivity to cisatracurium/benzylisoquinoliniums
CI (pancuronium): hypersensitivity to pancuronium or bromide products
CI (rocuronium, vecuronium): hypersensitivity to product ingredients

Atracurium	EHL 20min, PRC C, Lact ?
Generics *Inj 10mg/ml*	**General anesthesia:** ini 0.4-0.5mg/kg IV bolus, maint. 0.08-0.1mg/kg IV boluses

Cisatracurium	EHL 22-31min, PRC B, Lact ?
Nimbex *Inj 2mg/ml, 10mg/ml*	**General anesthesia:** ini 0.15mg/kg IV maint. 1-2mcg/kg/min IV; **ICU long-term use:** 3mcg/kg/min IV; **CH 2-12y:** **general anesthesia:** ini 0.1mg/kg IV

Mivacurium	EHL 1.8-2min, PRC C, Lact ?
Mivacron Inj 2mg/ml	**General anesthesia:** ini 0.15-0.25mg/kg IV, maint 0.1mg/ kg q15min or 4mcg/kg/min; **CH** 2-12y: **general anesthesia:** ini 0.2mg/kg IV, maint 0.1mg/kg q10-15min or 10-15mcg/kg/min
Pancuronium	EHL 89-140min, PRC C, Lact ?
Pancuronium Inj 1mg/ml, 2mg/ml **Generics** Inj 1mg/ml, 2mg/ml	**General anesthesia:** 0.06-0.1mg/kg IV, maint 0.01- 0.06mg/kg q80-150min; DARF: GFR (ml/min) >10: 100%, <10: not rated
Rocuronium	EHL 84-131min, PRC B, Lact ?
Zemuron Inj 10mg/ml	**General anesthesia:** ini 600mcg/kg IV, maint 75- 225mcg/kg prn
Vecuronium	EHL 65-80min, PRC C, Lact ?
Norcuron Inj 10mg/vial, 20mg/vial **Generics** Inj 10mg/vial	**General anesthesia:** 0.075-0.1mg/kg IV, maint 0.01- 0.015mg/kg, rep q15-40min prn

10.3 Local Anesthetics

MA/EF: membrane permeability for cations , especially Na+ ⇒ excitability of nerve fibers↓ ;
AE: dizziness, vomiting, drowsiness, convulsions, bradycardia, dysrhythmias, shock
AE (bupivacaine): arterial hypotension, ventricular arrhythmias, CNS excitation
AE (lidocaine): seizures, drowsiness, tremors, hypotension
AE (mepivacaine): fetal bradycardia, respiratory arrest, seizures, allergic reaction, porphyria
CI (topical anesthetics): severe conduction disturbances, acute decompensated coronary insufficiency, shock, infections around injection site, known allergy
CI (bupivacaine): regional IV anesthesia, paracervical block, shock or myasthenia gravis, hypersensitivity to bupivacaine products
CI (lidocaine, mepivacaine): hypersensitivity to product ingredients/amide-type anesthetics

Articaine + Epinephrine	EHL 25min, PRC C, Lact +
Astracaine *Inj 40mg + 5mcg/ml* **Astracaine forte** *Inj 40mg + 10mcg/ml*	**Local anesthesia, nerve block:** 0.5-3.6ml; oral surgery: 1-5.4ml; max 7mg/kg
Bupivacaine	EHL no data
Marcaine with epinephrine *1:200 000 Inj 0.25%, 0.5%* **Marcaine** *Inj (spinal) 0.75%* **Sensorcaine** *Inj 0.25%, 0.5%* **Sensorcaine with epinephrine 1:200 000** *Inj 0.25%, 0.5%* **Sensorcaine Forte with epinephrine 1:200 000** *Inj 0.5%* **Generics** *Inj 0.25%, 0.5%, 0.75%*	**Local infiltration:** 175mg (0.25% sol.); complete motor blockade, epidural: 75-150mg (0.5-0.75% sol.); **dental anesthesia:** 9-18mg (0.5% sol.)
Chloroprocaine	PRC C, Lact ?
Nesacaine-CE *Inj 2%, 3%*	**Mandibular nerve block:** 2-3ml (2% sol); infraorbital: 0.5-1ml (2% sol); brachial plexus: 30-40ml (2% sol); pudendal block: 10ml (2% sol); caudal and epidural block: 15-25ml (2-3% sol)
Lidocaine	EHL 1.5-2h, PRC B, Lact +
Xylocaine CO2 *Inj 17.3mg/ml* **Xylocaine** *Inj 0.5%, 1%, 1.5%, 2.0%, 4.0%* **Xylocaine (with epinephrine)** *Inj 0.5%, 1%, 1.5%, 2.0%* **Xylocaine Spinal** *Inj 5.0%* **Generics** *Inj 1%, 2.0%, Inj (with epinephrine) 1%, 2.0%*	**Caudal anesthesia:** 200-300mg (1% sol.) **epidural anesthesia:** 250-300mg (1-2% sol.); **arrhythmias**
Mepivacaine	EHL 1.9-3.2h, PRC C, Lact ?
Carbocaine *Inj 1%, 2%* **Isocaine** *Inj 3%* **Isocaine (with levonordefrin)** *Inj 2%* **Scandonest** *Inj 3%* **Scandonest (with epinephrine)** *Inj 2%* **Polocaine** *Inj 3%* **Polocaine (with levonordefrin)** *Inj 2%*	**Brachial nerve block:** 50-400mg (1-2% sol); **epidural nerve block:** 150-300mg (1-2% sol); **local infiltration:** up to 400mg (0.5-1% sol.)

Prilocaine	EHL 1.6h, PRC C, Lact +
Citanest 4% Forte *Inj (with epinephrine)* 4% **Citanest 4% Plain** *Inj* 4%	**Dental procedures:** ini 1-2ml

Procaine	EHL 7.7min, PRC C, Lact ?
Novocain *Inj* 2%	**Nerve block:** up to 50 mL (2% sol)

Ropivacaine	EHL 4h, PRC B, Lact ?
Naropin *Inj* 2mg/ml, 5mg/ml, 7.5mg/ml, 10mg/ml	**Epidural block:** 250mg

11. Neurology

11.1 Anticonvulsants

MA (carbamazepine): repeated stimulation of afferences ⇒ stimulus answer ↓
MA (benzodiazepines; clonazepam, diazepam, lorazepam): opening of chloride channels ⇒ inhibiting function of GABA neurons ↑, especially in the limbic system
MA (fosphenytoin, phenytoin): ion permeability ↓ ⇒ membrane stabilization
MA (lamotrigine): blockage of presynaptic Na+ channels ⇒ release of excitatory amino acids ↓
MA (phenobarbital): reinforcement of inhibitory effect of GABA in the CNS
MA (oxcarbazepine, topiramate): membrane stabilization by blockage of Na- channels, antagonization of the excitatory effect of glutamate, reinforcement of the inhibitory effect caused by GABA
MA (valproic acid, vigabatrin): enzymatic breakdown of GABA ↓
EF (benzodiazepines; diazepam, phenobarbital): sedative, sleep inducing, anxiolytic, anti-aggressive, anti-convulsive, muscle relaxing
AE (carbamazepine): headache, dizziness, ataxia, dysopias, cholestatic hepatitis, disturbances of haematopoiesis, bradycardic cardiac arrhythmias, allergic reactions
AE (benzodiazepines; clonazepam, diazepam, lorazepam): tiredness, sleepiness, drowsiness, confusion, paradox reactions, anterograde amnesia, respiratory depression, psychic and physical addiction
AE (fosphenytoin, phenytoin): gingival hyperplasia, hypertrichosis, dizziness, ataxia, complete blood count changes
AE (oxcarbazepine): tiredness, dizziness, headache, nausea, diplopia, hyponatremia, acne, alopecia, exanthema
AE (phenobarbital): tiredness, dizziness, anterograde amnesia, dizziness, ataxia, dysopias, porphyria, N/V, hepatic dysfunction, bradycardia, respiratory depression, skin reactions, complete blood count changes, enzyme ind., addiction
AE (valproic acid): tiredness, tremors, hair loss, hepatic damage, coagul. DO
CI (carbamazepine): AV block, severe hepatic dysfunction, combination with MAO-inhib.
CI (benzos; clonazepam, diazepam, lorazepam): myasthenia gravis, severe hepatic damage, respiratory insufficiency, ataxia
CI (fosphenytoin, phenytoin): AV block II° - III°, sick sinus, cardiac insufficiency
CI (phenobarbital): porphyria, severe hepatic and renal dysfunction, status asthmaticus, respiratory insufficiency
CI (valproic acid): liver diseases in family history, see also: sedatives/barbiturates →228 and sedatives/benzodiazepines →225

Carbamazepine	EHL 12-17h (mult. dose), 25-65h (1x dose), PRC D, Lact +, serum-level (mcg/ml): 4-12
Novo-Carbamaz *Tab 200mg* **Tegretol** *Tab (chew) 100mg, 200mg, Tab 200mg, Susp 100mg/5ml* **Tegretol CR** *Tab sust. rel. 200mg, 400mg* **Generics** *Tab 200mg, Tab sust. rel. 200mg, 400mg, Tab (chew) 100mg, 200mg*	**Mania:** 200mg PO qd-bid, incr by 200mg/d q2-4d, maint 600-1600mg/d, max 2,000-3,000mg/d; **epilepsy:** ini 200mg PO bid, incr by 200mg/d q wk div tid-qid or bid (ext.rel.); maint 800-1,200mg/d, max 1,200mg/d, max 1,600mg/d; **CH** >12 y: ini 200 mg PO bid, or 100mg PO qid (susp), incr by 200mg/d q wk div tid-qid or bid (ext.rel.), max 1,000 mg/d (age 12-15 y), max 1,200 mg/d (age >15 y); **CH** 6-12 y: 100mg PO bid or 50mg PO qid (susp), incr by 100mg/d q wk div tid-qid or bid (ext.rel.), 15-30 mg/kg/d PO div bid-qid, maint 400-800mg/d, max 1,000mg/d; **CH** <6 y: 10-20mg/kg/d PO div bid-qid, max 35 mg/kg/d; **trigeminal neuralgia:** ini 100mg PO bid or 200mg PO qd (ext. rel.) or 50mg PO qid (susp), incr by 200mg/d prn, maint 400-800mg/d, max 1,200mg/d; **migraine PRO:** 600 mg/d, 10-20mg/kg/d PO div bid; DARF: not req
Clobazam	EHL 18h, PRC X(1st), D(2nd, 3rd), Lact -
Frisium *Tab 10mg* **Generics** *Tab 10mg*	**Epilepsy:** ini 5-15mg/d, max 80mg/d; **CH** <2yrs ini 0.5-1mg/kg /d; 2-16yrs ini 5mg/d, max 40mg/d; DARF required, reduced dose required for impared liver function
Clonazepam	EHL 30-40h, PRC C, Lact ?, serum-level (ng/ml): 25-30
Clonapam *Tab 0.5mg, 1mg, 2mg* **Rivotril** *Tab 0.5mg, 2mg* **Generics** *Tab 0.25mg, 0.5mg, 1mg, 2mg*	**Epilepsy:** ini 0.5mg PO tid, incr by 0.5-1mg q3d, max 20mg/d; **CH** <10 y or <30kg: ini 0.01-0.03mg/kg/d (max 0.05mg/kg/d) PO div bid-tid, incr by 0.25- 0.5mg q3d up to 0.1-0.2mg/kg/d div tid, **neuralgias:** 2-4mg/d PO; **anxiety, panic DO:** →225

Diazepam	EHL 22-54h, PRC D, Lact ?
Diastat *Gel (rectal) 5mg/ml* **Diazemuls** *Conc (oral) 5mg/ml* **E Pam** *Tab 2mg, 5mg, 10mg* **Novo-Dipam** *Tab 2mg, 5mg, 10mg* **Valium** *Tab 5mg* **Generics** *Tab 2mg, 5mg, 10mg* *Inj 1mg/ml, 5mg/ml*	**Status epilepticus:** 5-10mg IV, rep in 10-15min, max 30mg; **CH** 1 mo-5 y: 0.2-0.5mg/kg IV slowly q2-5min to max 5mg, >5 y: 1mg IV slowly q2-5min to max 10mg, rep q2-4h prn; **epilepsy, adj** Tx: 2-10mg PO bid-qid; **CH** >6 mo: 1-2.5mg PO bid-qid, <5 y: max 5mg/d, >5 y: max 10mg; **seizure activity↑:** 0.2-0.5 mg/kg PR or 14-27kg: 5mg, 28-50kg: 10mg, 51-75kg: 15mg, 76-111kg: 20mg, rep prn in 4-12h, max 20 mg/d or ch 2-5 y: 0.5 mg/kg PR, 6-11 y: 0.3 mg/kg PR, <12 y: 0.2 mg/kg PR; **alcohol withdrawal:** ini 10mg PO tid-qid x 24h, then red to 5mg tid-qid prn; DARF: not req; **muscle spasm, sedation, anxiety: ;**
Divalproex Sodium	EHL 6-17h, PRC D, Lact + serum-level(mcg/ml): 70-120
Epival *Tab 125mg, 250mg, 500mg VAE,* *Tab ext. rel 500mg VAE* **Generics** *Tab 125mg, 250mg, 500mg VAE* *(VAE=valproic acid equivalents)*	**Migraine PRO:** 250mg PO bid, titrate to max 1,000mg/d; DARF: not req
Ethosuximide	PRC C, Lact ? serum-level (mcg/ml): 40-100
Zarontin *Cap 250mg, Syr 250mg/5ml*	**Epilepsy:** 500mg PO qd or div bid, incr by 250 mg/d q4- 7d, maint 20-30mg/kg/d div qd-bid, max 1.5 g/d; **CH** 3-6 y: 250mg PO qd, incr by 250mg/d q4-7d, maint 20-30mg/ kg/d, >6 y: 500mg PO qd, incr by 250mg/d q4-7d, maint 20-30mg/kg/d, max 1.5g/d
Fosphenytoin	EHL (Phenytoin): 12-29h, PRC D, Lact ? serum-level (mcg/ml): 10-20
Cerebyx *Inj 50mg mg PE/ml* *(PE = phenytoin equivalents)*	**Status epilepticus:** 15-20mg PE/kg IV, max IV rate100- 150mg PE/min; **CH** 15-20mg PE/kg IV at rate <2mg PE/ kg/min; **seizure PRO:** 10-20mg PE/kg IM; maint 4-6mg PE/kg/d

Gabapentin

EHL 5-7h, PRC C, Lact ?

Neurontin Tab 600mg, 800mg,
Cap 100mg, 300mg, 400mg
Generics Cap 100mg, 300mg, 400mg

Epilepsy (adj Tx): ini 300mg PO tid, incr by
300mg/d q3- 5d, maint 300-600mg PO tid,
max 3,600mg/d;
CH >12 y: adult dose;
neuropathic pain: 300mg PO tid, max
3,600mg/d;
restless leg syndrome: 300-2,700mg/d PO;
mania: ini 300mg PO hs, titrate to 900-
2,400 mg/d in div doses; DARF: CrCl(ml/min)
30-60: 300mg PO bid, 15-30: 300mg PO qd,
<15: 300mg PO qod

Lamotrigine

EHL 25-30h, PRC C, Lact ?

Lamictal Tab (chew) 5mg, Tab 25mg,
100mg, 150mg

Epilepsy (adj Tx with valproic acid): ini
25mg PO qod x 2wk, then 25mg PO qd x
2wk, incr by 25-50mg/d q1-2wk, maint
100-400mg/d div qd-bid, maint with
valproic acid alone: 100-200mg/d div
qd-bid;
**epilepsy (adj Tx with enzyme-inducing
antiepileptic drugs):** ini 50mg PO qd x 2wk,
then 50 mg PO bid x 2wk, incr by 100 mg/d
q1- 2wk, maint 150-250mg PO bid;
**Lennox-Gastaut (adj Tx with valproic
acid)** ch 2-12 y: ini 0.15mg/kg/d PO div
qd- bid x 2wk, then 0.3mg/kg/d PO div
qd-bid x 2wk, incr q1- 2wk,
maint 1-5mg/kg/d, max 200mg/d;
**Lennox-Gastaut (adj Tx with
enzyme-inducing antiepileptic drugs)**
CH 2-12 y: ini 0.6mg/kg/d PO div bid x 2wk,
then 1.2mg/kg/d PO div bid x 2wk, incr
q1-2wk, maint 5-15mg/kg/d, max 400mg/d;
bipolar depression: ini 25-50mg/d PO qd, incr
to 100-500mg/d div bid;
DARF: reduce maint dose

Lorazepam

EHL 10-20h, PRC D, Lact ?

Ativan Tab 0.5mg, 1mg, 2mg,
Tab (subling.) 0.5mg, 1mg, 2mg, Inj 4mg/ml
Novo-Lorazem Tab 0.5mg, 1mg, 2mg
Nu-Loraz Tab 0.5mg, 1mg, 2mg
Generics Tab 0.5mg, 1mg, 2mg

Status epilepticus: 0.05-0.1mg/kg IV x 2-5min or 4mg IV, rep prn 0.05mg/kg in 5-15min, max single dose 4mg/ kg, max 8mg/12h;
anxiety: 0.05mg/kg IV, max IV dose 4mg, max 2mg (preop), ini 1-2mg PO bid-tid, maint 2- 6mg/d, max 10mg/d;
insomnia: 2-4mg PO hs; DA in mild and moderate RF: use lowest effective dose in severe RF: contraind.

Methsuximide

EHL 3h, PRC D, Lact -

Celontin Cap 300mg

Absense seizures: ini 300mg PO qd, incr by 300mg/wk, maint 1200mg/d

Nitrazepam

EHL 30h, PRC D, Lact -

Mogadon Tab 5mg, 10mg
Nitrazadon Tab 5mg, 10mg
Generics Tab 5mg, 10mg

Insomnia: 2.5-10mg PO qhs; myoclonic seizures: **CH** (up to 30kg) 0.3-1mg/kg/d in 3 div doses

Oxcarbazepine

EHL 1-2.5h, metabolites 8-11h, PRC C, Lact ?

Trileptal Tab 150mg, 300mg, 600mg,
Susp (oral) 60mg/ml

Epilepsy, monotherapy: ini 300mg PO bid, incr by 300mg/d q3d, maint 1,200mg/d, max 2,400mg/d;
epilepsy, adj: ini 300mg PO bid, incr by 600mg/d q wk, maint 1,200mg/d, max 2,400mg/d;
CH 4-16 y: ini 8-10 mg/ kg/d div bid, max loading dose 600mg/d, maint 900mg/d (20-29kg), 1,200mg/d (29.1-39kg), 1,800mg/d (>39kg); DARF: CrCl (ml/min) <30: reduce ini dose by 50%, titrate carefully

Paraldehyde

Generics Inj 1ml/ml

Sedation: 0.15 ml/kg/dose PO or PR, max 5ml; seizures: 0.2-0.4ml/kg IV over 2h, max 0.4 ml/kg/d IV; 0.3ml/kg/dose PO/PR, max 5.0ml PO/PR, diluted with equal volumes of mineral or veget. oil, may repeat q4-6 h prn

Phenobarbital	EHL 1.5-4.9d, PRC D, Lact -, serum-level (mcg/ml): 15-40
Barbilixir *Elix 4mg/ml* **Generics** *Tab 15mg, 30mg, 60mg, 100mg,* *Elixir 5mg/ml,* *Inj 30mg/ml, 120mg/ml*	**Epilepsy:** 60-250mg/d PO qd or 2-3mg/kg/d; **CH** 1-5 y: 6- 8mg/kg/d PO/IV, 6-12 y: 4-6mg/kg/d PO/IV, >12 y: 1-3mg/ kg/d IV/PO; **status epilepticus:** 15-20mg/kg IV, max IV rate 60mg/min, max 20mg/kg; **sedation:** 30-120mg PO qd/bid/tid, max 400mg/d; DARF: not req in mild/moderate RF, reduce in severe RF, no long term use
Phenytoin	EHL 22h, PRC D, Lact +, serum-level (mcg/ml): 10-20
Dilantin *Cap 30mg, 100mg, Susp (oral)* *30mg/5ml, 125mg/ml* **Dilantin Infatabs** *Tab (chew) 50mg* **Generics** *Inj 50mg/ml*	**Epilepsy:** ini 400mg PO, then 300mg in 2h and 4h, after 1d maint 300mg PO qd (ext.rel.)/div tid; **CH** >6 y: 5mg/kg/ d PO div bid-tid, maint 4-8mg/kg/d, max 300mg/d; **status epilepticus:** 10-15mg/kg IV, max rate 50mg/min, then 100mg IV/PO q6-8h; **CH** >6 y: 10-20mg/kg IV, max 1-3mg/kg/min; DARF: no loading dose
Primidone	EHL 3.3-7h, metabol. 29-150h, PRC D, Lact ? serum-level(mcg/ml): 5-12
Generics *Tab 125mg, 250mg*	**Epilepsy:** 125mg PO qhs, incr x 10d, maint 250mg PO tid-qid, max 2g/d; **CH** <8 y: ini 50mg PO qhs x 3d, incr to 50mg PO bid x 3d, incr to 100mg PO bid x 3d, then incr to maint 125-250mg PO tid or 10-25 mg/kg/d div tid-qid, **CH** >8 y: ini 100- 125mg PO qhs x 3d, incr to 100-125mg PO bid x 3d, incr to 100-125mg PO x 3d, incr to maint 250mg tid-qid or 750-1,000mg/kg/d div tid-qid; **essential tremor:** incr to 250mg PO tid DARF: GFR (ml/min) >50: dosing q8h, 10-50: dosing q8- 12h, <10: dosing q12-24h

Topiramate	EHL 18-24h, PRC C, Lact ?
Topamax *Cap 15mg, 25mg, Tab 25mg, 100mg, 200mg*	**Epilepsy, adj Tx:** ini 50mg PO qhs, incr by 5mg/d q wk, maint 200mg PO bid, max 1,600mg/d; **CH** 2-16 y: ini 1- 3mg/kg/d (or 25mg/d) PO qhs, incr by 1-3mg/kg/d q 1- 2wk up to 5-9mg/kg/d div bid; DARF: CrCl (ml/min) <70: 50%
Valproic Acid	EHL 6-17h, PRC D, Lact + serum-level (mcg/ml): 50-100 (epilepsy), 25-125 (mania)
Depakene *Cap 250mg, 500mg, Syr 250mg/5ml* **Epiject IV** *Syr 100mg/ml* **Generics** *Cap 250mg, 500mg, Syr 250mg/5ml*	**Seizures:** 10-15mg/kg/d PO or IV inf x 60min, max 20mg/ min, incr by 5-10mg/kg/d q wk, max 60mg/kg/d, div doses >250mg/d into bid-qid; **CH** >10 y: 10-15mg/kg/d PO or IV inf x 60min, max 20mg/min, incr by 5-10mg/kg/d q wk, max 60mg/kg/d, div doses >250 mg/d into bid-qid; **absence seizures:** 10-24.9kg: 250mg/d, 25-39.9kg: 500mg/d, 40-59.9kg: 750mg/d, 60-74.9kg: 1,000mg/d, 75-89.9kg: 1,250mg/d, div doses <250mg/d into bid-qid; **migraine: mania:**
Vigabatrin	EHL 5-8h, PRC C, Lact ?
Sabril *Powder (oral) 0.5g/sachet, Tab 500mg*	**Epilepsy:** ini 1-2g/d PO in one to two doses, maint. 2-4g/d; **CH** ini 40mg/kg/d PO in one to two doses, maint. 80-100mg/kg/d

11.2 Migraine Therapy
11.2.1 5-HT₁ Agonists

MA/EF: serotonin agonism (5-HT1D-Rec) ⇒ vasoconstriction; Tx of migraine attack
AE: heaviness, feeling of pressure, tiredness, dizziness, flush
CI: hypersensitivity to sumatriptane, ischemic coronary diseases, heart attack, vasospastic angina, M. Raynaud, HTN, not with (dihydro-)ergotamine

Eletriptan	EHL 4h, PRC C, Lact +
Replax Tab 20mg, 40mg	**Migraine Tx:** 20-40mg PO, rep prn in 2h, max 80mg/d
Naratriptan	EHL 5-6h, PRC C, Lact ?
Amerge Tab 1mg, 2.5mg	**Migraine Tx:** 1-2.5mg PO, rep prn in 4h, max 5mg/24h; >4 Tx/mo not established; DARF: CrCl (ml/min) <15: contraind., mild RF: max 2.5mg/d, reduce ini dose
Rizatriptan	EHL 2-3h, PRC C, Lact ?
Maxalt Tab 5mg, 10mg *Maxalt RPD* Tab (orally disint) 5mg, 10mg	**Migraine Tx:** 5-10mg PO, rep prn in 2h, max 30mg/24h, >4 Tx/mo not established, under propranolol Tx max 5mg PO tid
Sumatriptan	EHL 2h, PRC C, Lact -
Imitrex Spray (nasal) 5mg/Spray, 20mg/Spray, Inj 6mg/0.5ml *Imitrex DF* Tab 25mg, 50mg, 100mg	**Migraine Tx:** 6mg SC, rep prn in 1h, max 12mg/d or 25mg PO, rep q2h 25-100mg, max 200mg (if 1st dose was SC), max 300mg/d (if 1st dose was PO) or 5-20mg intranasally, rep prn q2h, max 4mg/d, >4 Tx/mo not established; **cluster headache:** 6mg SC, rep. prn in 1h, max 12mg/d
Zolmitriptan	EHL 2.5-3h, PRC C, Lact ?
Zomig Tab 2.5mg, Nasal spray 2.5mg/spray, 5mg/spray *Zomig Rapimelt* Tab (dispersable) 2.5mg	**Migraine Tx:** 1.25-2.5 mg PO, rep prn q2h, max 10mg/ 24h; DARF: not req

11.2.2 Ergot Derivates

MA/EF (dihydroergotamine): stimulation of serotonin rec. ⇒ constriction of venous capacity vessels; interval Tx;
MA/EF (ergotamine): mostly a-receptor agonism⇒ vasoconstriction; migraine attack Tx;
AE (dihydroergotamine): N/V, peripherally inadequate circulation;
CI (dihydroergotamine): hypersensitivity to seca alkaloids, severe coronary insufficiency, vascular diseases, severe hepatic dysfunction

Caffeine + Ergotamine	EHL 3-6 (C.), 1.5-2.5h (E.), PRC X, Lact -
Cafergot *Supp 100mg+2mg, Tab 100mg + 1mg*	**Migraine, cluster headache:** ini 2 tab PO, then 1 tab q30min prn, max 6 tab/attack, max 10 tab/wk or max 2 supp/attack, max 5 supp/wk; DARF: contraind.
Dihydroergotamine	EHL 7-9h, PRC X, Lact -
D.H.E. 45 *Inj 1mg/ml* **Migranal** *Spray (nasal) 4mg/ml* **Generics** *Inj 1mg/ml*	**Migraine:** 1mg IV/IM/SC, rep prn q1h, max 2mg(IV) or 3mg(IM/SC)/24h or 1 spray (0.5mg) in each nostril, rep in 15min, max 4 sprays (2mg)/24h or 8 sprays (4mg)/wk; DARF: contraind. in severe RF
Methysergide	EHL 45-62min, PRC X, Lact -
Sansert *Tab 2mg*	**Migraine/cluster headache PRO:** ini 2mg PO qd, titrate to 4-8mg/d PO div bid-qid with meals, taper dose x 2-3 wk prior to discontinuation, 3-4 wk of drug-free interval after 6-mo Tx; DARF: contraind.

11.2.3 Migraine Therapy - Other Drugs

MA/EF (divalproex, valproic acid): potassium conductance↑ ⇒ neuronal activity↓
AE, CI (divalproex, valproic acid)

Divalproex Sodium	EHL 6-17h, PRC D, Lact + serum-level(mcg/ml): 70-120
Epival *Tab 125mg, 250mg, 500mg VAE, Tab ext. rel 500mg VAE* **Generics** *Tab 125mg, 250mg, 500mg VAE (VAE=valproic acid equivalents)*	**Migraine PRO:** 250mg PO bid, titrate to max 1,000mg/d; DARF: not req

Flunarizine	EHL 19d, PRC ?, Lact ?
Sibelium *Cap 5mg*	**Migraine PRO:** 10mg/d
Pizotifen	EHL 26h, PRC C, Lact ?
Sandomigran *Tab 0.5mg* Sandomigran DS *Tab 1mg*	**Migraine PRO:** ini 0.5mg PO qhs, incr to 0.5mg PO tid, maint 1-6mg/d
Propranolol	EHL 3-4h, PRC C, Lact ?
Inderal *Tab 10mg, 20mg, 40mg, 80mg, 120mg, Inj 1mg/ml* Inderal LA *Cap ext.rel 60mg, 80mg, 120mg, 160mg* Generics *Tab 10mg, 20mg, 40mg, 80mg, 120mg*	**Migraine:** ini 80mg/d PO, maint 160-240mg/d
Tanacetum	PRC X, Lact -
Feverfew *Cap 125mg, 400mg*	**Migraine:** 125-400mg PO daily
Valproic Acid	EHL 6-17h, PRC D, Lact + serum-level(mcg/ml): 70-120
Depakene *Cap 250mg, 500mg, Syr 250mg/5ml* Epiject IV *Syr 100mg/ml* Generics *Cap 250mg, 500mg, Syr 250mg/5ml*	**Migraine PRO:** 250mg PO bid, titrate to max 1,000mg/d; DARF: not req; epilepsy; mania:

11.3   Alzheimer's – Cholinesterase Inhibitors

MA/EF: reversible and noncompetitive inhibition of centrally-active acetylcholinesterase ⇒ concentration of acetylcholine ↑ ⇒ synaptic transmission ↑ ⇒ cognitive function ↑
AE (donepezil, rivastigmine): N/V, diarrhea, anorexia, muscle cramps, insomnia, fatigue, urinary incontinence, psychiatric disturbances, hypotension;
CI: hypersensitivity to one of the substances or other cholinesterase inhibitors, GI disease, concurrent use of NSAIDs, asthma, obstructive pulmonary disease, sick sinus syndrome, SV cardiac conduction conditions, history of seizures, major surgery
CI (rivastigmine): DM, CVS/pulmonary disease, urogenital tract obstruction, Parkinson's disease (exacerbation), renal/hepatic insufficiency

Donepezil	EHL 70h, PRC C, Lact ?
Aricept *Tab 5mg, 10mg*	**Alzheimer's dementia:** ini 5mg PO qhs, incr prn to 10mg PO qhs after 4-6wk, max 10mg/d; DARF: limited data

Galantamine	EHL 7-8h, PRC B, Lact -
Reminyl *Tab 4mg, 8mg, 12mg*	**Alzheimer's dementia:** ini 4mg PO bid, incr prn to 4mg prn by 4mg q4wk to 8-12mg PO bid, max 32mg/d; DARF: moderate RF: max 16mg/d; severe RF: not rec

Rivastigmine	PRC B, Lact ?
Exelon *Cap 1.5mg, 3mg, 4.5mg, 6mg*	**Alzheimer's dementia:** ini 1.5mg PO bid, incr to 3mg PO bid >2wk, prn incr to 4.5mg PO bid up to 6mg PO bid q2wk, max 12mg/d; DARF: not req

11.4 Parkinsonian Drugs
11.4.1 Anticholinergic Parkinsonian Drugs

MA/EF: inhibition of central cholinergic neurons ⇒ plus symptoms rigor and tremor ↓
AE: confusion to psychosis, mydriasis, accommodation disturbances, glaucoma, oral dryness, micturition disturbances, fatigue, tachycardia, thermostatic dysregulation
CI: glaucoma, micturition disturbances, tachyarrhythmia, cognitive impairment; use in patients over 65 only if strictly indicated

Benztropine Mesylate	PRC C, Lact ?
Benztropine Omega *Inj 1mg/ml* **Generics** *Tab 2mg*	**Parkinsonism:** ini 0.5-2mg/qhs PO/IM/IV, incr by 0.5mg q wk, max 6mg/d, div qd-qid; **drug-induced extrapyramidal DO:** 1-4mg PO/IM/IV qd-bid; **CH** >3 y: 1- 2mg/d IM/IV div qd-bid

Biperiden	EHL 18.4-24.3h, PRC C, Lact ?
Akineton *Tab 2mg*	**Parkinsonism:** 2mg PO bid-tid, incr prn to max 16mg/d; **(drug-induced) extrapyramidal DO:** 2mg PO qd-tid or 2mg IM/IV q30min prn, max 8mg/24h; **CH** 0.04mg/kg/dose IM, rep prn q30min, max 4 doses/d

12.1.7 Selective Serotonin Reuptake Inhibitors (SSRI)

MA: selective inhibition of serotonin reuptake ⇒ serotonin levels in synaptic cleft ↑
EF: antidepressant, psychomotor activation
AE (SSRIs): sleeplessness, agitation, somnolence, headache, N/V, diarrhea, arrhythmias, ejaculation disturbances
AE (citalopram): nausea, dry mouth, sweating, somnolence, ejaculation DO
AE (fluoxetine): insomnia, asthenia, tremor, headache, GI complaints
AE (fluvoxamine): somnolence, headache, agitation, N/V, insomnia
AE (paroxetine): headache, sedation, dry mouth, insomnia, dizziness, nausea
AE (sertraline): GI complaints, tremor, headache, insomnia, male sexual dysfunction
CI (SSRIs): simultaneous treatment with MAO inhibitors, triptophan and oxitriptan; caution in children and adolescents < 18, hypersensitivity to product ingredients
CI (fluoxetine, in addition): present or recent treatment with thioridazine
CI (fluvoxamine, in addit.): coadministration of fexofenadine, astemizole or cisapride

Citalopram	EHL 33-37h, PRC C, Lact ?
Celexa *Tab 20mg, 40mg* Generics *Tab 20mg, 40mg*	**Depression:** ini 20mg PO qd, incr to 40mg/d at an interval of >1wk, max 60mg/d; DARF: to be used cautiously in renal impairment; see Prod Info

Fluoxetine	EHL 4-6d (chronic); 1-3d (acute), PRC C, Lact -
FXT *Cap 10mg, 40mg* Prozac *Cap 10mg, 20mg, Sol (oral) 20mg/5ml* Generics *Cap 10mg, 90mg, Sol (oral) 20mg/5ml*	**Depression/obsessive compulsive DO:** ini 20mg PO qam, incr prn q several wk, max 80mg/d; ext.rel.: 90mg PO once weekly; **bulimia:** 60mg PO qam; DARF: see Prod Info

Fluvoxamine	EHL 15.6h, PRC C, Lact ?
Luvox *Tab 50mg, 100mg* Generics *Tab 50mg, 100mg*	**Obsessive compulsive DO, depression:** ini 50mg PO hs, incr prn by 50mg q4-7d (doses opf > 100mg/d div bid); max 300mg/d; **8-17y + obsessive compulsive DO:** ini 25mg PO hs, incr prn by 25mg q4-7d (doses of > 50mg/d div bid), max: 200mg/d; DARF: low starting dosage + careful monitoring; see Prod Info

Paroxetine	EHL 17-22h, PRC C, Lact ?
Paxil Tab 10mg, 20mg, 30mg **Paxil CR** Tab cont. rel. 12.5mg, 25mg **Generics** Tab 10mg, 20mg, 30mg	**Depression:** ini 20mg PO qam, incr prn by 10mg/d q ≥ 1wk, max 50mg/d; ext.rel.: ini 25mg PO qam, incr prn by 12.5mg/d q ≥ 1wk, max 62.5mg/d; **obsessive compulsive DO:** ini 20mg PO qam, incr by 10mg/d q ≥ 1wk, rec dosage 40mg/d, max 60mg/d; **panic DO:** ini. 10mg PO qam; incr by 10mg/d, q ≥ 1wk, rec dosage 40mg/d, max 60mg/d; **social anxiety DO:** 20mg/d PO qam; DARF: ini 10mg/d, max 40mg/d; for paroxetine ext. rel. ini 12.5mg/d, max 50mg/d
Sertraline	EHL 24h, PRC C, Lact ?
Zoloft Cap 25mg, 50mg, 100mg **Generics** Cap 25mg, 50mg, 100mg	**Depression/obsessive compulsive DO:** ini 50mg/d PO, prn gradually incr at ≥ 1wk intervals, max 200mg/d; **6-12 y/OCD:** 25mg/d PO, **13-17 y/OCD:** 50mg/d PO; **panic/ postrraumatic stress DO:** ini 25mg/d PO, incr after 1wk to 50mg/d, prn further incr q ≥1wk, max 200mg/d; DARF: not req

12.1.8 Serotonin Antagonists and Reuptake Inhibitors (SARI)

MA: serotonin antagonists and reuptake inhibitors (serotonin-5-HT2 antagonists); trazodone: selective serotonin reuptake inhibitor, at low doses, trazodone appears to act as a serotonin antagonist and at higher doses as an agonist
AE (nefazodone): dry mouth, nausea, somnolence, dizziness, blurred vision
AE (trazodone): dry mouth, dizziness, drowsiness, N/V, hypotension
CI (nefazodone): hypersensitivity to phenylpiperazine antidepressants, administration of fexofenadine/astemizole/cisapride/ **MAOIs**/pimozide/triazolam, caution with alprazolam, many other drug interactions
CI (trazodone): hypersensitivity to trazodone, carcinoid syndrome, initial recovery phase of myocardial infarction

Nefazodone	EHL 1.9-5.3h, PRC C, Lact ?
Generics *Tab 50mg, 100mg, 150mg, 200mg*	**Depression:** ini 100mg PO bid, incr prn by 100-200mg/d, div bid, at >1wk intervals, maint 300-600mg/d div bid-tid

L-Tryptophan	
Tryptan *Cap 500mg, Tab 250mg, 500mg, 750mg, 1g* **Generics** *Cap 500mg, 1000mg*	**Depression:** ini 12g/d (div tid-qid)

Trazodone	EHL 7.1h, PRC C, Lact ?
Desyrel *Tab 50mg, 100mg* **Desyrel Dividose** *Tab 150mg* **Generics** *Tab 50mg, 75mg, 100mg, 150mg*	**Depression:** 50-150mg/d PO in div doses, incr gradually prn by 50mg q3-4d, max 400mg/d div (outpatients), 600mg/d div (inpatients); DARF: not req

12.1.9 Norepinephrine Antagonist and Serotonin Antagonists (NASA)

MA: norepinephrine antagonist and serotonin antagonist (norepinephrine, serotonin 5-HT2 and 5-HT3)
AE (Mirtazapine): drowsiness, dizziness, constipation, appetite ↑, weight gain ↑, dry mouth, agranulozytosis (0,1%)
CI (Mirtazapine): hypersensitivity to mirtazapine. Don't use with **MAOIs**

Mirtazapine	EHL 20-40h, PRC C, Lact ?
Remeron *Tab 30mg* **Remeron RD** *Tab (oral disint.) 15mg, 30mg, 45mg*	**Depression:** ini 15mg/d PO, incr prn in intervals of >1- 2wk to 15-45mg/d; DARF: see Prod Info

12.2 Antimanic (Bimodal) Drugs

MA/EF (lithium): influence on phosphatidylinositol metabolism → Tx/PRO of manic depressive states, PRO of schizoaffective psychoses
MA (valproic acid): inhibition of the enzymatic breakdown of GABA
AE (lithium): polydipsie, polyuria, GI disturbances, tremors, goiter, hypothyroidism, renal damage
AE (valproic acid): tiredness, tremors, hair loss, hepatic damage, coagulation DO
CI (lithium): severe coronary dysfunction, M. Addison, RF
CI (valproic acid): liver diseases in family, hypersensitivity to valproic acid

Lithium	EHL 14-24h, PRC D, Lact -, serum level(mEq/l): 1-1.5 (acute), 0.6-1.2 (chronic)
Carbolith *Cap 150mg, 300mg, 600mg* **Duralith** *Tab ext.rel. 300mg* **Lithane** *Cap 150mg, 300mg* **Generics** *Cap 150mg, 300mg, 600mg, Syr 300mg/5ml*	**Acute mania:** 900-1800mg/d PO div bid-tid; **long-term use:** maint 300mg PO tid-qid; ext.rel. 600mg bid; DARF: GFR (ml/min): > 50: 100%, 10-50: 50-75%, < 10: 25-50%
Valproic Acid	EHL no data, PRC D, Lact + serum level: trough: 50-100mcg/ml
Depakene *Cap 250mg, 500mg, Syr 250mg/5ml* **Epiject IV** *Syr 100mg/ml* **Generics** *Cap 250mg, 500mg, Syr 250mg/5ml*	**Mania:** 250mg PO tid (Depakote), adjust dose rapidly to lowest therapeutic dose; DARF: see Prod Info; **epilepsy** →193; **migraine** →200

see Carbamazepine →193

Methotrimeprazine	PRC C, Lact ?
Apo-Methoprazine Tab 2mg, 5mg, 25mg, 50mg Nozinan Inj 25mg/ml, Liq (oral) 25mg/5ml, Oral drops 40mg/ml, Tab 2mg, 5mg, 25mg, 50mg	**Sedation, anxiolytic**: ini 6-25mg/d PO/IM (div tid) or 10-25mg PO/IM qhs prn; **psychotic DO**: ini 50-75mg/d PO/IM (div bid-tid) ; **CH** PO: ini 1/4mg/kg/d PO (div bid-tid), max 40mg/d; IM: 1/16-1/8mg/kg/d IM (qd or div bid)
Pericyazine	PRC C, Lact ?
Neuleptil Cap 5mg, 10mg, 20mg, Oral drops 10mg/ml	**Psychotic DO:** 5-20mg PO qam and 10-40mg PO qpm; **CH** (>5yrs): 2.5mg-10mg PO qam and 5-30mg PO qm
Pipotiazine	PRC C, Lact ?
Piportil L4 Inj 25mg/ml, 50mg/ml	**Schizophrenia:** ini 50-100mg IM q3-6wks, maint 75-150mg IM q4wks
Promazine	PRC C, Lact?
Promazine Inj 50mg/ml	**Schizophrenia:** ini 50-150mg IM; repeat q30min PRN, maint 10-200mg IM q4-6h PRN; **CH** (>12yrs) 10-25mg IM q4-6 h, max 1 g/d
Thioproperazine	PRC C, Lact ?
Majeptil Tab 10mg	**Schizophrenia, manic syndromes:** ini 5mg PO (qd or div bid), maint 30-40mg/d PO; **CH** (>10yrs): ini 1-3mg PO qd
Thioridazine	EHL 21-24h , PRC C, Lact ?
Mellaril Susp (oral) 10mg/5ml Generics Tab 10mg, 25mg, 50mg, 100mg	**Psychotic DO:** ini 50-100mg PO tid, gradual incr prn, maint 200-800mg/d div bid-qid, max 800mg/d; doses > 300mg/d are only rec for patients with severe psychoses; **CH** 2-12y (if unresponsive to other agents): 0.5mg/kg/d PO div bid-tid, titrate to optimum clinical response or to max 3mg/kg/d

12.3.3 Antipsychotics: D$_2$ Antagonists – Mid Potency

MA, EF, AE, CI (D$_2$ Antagonists): see: low potency neuroleptic drugs →221
AE (loxapine): hypotension, extrapyramidal effects, blurred vision, weight gain, sedation
CI (loxapine): coma, hypersensitivity to loxapine products

Droperidol	PRC C, Lact -
Generic *Inj 2.5mg/ml*	**Psychosis:** 5mg IM/IV; nausea: 0.675mg IM/IV
Loxapine	EHL 4h (oral), 12h (IM), PRC C, Lact ?
Generics *Tab 2.5mg, 5mg, 10mg, 25mg, 50mg*	**Psychosis:** ini 10mg PO bid or up to 50mg/d in severe cases, maint 60-100mg/d div bid-qid, max 250mg/d; IM: 12.5-50mg IM q4-12h, according to response

12.3.4 Antipsychotics: D$_2$ Antagonists – High Potency

MA, EF, AE, CI (D$_2$ Antagonists): see: low potency neuroleptic drugs →221
AE (fluphenazine hydrochloride): agranulocytosis, akathisia, weight gain, hepatotoxicity, extrapyramidal effects, neuroleptic malignant syndrome
AE (haloperidol): sedation, dystonic/extrapyramidal reactions, hypotension, arrhythmias
AE (perphenazine): extrapyramidal, anticholinergic + CVS effects, seizures, sedation
AE (pimozide): extrapyramidal + CVS effects, nausea, seizures
AE (thiothixene): restlessness, blurred vision, extrapyramidal effects, N/V, myelosuppression
AE (trifluoperazine): seizures, NMS, extrapyramidal effects, blood dyscrasias
CI (fluphenazine): coma, hypersensitivity to fluphenazine products;
CI (haloperidol): hypersensitivity to haloperidol products, Parkinson's disease
CI (perphenazine): blood dyscrasias, subcortical brain damage, coma, hypersensitivity to perphenazine products, severe liver disease
CI (pimozide): QT interval ↑, concomitant macrolides, hypersensitivity to pimozide, coma
CI (thiothixene): hypersensitivity to thiothixene products
CI (trifluoperazine): coma, bone marrow depression, hypersensitivity to trifluoperazine

Flupenthixol	PRC C, Lact ?
Fluoxnol Depot *Inj 20mg/ml, 100mg/ml* **Fluoxnol Tablets** *Tab 0.5mg, 3mg*	**Schizophrenia:** IM: ini 5mg IM test dose then 20-40mg IM, maint 20-40mg IM q2-3wks; PO: ini 1mg PO tid, maint 3-6mg/d

Fluphenazine	EHL 33h, PRC C, Lact ?
Modecate *Inj 25mg/ml, 100mg/ml* **Generics** *Tab 1mg, 2mg, 5mg* *Inj 25mg/ml, 100mg/ml*	**Psychosis:** 0.5-10mg/d PO div q6-8h; usual effective doses 1-20mg/d, max 40mg/d PO; IM: 1.25-10mg/d IM div q6-8h, max 10mg/d IM
Haloperidol	EHL 21h, IM: approx. 3wk; PRC C, Lact ?
Haldol *Inj 5mg/ml* **Haloperidol Long Acting** *Inj 50mg/ml, 100mg/ml* **Novo-Peridol** *Tab 0.5mg, 1mg, 2mg, 5mg, 10mg, 20mg* **Generics** *Tab 0.5mg, 1mg, 2mg, 5mg, 10mg* *Sol (oral) 2mg/ml* *Inj 50mg/ml, 100mg/ml*	**IM (non depot): acutely agitated patients:** ini 2-5mg IM, may repeat q1-8h; **psychotic DO:** ini 1-6mg/d PO (moderate) and 6-15mg/d (severe symptoms) div bid-tid; usual range 1-15mg/d, max 100mg/d; **Haldol decanoate** (oral to depot convers.): ini: 10-20 x the previous daily oral dose, but 100mg max ini dose, at monthly intervals; **CH 3-12 y psychotic DO:** 0.05-0.15mg/kg/d PO div bid- tid, **non-psychotic DO:** 0.05-0.075mg/kg/d PO div bid-tid; DARF: not req
Perphenazine	EHL 8.4-12.3h, PRC C, Lact -
Trilafon *Inj 5mg/ml* **Generic** *Tab 2mg, 4mg, 8mg, 16mg*	**Psychotic symptoms:** ini 4-8mg PO tid (moderately disturbed outpatients) or 8-16mg PO bid-qid (inpatients); IM: ini 5-10mg IM, then 5mg IM q6h prn, max 15mg/d IM (out-), max 30mg/d IM (inpatients)
Pimozide	EHL 53-55h, PRC C, Lact ?
Orap *Tab 2mg, 4mg* **Generics** *Tab 2mg, 4mg*	**Tourette's syndrome:** ini 1-2mg/d PO in div doses, incr q2d prn; max 0.2mg/kg/d up to 10mg/d; **Tourette's syndrome + CH >12y:** ini 0.05mg/kg PO hs, incr prn q3d to max 0.2mg/kg up to 10mg/d; DARF: probably not req; see Prod Info
Thiothixene	EHL 34h, PRC C, Lact ?
Navane *Cap 2mg, 5mg, 10mg*	**Schizophrenia:** ini 6mg PO div tid (milder conditions) and 5mg bid (severe conditions); usual effective dose range 20-30mg/d, max 60mg/d; IM: ini 4mg bid-qid, max 30mg/d

Trifluoperazine	EHL 24h, PRC C, Lact ?
Generic *Tab 1mg, 2mg, 5mg, 10mg, 20mg*	**Non-psychotic anxiety:** 1-2mg PO bid for up to 12wk, max 6mg/d; **psychotic DO:** ini 2-5mg PO bid, usual dose is 15-20mg/d, sometimes up to 40mg/d; IM: 1-2mg q4-6h prn; **CH** 6-12y (hospitalized or under close supervision): 1mg PO qd-bid, prn gradually incr, max 15mg/d; IM: 1mg IM qd-bid

Zuclopenthixol	EHL 20h(PO), 19d(depot), PRC C, Lact -
Clopixol *Tab 10mg, 25mg, 40mg* **Clopixol-Acuphase** *Inj 50mg/ml* **Clopixol Depot** *Inj 200mg/ml*	**Schizophrenia:** Clopixol: ini 10-50mg/d PO, maint 20-60mg/d; Clopixol-Acuphase: ini 50-150mg IM, repeat q2-3d; Clopixol-Depot: 150-300mg IM q2-4wks

12.4 Anxiolytics, Hypnotics
12.4.1 Benzodiazepines

MA: opening of Cl- channels $\Rightarrow$ inhibition of GABA neurons$\uparrow$, especially in limbic system
EF: sedative, sleep inducing, anxiolytic, anti-aggressive, anti-convulsive, muscle relaxing
AE: tiredness, sleepiness, drowsiness, confusion, paradox reactions, anterograde amnesia, respiratory depression, psychic and physical addiction
CI: myasthenia gravis, severe hepatic damage, respiratory insufficiency, ataxia

Alprazolam	EHL 11.2h, PRC D, Lact ?
Apo-Alpraz *Tab 0.25mg, 0.5mg* **Novo-Alprazol** *Tab 0.25mg, 0.5mg* **Nu-Alpraz** *Tab 0.25mg, 0.5mg* **Xanax** *Tab 0.25mg, 0.5mg, 1mg, 2mg* **Generics** *Tab 0.25mg, 0.5mg, 1mg, 2mg*	**Anxiety:** ini 0.25-0.5mg PO tid, incr prn q3-4d to max 4mg/d, usual effective dose 0.5-4mg/d in div doses; **panic DO** ini 0.5mg PO tid, incr prn by max 1mg/d q3-4d, slower titration may be needed at doses > 4mg/d, usual effective dose 1-10mg/d (mean 5-6mg/d),max 10mg/d

Bromazepam	EHL 20h, PRC C, Lact -
Lectopam *Tab 1.5mg, 3mg, 6mg* **Generics** *Tab 1.5mg, 3mg, 6mg*	**Anxiety:** ini 6-18 mg/d in div doses, maint 6-30mg/d in div doses

Chlordiazepoxide	EHL 10-48h, PRC D, Lact ?
Generics *Cap 5mg, 10mg, 25mg*	**Anxiety:** usual oral dose range is 5-10mg PO tid-qid (mild to moderate anxiety + tension) or 20-25mg tid-qid (sev. anxiety + tension); **IV/IM: acute or severe anxiety:** 25-50mg IM/IV tid-qid; **CH > 6y + anxiety:** ini with lowest dose, incr prn, maint 5mg PO bid-qid, max 10mgbid-tid; **acute alcohol withdrawal:** 50-100mg IM/IV, repeat q2-4h prn up to 300mg/d; DARF: mild to moder. RF: not req; CrCl (ml/min)<10: 50%; see Prod Info
Clonazepam	EHL 30-40h, PRC C, Lact - serum-level (ng/ml): 25-30
Clonapam *Tab 0.5mg, 1mg, 2mg* Rivotril *Tab 0.5mg, 2mg* Generics *Tab 0.25mg, 0.5mg, 1mg, 2mg*	**Panic DO:** ini 0.25mg PO bid, gradually incr prn after 3d, max 4mg/d; (gradually decr by 0.125mg bid, q3d); **epilepsy, neuralgias**
Clorazepate	EHL 2.29h, PRC D, Lact ?
Novo-Clopate *Cap 3.75mg, 7.5mg, 15mg* Generics *Cap 3.75mg, 7.5mg, 15mg*	**Anxiety:** ini 7.5-15mg/d PO, maint. 15-60mg/d according to patients response; DARF: not req
Diazepam	EHL 0.83-2.25d, PRC D, Lact ?
Diastat *Gel (rectal) 5mg/ml* Diazemuls *Conc (oral) 5mg/ml* E Pam *Tab 2mg, 5mg, 10mg* Novo-Dipam *Tab 2mg, 5mg, 10mg* Valium *Tab 5mg* Generics *Tab 2mg,5mg,10mg;Inj 1;5 mg/ml*	**Anxiety:** 2-10mg PO bid-qid; I M/IV: 2-5mg IM/IV, repeat in 3-4h prn (moderate anxiety); 5-10mg IM/IV, repeat q3-4h prn (severe DO); DARF: see Prod Info; **epilepsy ; muscle spasm**
Flurazepam	EHL 2.3h, PRC X, Lact ?
Generics *Cap 15mg, 30mg*	**Short term Tx of insomnia:** 15-30mg PO hs; DARF: see Prod Info
Lorazepam	EHL 10-20h (mean 12h) , PRC D, Lact ?
Ativan *Tab 0.5mg, 1mg, 2mg, Tab (subling.) 0.5mg, 1mg, 2mg, Inj 4mg/ml* Novo-Lorazem *Tab 0.5mg, 1mg, 2mg* Nu-Loraz *Tab 0.5mg, 1mg, 2mg* Generics *Tab 0.5mg, 1mg, 2mg*	**Anxiety:** ini 0.5-1mg PO bid-tid, maint 2-6mg/d in div doses, max 10mg/d (div) **insomnia:** 2-4mg PO hs prn; DARF: see Prod Info

Oxazepam	EHL 2.8-8.6h, PRC D, Lact ?
Generics *Cap 10mg, 15mg, 30mg*	**Anxiety:** 10-15mg PO tid-qid (mild-to-moderate anxiety),15-30mg tid-qid (severe anxiety and agitat. with depression); **alcoholics with acute inebriation, tremulousness, or anxiety on alcohol withdrawal:** 15- 30mg tid-qid; DARF: not req, see Prod Info
Temazepam	EHL 3.5-18.4h, PRC X, Lact ?
Restoril *Cap 15mg, 30mg* **Generics** *Cap 15mg, 30mg*	**Insomnia:** 7.5-30mg PO hs
Triazolam	EHL 2.3h, PRC X, Lact ?
Apo-Triazo *Tab 0.125mg, 0.25mg* **Halcion** *Tab 0.25mg* **Generics** *Tab 0.125mg, 0.25mg*	**Insomnia:** 0.125-0.25mg PO hs prn, max 0.5mg/d

12.4.2 Sedating Antihistamines

MA (diphenhydramine): antihistamine with sedative and hypnotic effect (see other antihistamines →82, →265, →266); **AE** (diphenhydramine): dizziness, headache, convulsions, cardiac arrhythmia, oral dryness, micturition disturbances, paralytic ileus **CI** (diphenhydramine): glaucoma, prostate hypertrophy with residual urine, acute asthma attacks, pheochromocytoma, epilepsy

Diphenhydramine	EHL 4-8h (prolonged with age), PRC B, Lact -
Allerdryl *Cap 25mg, 50mg* **Allernix** *Cap 25mg, 50mg, Elixir (oral) 12.5mg/5ml* **Benadryl** *Cap 25mg, 50mg, Cream 2%, Elixir (oral) 12.5mg/5ml, Liq (oral) 6.25mg/5ml, Tab (chew) 12.5mg* **Nytol** *Cap 25mg* **Nytol Extra Strength** *Cap 50mg* **Simply Sleep** *Cap 25mg* **Unisom Extra Strength/Extra Strength Sleepgels** **Generics** *Cap 25mg, 50mg, Elixir (oral) 2.5mg/ml, Inj 50mg/ml*	**Insomnia:** 50mg PO hs; **anaphylaxis , allergic rhinitis, rhinorrhea,** DARF: GFR (ml/min) >50: q6h, 10-50: q6-12h, < 10: q12- 18h; see Prod Info

12.4.3 Barbiturates

MA (barbiturat.): reinforcement of the inhibitory effect caused by GABA in the CNS
EF (barbiturates): sedative, sleep inducing, anxiolytic, anti-aggressive, anti-convulsive, muscle relaxing; **AE** (barbiturates): tiredness, dizziness, anterograde amnesia, dizziness, ataxia, dysopias, porphyria, N/V, hepatic dysfunction, bradycardia, respiratory depression, skin reactions, complete blood count changes, enzyme induction, addiction
AE (pentobarbital): respiratory depression, tachycardia, myasthenia gravis, drowsiness
AE (secobarbital): vertigo, excitation, respiratory depression, CNS depression
CI (barbiturates): porphyria, severe hepatic and renal dysfunction, status asthmaticus, respiratory insufficiency, barbiturate sensitivity

Pentobarbital	EHL 15-48h, PRC D, Lact ?
Nembutal Sodium *Inj 50mg/ml* **Novo-Pentobard** *Cap 100mg*	**Hypnotic:** 100mg PO hs; 120mg or 200mg PR (for patients < 110 lb.); 150-200mg IM; **CH hypnotic:** 10-20 lb. (2mo-1y): 30mg PR; 20-40 lb. (1-4y): 30mg or 60mg PR; 40-80 lb. (5-12y): 60mg PR; 80-110 lb. (12-14y): 60mg or 120mg PR; IM (**CH** hypnotic): 2-6mg/kg/dose IM, not to exceed 100mg; DARF: see Prod Info

Secobarbital	EHL 19-34h, PRC D, Lact +
Novo-Secobarb *Cap 100mg* **Seconal Sodium** *Cap 100mg*	**Hypnotic:** 100mg PO hs prn; 100-200mg IM hs prn ; DARF: not req

12.4.4 Other Anxiolytics, Hypnotics

MA (chloral hydrate): hypnotic without influence on REM sleep; **MA** (zaleplon, zolpidem): benzodiazepin-like effect; **AE** (buspirone): sedation, dizziness; **AE** (chloralhydrate): arrhythmias, hallucinations, disorientation, N/V, diarrhea; **AE** (zaleplon): allergic reactions, tiredness, headache, dizziness, somnolence, nausea, development of addiction; **CI** (buspirone): hypersensitivity to buspirone products; **CI** (chloral hydrate): hypersensitivity to chloral hydrate products ; **CI** (zaleplon): Myasthenia gravis, severe liver impairment, hypersensitivity to product ingredients

Buspirone	EHL 2.4-2.7h, PRC B, Lact ?
Buspar *Tab 10mg* **Generics** *Tab 5mg, 10mg*	**Anxiety:** ini 7.5mg PO bid, incr by 5mg/d q2-3d prn, usual effective dose 20-30mg/d (in div doses), max 60mg/d DARF: see Prod Info

Chloral Hydrate
Generics *Syr 100mg/ml*

EHL no data, PRC C, Lact ?

Alcohol withdrawal: 0.5g-1g PO q6h prn; **insomnia (short-term Tx):** 0.5g-1g PO/PR hs; **sedation:** 250mg PO/PR tid pc; **CH insomnia (short-term Tx):** 50mg/kg/d PO/PR, max 1g/ single dose; **CH sedation:** 8mg/kg/d PO/ PR tid, max 0.5g tid; DARF: GFR (ml/min): >50: 100%, < 50: not recommend.; see Prod Info

Doxylamine
Unisom-2 *Tab 25 mg*

Insomnia: 25 mg po qhs PRN

Hydroxyzine
Atarax *Syr 10mg/5ml, Inj 50mg/ml*
Generics *Cap 10mg, 25mg, 50mg, Syr 10mg/5ml, Inj 50mg/ml*

PRC C, Lact ?

Anxiety: 25-100mg PO tid-qid; **CH** (<6yrs) 30-50mg/d PO in div doses, (>6yrs) 50-100mg/d PO in div doses; IM: 50-100mg IM q4-6h; **CH** 1mg/kg IM

Zaleplon
Starnoc *Cap 5mg, 10mg*

EHL 1h, PRC C, Lact –

Short-term Tx of insomnia: 5-10mg PO hs prn; DARF: see Prod Info

Zopiclone
Generics *Tab 7.5mg*

EHL 5 h, PRC D, Lact +

Insomnia: 3.75-7.5 mg po qhs

12.4.5 Anxiolytics, Hypnotics - Combinations

AE (amitriptyline): drowsiness, anticholinergic + CVS effects, seizures, myelosuppression
AE (perphenazine): extrapyramidal, anticholinergic + CVS effects, sedation, seizures
CI (amitriptyline + chlordiazepoxide): hypersensitivity to benzodiazepines or TCAs, concomitant use with MAO inhibitors, recovery following an MI
CI (amitriptyline + perphenazine): CVS disease, recovery period after MI, MAO Inhibitor usage, large doses of other CNS depressants, blood dyscrasias, bone marrow depression or hepatic damage, hypersensitivity to perphenazine, other piperazine phenothiazines, amitriptyline, or other TCA, subcortical brain damage, coma

Perphenazine + Amitriptyline
Etrafon *Tab 2mg + 10mg, 4mg + 10mg, 2mg + 25mg, 4mg + 25mg*

Depression/anxiety: ini 2-4mg perphen. + 25mg amitript. tid-qid, use lowest effective level for maint; max daily dose 16mg perphenazine + 200mg amitriptyline

12.5 Drugs used in Substance Dependence
12.5.1 Smoking Cessation

MA/EF (bupropion): catecholamine reuptake in CNS↓ ⇒ local concentrations of noradrenaline + dopamine ↑ ⇒ nicotine withdrawal symptoms ↓, urge to smoke ↓
MA/EF (nicotine products): ganglionic (nicotinic) cholinergic-receptor agonists; used for nicotine replacement therapy as temporary adjunct in cessation of cigarette smoking
AE (nicotine products): tachycardia, diarrhea, nausea/indigestion, dizziness, insomnia, headache, nasal irritation with spray, skin irritation with patch, mouth irritation (gum)
AE (bupropion): fever, oral dryness, N/V, stomachache, constipation, insomnia, difficulty concentrating, headache, tachycardia, BP↑, depression, restlessness, fear, seizures/tremors, agitation, insomnia, hypersensitivity reactions; **CI** (nicotine products): angina, arrhythmias, active temporomandibular joint disease (gum), immediately post-MI, continued use of tobacco products, gastric ulcer, uncontrolled HTN, hypersensitivity to nicotine products
CI (bupropion): epilepsy, bulimia, anorexia, bipolar psychosis, severe liver cirrhosis, combination with MAO inhibitors, children and adolescents < 18, hypersensitivity to bupropion products, concomitant use of other bupropion products

Bupropion	EHL 14h (chronic dosing 21h), PRC B, Lact ?
Wellbutrin SR *Tab ext.rel. 100mg, 150mg* **Zyban** *Tab ext.rel. 150mg*	**Smoking cessation:** ini 150mg PO qd x 3d, incr to 150mg PO bid x 7-12wk, max 150mg PO bid; DARF: see Prod Info

Nicotine Gum	EHL 30-120min, PRC C, Lact ?
Nicorette *Gum (chew,buccal) 2mg* **Nicorette Plus** *Gum (chew,buccal) 4mg* **Nicorette Inhaler** *Inh 4mg/inh.*	**Smoking cessation:** 1 piece (2mg) q1-2h for 6wk, then 1 piece (2mg) q2-4h for 3wk, then 1 piece (2mg) q4-8h for 3wk,max 30 pieces/d of 2mg or 24 pieces/d of 4mg; 4mg pieces for high cigarette use (> 24 cigarettes/d)

Nicotine Patches	PRC (nicotine): D, Lact (nicotine): ?
Habitrol *Film (ext.rel, TD) 7mg/24h,* *14mg/24h, 21mg/24h* **Nicoderm** *Film (ext.rel, TD) 7mg/24h,* *14mg/24h, 21mg/24hr* **Nicotrol** *Film (ext.rel, TD) 5mg/16h,* *10mg/16h, 15mg/16h*	**Smoking cessation:** see Prod Info

12.5.2 Alcohol Dependence

see Diazepam→225, Chloral Hydrate→228, Chlordiazepoxide→225, Oxazepam→225

12.5.3 Opioid Dependence

AE (methadone): respiratory depression, dizziness, N/V, sweating, constipation
AE (naltrexone): opioid withdrawal-like syndrome, nausea, headache, dizziness, anxiety
CI (methadone): hypersensitivity to metha4done; **CI** (naltrexone): concomitant opioid analgesics, opioid dependency or withdraw., hypersensitivity to naltrexone, acute hepatitis or liver failure

Methadone	EHL 23h (IV), 22h (chronic PO), PRC C, Lact ?
Metadol *Sol (oral) 10mg/ ml*	**Narcotic addiction:** 40-180mg/d PO (div), taper dose as appropr. to avoid withdrawal symptoms; DARF: see Prod Info, GFR (ml/min): > 50: q6h; 10-50: q8h, severe RF: q8-12h)
Naltrexone	EHL 4h, PRC C, Lact ?
ReVia *Tab 50mg*	**Alcohol dependence:** 50mg PO qd **narcotic dependence:** ini 25mg PO qd, incr to 50mg PO qd if no signs of withdrawal

Isotretinoin	PRC X, Lact -
Accutane *Cap 10mg, 40mg* **Isotrex** *Gel (top) 0.05%*	**Severe, recalcitrant cystic acne:** PO: 0.5-2 mg/kg/d PO div bid x 15-20wk, rep prn 2nd course of Tx after >2mo; Topical: apply bid; **prevention of second primary tumors in pat. treated for squamous-cell CA of head/ neck:** 50-100mg/m²/dPO; **neuroblastoma** (maint Tx):100-250 mg/m²/dPO div bid
Tazarotene	PRC X, Lact ?
Tazorac *Crm 0.05%, 0.1%; Gel(top) 0.05,1%*	**Acne, psoriasis:** apply qhs, max x 3mo
Tretinoin	PRC X, Lact ?
Retin-A *Crm 0.01%, 0.025%, 0.05%, 0.1%, Gel 0.01%, 0.025%* **Vitamin A acid** *Crm 0.01%, 0.025%, 0.05%, 0.1%, Gel 0.01%, 0.025%, 0.05%*	**Acne:** apply qhs

13.1.4 Retinoid-Like Drugs

AE (adapalene): skin irritation ; **CI** (adapalene): hypersensitivity to adapalene

Adapalene	PRC C, Lact ?
Differin *Sol (top) 0.1%, Gel (top) 0.1%, Crm (top) 0.1%*	**Acne:** apply qhs, therapeutic results in 8-12wk

13.2 Anti-Infectives

13.2.1 Antibacterials (topical)

AE (bacitracin): contact dermatitis;
AE (mafenide): burning sensation, rash/pruritus
AE (mupirocin): headache (nasal), rhinitis/pharyngitis (nasal), taste DO (nasal), stinging/ burning, pruritus;
AE (silver sulfadiazine): local skin irritat., skin rash, itch.; **CI** (bacitracin): hypersensit. to bacitracin products;
CI (mafenide): hypersens. to mafenide prod., hypersensiti. to sulfites (metabisulfite in cream);
CI (mupirocin): hypersensit. to mupirocin products, avoid contact with the eyes, avoid prod. with polyethylene glycol on open wounds ;
CI (silver sulfadiazine): hypersens. to silver or sulfonamide prod., preterms, newborns<2mo

| **Bacitracin** | PRC C, Lact ? |
| **Baciquent** *Oint 500 U/g* | **Minor cuts, wounds, burns, skin abras.:** apl. apply qd-tid |

| **Gentamicin** | PRC C, Lact ? |
| **Garamycin, Generics** *Crm 0.1%, Oint 0.1%* | **Skin infx:** apply tid-qid, **CH** >1y: apply tid-qid |

| **Mafenide** | PRC C, Lact ? |
| **Sulfamylon** *Crm 8.5%* | **Adj Tx of burns:** apply qd-bid |

| **Metronidazole** | PRC B/X in 1st trimester Lact - |
| **MetroCream** *Crm 0.75%*
 MetroGel *Gel (top) 0.75%*
 Nidagel *Gel (top) 0.75%*
 Noritate *Crm (top) 1%* | **Rosacea:** apply bid, therapeutical effects in 3-9wk |

| **Mupirocin** | PRC B, Lact - |
| **Bactroban** *Crm (augmented) 2%, Oint (nasal) 2%* | **Impetigo:** apply tid x 3-5d; **wound infx:** tid x 10d; **nasal MRSA eradication:** 1g div between nostrils bid x 5 d |

| **Neomycin + Polymyxin + Bacitracin Zinc** | PRC C, Lact ? |
| **Neosporin Ointment** *Oint 5mg/g + 5,000 U/g + 400U/g* | **Minor cuts, wounds, burns or skin abrasions:** apply qd-tid |

| **Silver Sulfadiazine** | PRC B, Lact - |
| **Dermazin, Flamazine** *Crm 1%* | **Burns:** apply qd-bid; **DARF:** measurement of sulfadiazine levels in severe RF |

13.2.2 Antifungals (topical) - Polyene Group

see systemic Antifungals →152

| **Nystatin** | PRC C, Lact ? |
| **Candistatin** *Crm 100,000 U/g*
 Mycostatin *Oint 100,000U/g, Crm 100,000 U/g, Crm (vag) 25,000U/g*
 Nyaderm *Crm 100,000 U/g, Oint 100,000 U/g*
 Generics *Powder 1 billion U/bottle, Crm 100,000 U/g, Oint 100,000U/g* | **Cutaneous or mucocutaneous Candida infx:** apply bid-tid; **fungal infx of the feet, dust feet and footwear:** powder applied bid-tid; **thrush:** 4-6ml PO swish and swallow qid or suck on 1-2 troches 4-5 x/d; infants: 2ml/ dose PO with 1ml in each cheek qid |

13.2.3   Antifungals (topical) - Azole Group

see systemic Antifungals →152

Clotrimazole   PRC B, Lact ?

Canesten *Crm 1%*
Clotrimaderm *Crm 1%, Sol (top) 1%*   **Tinea pedis, cruris, corporis, versicolor/
cutaneous candidiasis: apply bid**

Econazole   PRC C, Lact ?

Ecostatin *Crm 1%, Ovule 150mg*   **Tinea pedis, cruris, corporis, versicolor:
apply qd x 2wk, tinea pedis x 4wk;
cutaneous candidiasis: apply bid x 2wk**

Ketoconazole   PRC C, Lact ?

Ketoderm *Crm 2%*
Nizoral *Crm 2%, Shampoo 2%*   **Tinea versicolor: apply shampoo 2% to
affected area, leave on x 5min, rinse, treat x
2wk; cutaneous candidiasis, tinea coporis,
cruris, versicolor:** apply crm qd, treat x 2wk,
tinea pedis x 6wk;
seborrheic dermatitis: apply crm (2%) bid x
4wk; 3 apply shampoo (1%) 2x/wk

Miconazole   PRC, Lact ?

Micatin *Crm 2%, Spray 2%*
Monistat *Crm 2%*   **Tinea pedis, cruris, corporis, versicolor/
cutaneous candidiasis: apply bid x 2wk,
tinea pedis x 1mo**

Oxiconazole   PRC B, Lact ?

Oxizole *Crm 1%*   **Tinea pedis, cruris, corporis:** apply qd-bid;
tinea versicolor: apply cream qd

13.2.4   Antifungals (topical) - Allylamine Group

AE (naftifine): local burning or stinging, contact dermatitis
AE (terbinafine): local irritation, N/V, LFT's↑
CI (naftifine, terbinafine): hypersensitivity to product ingredients

Naftifine   PRC B, Lact ?

Naftin *Gel 1%, Crm 1%*   **Tinea pedis, cruris, corporis:** apply qd
(cream) or bid (gel)

Terbinafine	PRC B, Lact -
Lamisil *Tab 250mg, Spray 1%, Crm 1%*	**Tinea pedis:** apply bid x 1-4wk; **tinea cruris, corporis:** apply qd-bid x 1-4wk; tinea versicolor: apply sol bid x 1- 4wk; **onychomycosis (fingernails):** 250mg PO qd x 6wk; **onychomycosis (toenails):** 250mg PO qd x 12wk; **CH** <20kg: 67.5mg PO qd, 20-40kg: 125mg PO qd, >40kg: 250 mg PO qd, x 6wk for fingernails, x 12wk for toenails; **onychomycosis "pulse dosing":** 500mg PO qd for 1st wk of mo x 2mo for fingernails, 4mo for toenails; DARF: CrCl (ml/min):<50: contraind.

13.2.5 Other Topical Antifungals

AE (butenafine): burning/stinging
AE (ciclopirox): periungual erythema, burning of surrounding skin
AE (haloprogin): dermal allergic reactions
AE (tolnaftate): irritation, contact dermatitis
CI (butenafine, ciclopirox, haloprogin, tolnaftate): hypersensitivity to product ingredients

Butenafine	PRC B, Lact ?
Dr. Scholl's Athlete's Foot Cream *Crm 1%*	**Tinea pedis:** apply qd x 4wk or bid x 7d; **tinea coporis/ cruris:** apply qd x 2wk

Ciclopirox	PRC B, Lact ?
Loprox *Lot (top) 1%, Crm 1%*	**Tinea pedis, cruris, corporis, versicolor/ candidiasis:** cream, lotion: apply bid; **onychomycosis of fingernails/ toenails:** apply nail sol qd to affected nails, over previous coat, remove with alcohol q7d

Tolnaftate	PRC N, Lact ?
Pitrex *Crm 1%* **ZeaSorb AF** *Powder 1%*	**tinea pedis, cruris, corporis, versicolor:** apply bid, **CH** >2y: apply bid; **prevention of tinea pedis:** apply powder/ aerosol prn

13.2.6 Antivirals

AE (acyclovir): N/V, headache, renal impairment, rash, phlebitis; **AE** (imiquimod): erosion, flaking, edema, erythema; **AE** (penciclovir): erythema; **AE** (podofilox): local irritation, inflammation, itching; **CI** (podophyllin): see Prod Info; **CI** (acyclovir, imiquimod, penciclovir, podofilox): hypersensitivity to product ingredients; **CI** (podophyllin): DM, patients using steroids or with poor blood circulation, not on bleeding warts, moles, birthmarks or unusual warts with hair growing from them

Acyclovir	PRC C (top)/B (oral) Lact +
Zovirax Tab 200mg, 400mg, 800mg, Susp 200mg/5ml, Crm 5%, Oint 5% **Generics** Tab 200mg, 400mg, 800mg	**Herpes genitalis** (ini episodes): apply q3h (6x/d) x 7d or 200mg PO q4h (5x/d) x 10d for 1st episode, x 5d for recurrent episodes, **CH** 80 mg/kg/d PO div tid (max 1.2g/ d) x 7-10d; **mucocutaneous herpes simplex in immunocompromised patients** (non-life threatening): apply q3h (6x/d) x 7d; **herpes PRO**: 400 mg PO bid; **herpes zoster**: 800mg PO q4h (5x/d) x 7-10d; **varicella**: 800mg PO qid x 5d, IV: 5-10mg/kg IV q8h, each dose x 1h, **CH** >2y: 20mg/kg PO qid x 5d, >40kg: adult dose; **primary gingivostomatitis**: 15mg/kg PO 5x/d x 7d; DARF: CrCl (ml/min) 10-25, 800mg: q8h, <10, 800mg: q12h, <10, 400mg: 50% q12h, <10, 200mg: q12h
Cantharidin	PRC C, Lact -
Canthacur Liq 0.7% **Cantharone** Liq 0.7%	**Warts, molluscum contagiosum**: apply to warts, allow to dry and remove necrotic tissue, repeat prn
Cantharidin + Podophyllin + Salicylic acid	PRC C, Lact -
Canthacur-PS Liq 1% + 5% + 30% **Cantharone Plus** Liq 1% + 2% + 30%	**Warts, molluscum contagiosum**: apply to warts, allow to dry and remove necrotic tissue, repeat prn
Imiquimod	PRC B, Lact ?
Aldara Crm 5%	**External genital and perianal warts**: apply 3 x/wk hs, wash off in 6-10h; **giant molluscum contagiosum**: apply 3x/wk x 6-10h

Podofilox	PRC C, Lact ?
Condyline *Sol (top) 0.5%* **Wartec** *Sol (top) 0.5%*	**External genital warts** (gel/sol)/ **perianal warts** (gel only): apply bid x 3 consecutive d/wk, rep x max 4wk

Podophyllin	PRC N, Lact -
Podofilm *Sol (top) 25%*	**Genital wart removal:** ini apply to wart and leave on x 30-40min to determine patient's sensitivity, then use minimum contact time necessary (1-4h), then remove dried podophyllin with alcohol or soap + water

13.2.7 Antiparasitics (topical)

AE (crotamiton): dermatitis, skin irritation; **AE** (lindane): dermatitis, anxiety, dizziness, insomnia, myelosuppression; **AE** (permethrin): pruritus, burning, stinging, rash
CI (crotamiton): hypersens. to crotamiton; **CI** (lindane): hypersens. to lindane, premature neonates, seizure DO; **CI** (permethrin): hypersens. to permethrin/chrysanthemums

Crotamiton	PRC C, Lact ?
Eurax *Crm 10%*	**Scabies:** massage cream/lotion into entire body from chin down, rep in 24h, then bathe in 48h; **pruritus:** massage into affected areas prn

Lindane	PRC B, Lact ?
Hexit *Shampoo 1%* **Lindane** *Lot (top) 1%, Shampoo 1%*	**Head/crab lice:** apply lotion 30-60ml to affected area, wash off in 12h or apply shampoo 30-60ml, wash off in 4min, then comb to remove nits, prn rep in 7d; **scabies:** apply lotion to total body from neck down, wash off in 8-12h

Permethrin	PRC B, Lact ?
Kwellada-P *Crm (rinse) 1%, Lot (top) 5%* **Nix** *Crm (rinse) 1%, Crm 5%*	**Scabies:** massage 30g (cream) into entire body, wash off in 8-14h, **CH** >2mo: <30g of cream needed; **head lice:** apply liquid to clean, towel-dried hair, saturate hair and scalp, wash off in 10min, **CH** >2mo: adult application

Pyrethrins, Piperonyl Butoxide	PRC C, Lact ?
R & C *Shampoo 0.33% + 3%* **R & C II** *Spray 0.3% + 1.5%*	**Head/crab/body lice:** apply shampoo/foam on dry hair, wash after 10min, rep in 5-7d

13.2.8 Anti-Infective Combinations

Betamethasone + Clotrimazole	PRC C, Lact ?
Lotriderm *Crm 0.05% + 1%*	**Tinea pedis, cruris, corporis:** apply bid x 2wk, tinea pedis x 4wk

Clioquinol + Hydrocortisone	
Vioform Hydrocortisone *Crm 3% + 1%*	**Skin infection:** apply 2-3 times daily

Framycetin + Gramicidin	
Soframycin Skin Ointment *Oint 15 + 0.05mg/g*	**Skin infection:** apply 2-4 times daily

Nystatin + Gramicidin + Neomycin + Trimacinolone	PRC C, Lact ?
Kenacomb *Crm 100,000U/g + 250mcg/g + 2.5mg/g + 0.025%, 100,000 U/g + 250mcg/g + 2.5mg/g + 1mg/g* *Oint 100,000U/g + 250mcg/g + 2.5mg/g + 0.025%, 100,000 U/g + 250mcg/g + 2.5mg/g + 1mg/g* **ratio-Triacomb** *Crm 100,000 U/g + 250mcg/g + 2.5mg/g + 1mg/g* **Viaderm-K.C.** *Crm 100,000U/g + 250mcg/g + 2.5mg/g + 1mg/g* *Oint 100,000U/g + 250mcg/g + 2.5mg/g + 1mg/g*	**Cutaneous candidiasis:** apply bid

Polymyxin + Bacitracin	PRC C, Lact ?
Polysporin Ointment *Oint 10,000U/g + 500U/g*	**Skin infx:** apply qd-tid

Polymyxin + Bacitracin + Gramicidin	PRC C, Lact ?
Polysporin Triple *Oint 10,000U/g + 500U/g + 250mcg/g*	**Skin infx:** apply qd-tid

Polymyxin B + Bacitracin + Lidocaine	PRC C, Lact ?
Ozonol Antibiotics Plus *Oint 10,000U + 500U + 40mg/g*	**Skin infection:** apply 1-3 times/d

Polymyxin + Bacitracin Zinc + Hydrocortisone + Neomycin	PRC C, Lact ?
Cortisporin *Oint 5,000U/g + 400U/g + 10mg/g + 5mg/g*	**Skin infx:** apply bid-qid

Polymyxin + Gramicidin	PRC C, Lact ?
Polysporin Cream *Crm 10,000U/g + 250mcg/g*	**Skin infx:** apply qd-tid

Polymyxin + Gramicidin + Lidocaine	PRC C, Lact ?
Lidosporin *Crm 10,000U/g + 250mcg/g + 50mg/g* **Polysporin Plus Pain Relief** *Crm 10,000U/g + 250mcg/g + 50mg/g*	**Skin infx:** apply qd-tid

Polymyxin + Gramicidin + Neomycin	PRC C, Lact ?
Neosporin Cream *Crm 10,000U/g + 250mcg/g + 5mg/g*	**Skin infx:** apply bid-5 times/d

13.3 Antipsoriatics

MA/EF (calcipotriene): vitamin D3 derivative;
AE (anthralin): skin inflammation, irritiation, rash;
AE (calcipotriene): skin irritation;
AE (coal tar): rash; **CI** (anthralin): hypersens. to anthralin, erythroderma, psoriasis pustul., type Zumbusch (full- body psoriasis), inflammatory + acute psoriasis, renal DO, flexures;
CI (calcipotriene): vitamin D toxicity, hypercalcemia, hypersensitivity to calcipotriene;
CI (coal tar): hypersensitivity to coal tar

Anthralin	PRC C, Lact ?
Anthraforte *Oint 1%, 2%* **Anthranol** *Crm 0.1%, 0.2%, 0.4%* **Anthrascalp** *Lot 0.4%* **Micanol** *Crm 1%, 3%*	**Quiescent/chronic psoriasis:** apply qd

Calcipotriol	PRC C, Lact ?
Dovonex *Sol (top) 0.05mg/ml, Crm 0.005%, Oint 0.005%*	**Moderate plaque psoriasis:** apply bid

Calcitriol + Betamethasone	PRC C, Lact ?
Dovobet *Oint 50mcg + 0.5mg/g*	**Psoriasis:** apply daily
Coal Tar	PRC N, Lact ?
Balnetar *Sol 2.5%* **Estar** *Gel 5%* **Liquor Carbonis Detergens** *Sol 20%*	**Dandruff, seborrheic dermatitis:** shampoo ≥ 2x/wk; **psoriasis:** apply cream qd-qid or shampoo affected areas, **CH** >2y: as adults
see Retinoids →235	

13.4   Corticosteroids (topical)
13.4.1   Topical Corticosteroids – Very High Potency

Augmented Betamethasone Dipropionate PRC C, Lact ?	
Diprolene Glycol *Lot (top) 0.05%, Oint 0.05%, Crm 0.05%* **Diprosone** *Lot (top) 0.05%, Oint 0.05%, Crm 0.05%* **Taro-Sone** *Lot (top) 0.05%, Oint 0.05%, Crm 0.05%* **ratio-Topilene** *Lot (top) 0.05%, Oint 0.05%, Crm 0.05%* **ratio-Topisone** *Lot (top) 0.05%, Oint 0.05%, Crm 0.05%*	**Dermatoses:** apply qd-bid, max x 2wk, max 50g/wk resp. 50ml/wk
Clobetasol Propionate	PRC C, Lact ?
Dermovate *Crm 0.05%, Oint (top) 0.05%, Lot 0.05%* **Generics** *Sol (top) 0.05%, Crm 0.05%, Oint 0.05%*	**Dermatoses:** apply bid, max x 2wk, max 50g/wk
Halobetasol Propionate	PRC C, Lact ?
Ultravate *Crm 0.05%, Oint 0.05%*	**Dermatoses:** apply qd-bid, max x 2wk, max 50g cream or oint/wk

13.4.2 Topical Corticosteroids - High Potency

Amcinonide — PRC C, Lact ?

Cyclocort *Lot (top) 0.1%, Crm 0.1%, Oint 0.1%*

Dermatoses: apply bid-tid

Betamethasone Dipropionate — PRC C, Lact ?

Diprolene Glycol *Lot (top) 0.05%, Oint 0.05%, Crm 0.05%*
Diprosone *Lot (top) 0.05%, Oint 0.05%, Crm 0.05%*
Taro-Sone *Lot (top) 0.05%, Oint 0.05%, Crm 0.05%*
Topilene *Lot (top) 0.05%, Oint 0.05%, Crm 0.05%*
Topisone *Lot (top) 0.05%, Oint 0.05%, Crm 0.05%*

Dermatoses: apply qd-bid

Desoximetasone — PRC C, Lact ?

Topicort *Crm 0.05%, 0.25%, Oint 0.25%, Gel (top) 0.05%*

Dermatoses: apply bid

Fluticasone — PRC C, Lact ?

Cutivate *Oint 0.005%, 0.05%*

Dermatoses: apply bid-qid

Fluocinonide — PRC C, Lact ?

Lidemol *Sol (top) 0.05%*
Lidex *Crm 0.05%, Oint 0.05%*
Lyderm *Crm 0.05%, Oint 0.05%*
Tiamol *Crm 0.05%*
Topsyn *Gel (top) 0.05%*

Dermatoses: apply bid-qid

Halcinonide — PRC C, Lact ?

Halog *Sol (top) 0.1%, Crm 0.1%, Oint 0.1%*

Dermatoses: apply bid-tid

Triamcinolone Acetonide — PRC C, Lact ?

Aristocort *Crm 0.1%, 0.5%, Oint 0.1%*
Kenalog *Crm 0.1%, Oint 0.1%*
Triaderm *Crm 0.025%, 0.1%, Oint 0.025%, 0.1%*

Dermatoses: apply tid-qid

13.4.3 Topical Corticosteroids – Medium Potency

Betamethasone Valerate
PRC C, Lact ?

Betaderm *Lot (top) 0.1%, Crm 0.05%, 0.1%, Oint 0.05%, 0.1%*
Betnovate *Crm (top) 0.1%, Oint 0.05%*
ratio-Ectosone *Crm 0.05%, 0.1%, Lot (top) 0.05%, 0.1%*
Prevex B *Crm 0.1%*
Valisone *Lot (top) 0.1%*

Dermatoses: apply qd-bid, for skalp: foam

Desoximetasone
PRC C, Lact ?

Topicort *Crm 0.05%, 0.25%, Oint 0.25%, Gel (top) 0.05%*

Dermatoses: apply bid

Fluocinolone Acetonide
PRC C, Lact ?

Capex Shampoo *Shampoo 0.1mg/ml*
Derma-Smoothe/FS *Oil (top) 0.01%*
Synalar *Sol (top) 0.01%, Oint 0.025%*

Dermatoses: apply bid-qid

Hydrocortisone Valerate
PRC C, Lact ?

Hydroval *Crm 0.2%, Oint 0.2%*
Westcort *Crm 0.2%, Oint 0.2%*

Dermatoses: apply bid-tid

Mometasone Furoate
PRC C, Lact ?

Elocom *Lot (top) 0.1%, Crm 0.1%, Oint 0.1%*

Dermatoses: apply qd, CH ≥ 2y: adult application

Prednicarbate
PRC C, Lact ?

Dermatop *Crm 0.1%, Oint 0.1%*

Dermatoses: apply bid, CH ≥ 1y: adult application

Triamcinolone Acetonide
PRC C, Lact ?

Aristocort *Crm 0.1%, 0.5%, Oint 0.1%*
Kenalog *Crm 0.1%, Oint 0.1%*
Triaderm *Crm 0.025%, 0.1%, Oint 0.025%, 0.1%*

Dermatoses: apply tid-qid

13.4.4 Topical Corticosteroids – Low Potency

Desonide | PRC C, Lact ?
Desocort *Lot (top) 0.05%, Crm 0.05%, Oint 0.05%* | **Dermatoses:** apply bid-tid

Hydrocortisone | PRC C (top) Lact ?
Aquacort *Lot (top) 2.5%*
Emo-Cort *Sol (top) 2.5%, Lot (top) 1%, 2.5%, Crm 1%, 2.5%*
Prevex HC *Crm 1%*
Sarna HC *Lot (top) 1%, 2.5%* | **Dermatoses:** apply bid-qid

Hydrocortisone Acetate | PRC C, Lact ?
Cortef Cream *Crm 0.5%*
Hyderm *Crm 0.5%, 1%* | **Dermatoses:** apply bid-qid

13.5 Antipruritics
13.5.1 Histamine Receptor Blockers and Combinations

AE (doxepin): burning/stinging (cream), drowsiness, CVS/anticholin. effects, seizures
CI (doxepin): hypersensitivity to doxepin products, glaucoma, urinary retention, concomitant MAO inhibitors

Calamine + Diphenhydramine | PRC N, Lact ?
Caladryl *Crm 8% + 1%, Lot 8% + 1%* | **Itching due to poison ivy/oak/sumac, insect bites, minor irritation:** apply prn, max tid-qid

Doxepin | PRC B (top) Lact -
Zonalon *Crm 5% v* | **Pruritus associated with atopic dermatitis, lichen simplex chronicus, eczematous dermatitis:** qid x max 8d

13.5.2 Other Antipruritics

Oatmeal | PRC N, Lact +
Equate, Nutra Soothe *Bath Packets 100% colloidal oatmeal* | **Pruritus from poison ivy/oak, varicella:** add packet to bath qd prn

13.6 Hemorrhoid Care

AE (dibucaine): contact dermatitis, photosensitivity reactions;
AE (witch hazel): mild itching or burning; **CI (dibucaine):** hypersensitivity to dibucaine
CI (witch hazel): hypersensitivity to Witch Hazel, internal consumption is not rec

Hydrocortisone + Framycetin + Cinchocaine + Esculin	
Proctomyxin *Oint 5 + 10 + 5 + 10mg/g, Supp 5 + 10 + 5 + 10mg/g*	**Hemorrhoids:** apply oint or supp prn
Dibucaine	PRC N, Lact ?
Nupercainal *Oint 1%*	**Hemorrhoids, other anorectal DO:** apply prn tid-qid, **CH** see adults
Hydrocortisone + Benzocaine + Zinc Sulfate	
Rectogel HC *Gel 1% + 10% + 0.5%*	**Hemorrhoids:** apply gel prn
Hydrocortisone + Zinc Sulfate	PRC C, Lact ?
Anodan-HC, Anusol-HC, ratio-Hemcort-HC, PMS-Egozinc-HC *Oint 0.5% + 0.5%, Supp 10mg + 10mg* **Rivasol HC** *Oint 0.5% + 0.5%*	**External anal itching:** apply cream tid-qid prn or supp PR bid
Pramoxine + Hydrocortisone	PRC C, Lact ?
Pramox HC *Crm 1% + 1%, Lot 1% + 1%* **Proctofoam-HC** *Foam 1% + 1%*	**Hemorrhoids:** apply oint prn, max 5 x/d
Pramoxine + Hydrocortisone + Zinc Sulfate	
Anugesic-HC *Oint 1% + 0.5% + 0.5%, Supp 20mg + 10mg + 10mg* **Anuzinc HC Plus** *Supp 20mg+10mg+10mg* **Proctodan-HC** *Oint 1% + 0.5% + 0.5%, Supp 20mg + 10mg + 10mg*	**Hemorrhoids:** apply oint or supp prn, max 5 x/d

Pramoxine + Zinc Sulfate	PRC N, Lact ?
Anusol Plus *Oint 1% + 0.5%, Supp 20mg + 10mg*	**Hemorrhoids:** apply oint or supp prn, max 5 x/d
Starch	PRC N, Lact +
Bum-Butt-R *Crm 50%*	**Hemorrhoids:** apply oint prn
Witch Hazel	PRC N, Lact +
Generics *Liq (top) 85%, 100%*	**Hemorrhoids:** apply to anus/perineum prn, max 6x/d
Zinc Sulfate	PRC C, Lact ?
Anuzinc *Oint 0.5%, Supp 10mg*	**Hemorrhoids:** apply oint or supp prn

13.7 Hair Restorers

MA/EF (finasteride): inhibition of 5-α-reductase ⇒ testosterone cannot be transformed to dihydro-testosterone ⇒ hair loss ↓, prostatic hyperplasia ↓
AE (finasteride): libido and erection disturbances, gynecomastia, lip swelling, skin rash; pregnant women may not touch tablet brittle!;
AE (minoxidil): hypertrichosis, pleural/pericard.effusion, reflex tachycardia, fluid retention;
CI (finasteride): women or children, hypersensitivity to finasteride products;
CI (minoxidil): hypersensitivity to minoxidil

Finasteride	EHL 6h, PRC X, Lact -
Propecia *Tab 1mg* **Proscar** *Tab 5mg*	**Androgenetic alopecia in men:** 1mg PO qd; **androgenetic alopecia in postmeno-pausal women:** 1mg PO
Minoxidil	EHL 2.3-28.9h, PRC C, Lact +
Apo-Gain *Sol (top) 2%* **Minox** *Sol (top) 2%* **Rogaine** *Sol (top) 2%*	**Androgenetic alopecia in men or women:** apply 1ml bid (to dry scalp)

13.8 Anesthetics

Lidocaine HCl	EHL 1.5-2h, PRC B, Lact +
Xylocaine *Jelly (top) 2%, Sol (top) 4%, 5%, Sol (viscous) 2%* **Generics** *Sol (viscous) 2%, Oint 5%*	**Topical anesthesia for minor dermal procedures** (eg, IV cannulation, venipuncture): apply 2.5g over 20-25cm² area or 1 disc ≥ 1h prior to procedure; **topical anesthesia for major dermal procedures** (ie, skin grafting harvesting): apply 2g per 10cm² area ≥ 2h prior to procedure; **topical anesthesia in CH** 1-3mo or <5kg: apply max 1g over max 10cm², 4-12mo and >5kg: apply max 2g over max 20cm², 1-6y and >10kg: apply max 10g over max 100cm², 7-12y and >20kg: apply max 20g over max 200cm²; **prior to circumcision in infants >37wk gestation:** apply ma 1g over max 10cm²;
Lidocaine + Prilocaine	PRC C, Lact +
EMLA *Crm 5% + 5%, Disc (top) 2.5% + 2.5%*	**Topical anesthesia for minor dermal procedures:** apply 2.5g/20-25cm² area or 1 disc ≥ 1h prior to procedure; **topical anesthesia for major dermal procedures** : apply 2g/10cm² area ≥ 2h prior to procedure; **topical anesthesia in CH** 1-3mo or <5kg: apply max 1g over max 10cm², 4-12mo and >5kg: apply max 2g over max 20cm², 1-6y and >10kg: apply max 10g over max 100cm², 7-12y and >20kg: apply max 20g over max 200cm²; **prior to circumcision in infants > 37 wk gestation:** apply max 1g over max 10cm²

see **Local Anesthetics**, →190

13.9 Other Dermatologic Agents

AE (alitretinoin): rash, pain (application site), exfoliative dermatitis, pruritus, edema;
AE (becaplermin): rash;
AE (capsaicin): cough with inhalation, local irritation;
AE (hydroquinone): urine discoloration, ochronosis, fingernail staining, local irritation;
AE (selenium sulfide): skin irritation, hair loss or disoloration, oily or dry scalp
CI (alitretinoin): hypersensitivity to retinoids or alitretinoin products; CI (becaplermin): hypersensitivity to bacaplermin or parabens, known neoplasm at application site;
CI (capsaicin, hydroquinone, selenium sulfide): hypersensitivity to product

Alitretinoin	PRC D, Lact -
Panretin *Gel (top) 0.1%*	**Cutaneous lesions of AIDS-related Kaposi's sarcoma:** apply bid-qid

Becaplermin	PRC C, Lact ?
Regranex *Gel 0.01%*	**Diabetic neuropathic ulcers:** apply qd (length x width x 0.6=amount of gel in inches), cover with saline- moistened gauze x 12h, then rinse and cover with saline gauze without medication

Botulinum Toxin Type A	PRC C, Lact ?
Botox *Inj 100U/vial* **Botox Cosmetic** *Inj 100U/vial*	**Cervical distonia:** **CH** >16y and adults: 198-300U IM; **blepharospasm:** ini 1.25-2.5U IM, max 5U/site; **strabismus:** 1.25-5U IM, max 25U/muscle; **reduction of glabellar line:** dose determined by gross evaluation

Capsaicin	PRC N, Lact ?
Zostrix *Crm 0.025%, 0.075%* **Generics** *Crm 0.025%, 0.075%*	**Pain due to rheumatoid arthritis, osteoarthritis, neuralgias (zoster):** apply prn, max tid-qid, **CH** >2y: adult application

Fluorouracil	PRC X, Lact -
Efudex *Crm 5%*	**Actinic/solar keratoses:** apply bid to lesions x 2-6wk; **superficial basal cell CA:** cover lesions with 5% bid x 3- 6wk, max 12wk

Hydroquinone	PRC C, Lact ?
Eldopaque, Eldoquin, Solaquin *Crm 2%, 4%* **Lustra** *Crm 4%* **Ultraquin** *Crm 4%, Gel (top) 4%*	**Temporary bleaching of hyperpigmented skin conditions** (i.e. chloasma, discoloration from oral contraceptives, pregnancy): apply bid to affected area
Hydroquinone + Octyl Methoxycinnamate + Avobenzone	PRC C, Lact ?
Lustra-AF *Crm 4% + 7.5%*	**Ultraviolet induced dyschromia and discoloration:** apply bid
Ammonium Lactate	PRC B, Lact ?
Dermalac *Crm 12%, Lot (top) 12%*	**Ichthyosis vulgaris, xerosis (dry, scaly skin):** apply bid to affected area
Lactic Acid + Glycerin	PRC C, Lact ?
Epi-Lyt AHA Medicated Lotion *Lot (top) 5% + 25%*	**Ichthyosis vulgaris, xerosis (dry, scaly skin):** apply bid to affected area
Salicylic acid + Urea	
Kerasal *Crm 5% + 10%*	**Foot xerosis:** apply 1-2 times daily
Mequinol + Tretinoin	PRC C, Lact ?
Solage *Sol (top) 2% + 0.01%*	**Solar lentigines:** apply bid separated >8h
Pimecrolimus	PRC C, Lact ?
Elidel *Crm 1%*	**Atopic dermatitis:** apply to lesions bid
Selenium Sulfide	PRC C, Lact ?
Head & Shoulders Shampoo *Shampoo 1%* **Selegel** *Lot (top) 1%* **Selsun** *Liq (top) 2.5%* **Selsun Blue** *Shampoo 1%* **Versel** *Lot (top) 2.5%*	**Dandruff, seborrheic dermatitis:** massage 5-10ml of shampoo into wet scalp, allow to remain 2-3min, rinse, apply 2x/wk x 2wk, maint 1x/wk; **tinea versicolor:** apply 2.5% shampoo/lotion to affected area, allow to remain on skin 10min, rinse, rep qd x 7d

14. Ophthalmology

14.1 Anti-Infectives
14.1.1 Antibacterials - Single Ingredient Drugs

S, R, AE, CI see Antibiotics →118

Bacitracin	PRC C, Lact ?
Generics *Oint 500 U/g*	**Ocular infx:** apply ½ inch ribbon of oint q3-4h or bid-qid
Ciprofloxacin	PRC C, Lact ?
Ciloxan *Sol/Gtt (oph) 0.3%* *Oint (oph) 0.3%*	**Corneal ulcers/keratitis:** 2 Gtt q15min x 6h, then 2 Gtt q30min x 1d, then 2 Gtt q1h x 1d and 2 Gtt q4h x 3-14d; **CH** adult dose, if ≧ 1 y use sol, ≧ 2 y use oint; **conjunctivitis:** 1-2 Gtt q2h while awake x 2d, then 1-2 Gtt q4h while awakefferve x 5d, or ½ inch ribbon of oint tid x 2d, then ½ inch ribbon bid x 5d; **CH** adult dose, if ≧ 1 y use sol, if ≧ 2 y use oint
Erythromycin	PRC B, Lact +
Diomycin *Oint 0.5%* **Generics** *Oint 0.5%*	**Ocular infx:** ½ inch ribbon of oint to affected eye(s) q3- 4h; **chlamydial infx:** ½ inch ribbon of oint bid x 2mo or bid x 5d/mo x 6mo; **ophthalmia neonatorum PRO:** ½ inch ribbon of oint to both eyes within 1h of birth
Framycetin	EHL n/a,
Soframycin Sterile Eye *Oint (oph) 5mg/ml, Sol/Gtt (oph) 5mg/ml*	**Ocular infx:** 1-2 gtts q 1-2 h in acute conditions (for 2-3 d), reducing to 1-2 gtts, tid-qid
Fusidic acid	PRC C, Lact +
Fucithalmic *Sol 10mg/1g*	**Ocular infx:** 1 gtts bid

Gentamicin	PRC C, Lact ?
Alcomicin *Sol/Gtt (oph)* 0.3% **Diogent** *Sol/Gtt (oph)* 0.3%, *Oint (oph)* 0.3% **Garamycin** *Sol/Gtt (oph)* 0.3%, *Sol/Gtt* *(otic)* 0.3% *Oint (oph)* 0.3% **Generics** *Sol/Gtt (oph)* 0.3%	**Ocular infx:** 1-2 Gtt q4h or ½ inch ribbon of oint bid- tid, for severe infx max 2 Gtt qh

Ofloxacin	PRC C, Lact -
Ocuflox *Sol/Gtt (oph)* 0.3%	**Corneal ulcers/keratitis:** 1-2 Gtt q30min while awake and 1-2 Gtt 4h and 6h after retiring x 2d, then 1-2 Gtt q1h while awake x 5d, then 1-2 Gtt qid x 3d; **conjunctivitis:** 1-2 Gtt q2-4h x 2d, then 1-2 Gtt qid x 5d; **CH ≥ 1 y:** adult dose

Sulfacetamide	PRC C, Lact -
Cetamide *Oint (oph)* 10% **Diosulf** *Sol/Gtt (oph)* 10%	**Ocular infx:** ini 1-2 Gtt q2-3h, then taper x 7-10d, or ini ½ inch ribbon of oint q3-4h, then taper x 7-10d; **CH ≥ 2 mo:** adult dose; **trachoma:** 2 Gtt q2h with systemic sulfonamide; **CH ≥ 2 mo:** adult dose

Tobramycin	PRC B, Lact -
Tobrex *Oint (oph)* 0.3%, *Sol/Gtt (oph)* 0.3% **Generics** *Sol/Gtt (oph)* 0.3%	**Ocular infx:** 1-2 Gtt q2h x 1-2d, then 1-2 Gtt q4-6h or ½ inch ribbon of oint bid-qid

14.1.2 Antibacterials - Combinations

Bacitracin + Polymyxin B	PRC C, Lact ?
LID-Pack *Oint (oph)* 500 U/g + 10,000 U/g **Optimyxin** *Oint (oph)* 500 U/g + 10,000 U/g **Polysporin** *Oint (oph)* 500 U/g + 10,000 U/g	**Ocular infx:** ½ inch ribbon of oint qd or q3-4h x 7-10d

Gentamicin + Betamethasone	PRC C, Lact ?
SAB-Pentasone Sol (oph) 3 + 1mg/ml	**Ocular infx:** 1-2 Gtt q4h
Polymyxin B + Bacitracin + Neomycin	PRC C, Lact ?
Neosporin *Oint* (oph) 10,000 U/g + 400 U/g + 5mg/g	**Ocular infx:** ½ inch ribbon of oint q3-4 h x 7-10d
Polymyxin B + Bacitracin + Neomycin + Hydrocortisone	PRC C, Lact ?
Cortisporin *Oint* (oph) 10,000 U/g + 400 U/g + 5mg/g + 10mg/g	**Ocular infx:** ½ inch ribbon of oint q3-4 h x 7-10d
Polymyxin + Gramicidin	PRC C, Lact ?
Optimyxin *Sol/Gtt* (oph/otic) 10,000U/ml + 0.025mg/ml	**Ocular infx:** 1-2 Gtt q3-4h; **otic infx:** 4 Gtt 3-4x/d
Polymyxin + Gramicidin + Neomycin	PRC C, Lact ?
Neosporin *Sol/Gtt* (oph) 10,000 U/ml + 0.025mg/ml + 2.5mg/ml **Optimyxin Plus** *Sol/Gtt* (oph) 10,000 U/ml + 0.025mg/ml + 2.5mg/ml	**Ocular infx:** 1-2 Gtt q1-6h x 7-10d, for severe infx max 1- 2 Gtt q1h
Polymyxin + Bacitracin + Gramicidin	PRC C, Lact ?
Polysporin Triple Antibiotic *Oint* (oph) 10,000 U/g + 500 U/g + 0.25mg/g	**Ocular infx:** ½ inch ribbon of oint q3-4 h x 7-10d
Polymyxin B + Trimethoprim	PRC C, Lact ?
Polytrim, Generics *Sol/Gtt* (oph) 10,000 U/ml + 1mg/ml	**Ocular infx:** 1 Gtt q3-6h x 7-10d, max 6 Gtt/d; **CH** ≥ 2 mo: adult dose

14.1.3 Antivirals

Trifluridine	EHL 12min, PRC C, Lact ?
Viroptic *Sol/Gtt* (oph) 1%	**HSV keratitis/keratoconjunctivitis:** 1 Gtt q2h, max 9 Gtt/d, after re-epithelialization, decr to 1 Gtt q4h (min 5 Gtt/d) while awake x 7-14d, max contin use: 21d; **CH** ≥ 6 y: adult dose

14.2 Ophthalmic Anti-Inflammatory Agents

14.2.1 Corticosteroids - Single Ingredient Drugs

AE (corticosteroids): glaucoma, cataracts, corneal ulcers, secondary infections
CI (corticosteroids): bacterial, viral and fungal diseases of the eyes, injuries, corneal ulcers

Fluorometholone	PRC C, Lact ?
Flarex *Susp/Gtt (oph) 0.1%* **Fml** *Susp/Gtt (oph) 0.1%* **Fml Forte** *Susp/Gtt (oph) 0.25%* **Generics** *Susp/Gtt (oph) 0.1%*	**Anti-inflammatory:** prn ini 1 Gtt q4h or ½ inch of oint q4h x 1-2d, then 1 Gtt bid-qid or ½ inch of oint qd-tid; **CH** ≥ 2 y: adult dose
Prednisolone	EHL 2.6-3h, PRC C, Lact -
Diopred *Susp/Gtt (oph) 1%* **Pred Forte** *Susp/Gtt (oph) 1%* **Pred Mild** *Susp/Gtt (oph) 0.12%* **Generics** *Susp/Gtt (oph) 0.5%, 1%*	**Anti-inflammatory:** ini 1-2 Gtt q1h during the day and q2h during the night, then 1-2 Gtt q3-12h
Rimexolone	EHL 1-2h, PRC C, Lact ?
Vexol *Susp/Gtt (oph) 1%*	**Postop inflammation:** 1-2 Gtt qid x 2wk, ini 24h after surgery; **uveitis:** 1-2 Gtt q1h while awake x 1wk, then 1 Gtt q2h while awake x 1wk, then taper

14.2.2 Corticosteroids - Combinations

Dexamethasone, Tobramycin	PRC C, Lact ?
Tobradex *Oint (oph) 0.1% + 0.3%* *Susp/Gtt (oph) 0.1% + 0.3%*	**Anti-inflammatory:** 1-2 Gtt q2h x 1-2d, then 1-2 Gtt q4- 6h or ½ inch ribbon of oint bid-qid, gradually taper when discontinuing
Neomycin, Polymyxin, Hydrocortisone, (Bacitracin Zinc) PRC C, Lact ?	
Cortisporin *Sol/Gtt (oph/otic) 10,000 U/ml + 3.5mg/ml + 10mg/ml*	**Anti-inflammatory:** 1-2 Gtt or ½ inch ribbon of oint q3- 4h, prn more frequently, gradually taper when discontinuing

Polymyxin, Dexamethasone, Neomycin	PRC C, Lact ?
Dioptrol Susp/Gtt (oph) 10,000 U/ml + 0.1% + 3.5mg/ml **Maxitrol** Oint (oph) 6,000 U/g + 0.1% + 3.5mg/g, Susp/Gtt (oph) 6,000 U/ml + 0.1% + 3.5mg/ml	**Anti-inflammatory:** ini 1-2 Gtt q1h during the day and q2h during the night, then 1 Gtt q4-8h or ini ½ -1 inch ribbon (oint) tid-qid, then qd-bid, gradually taper when discontinuing
Prednisolone Acetate + Sulfacetamide Sodium	PRC C, Lact -
Blephamide Susp (oph) 0.2% + 10% **Dioptimyd** Susp (oph) 0.5% + 10%	**Anti-inflammatory:** 2 Gtt q4h while awake and hs or ½ inch ribbon of oint tid-qid (during the day) and 1-2x during the night, gradually taper when discontinuing

14.2.3 Nonsteroidal Anti-Inflammatory Agents

Diclofenac	EHL 2h, PRC B, Lact ?
Voltaren Ophtha Sol/Gtt (oph) 0.1%	**Postop inflammation following cataract removal:** 1 Gtt qid x 2wk, ini 24h postop; **photophobia associated with incisional refractive surgery:** 1 Gtt to operative eye(s) 1h prior to surgery and 1 Gtt 15min postop, then 1 Gtt qid prn x max 3 d
Ketorolac	EHL 5.3h, PRC C, Lact ?
Acular Sol/Gtt (oph) 0.4%, 0.5%	**Allergic conjunctivitis:** 1 Gtt (0.25 mg) qid; **inflammation after cataract removal:** 1 Gtt (0.25 mg) to affected eye(s) qid, ini 24h postop x 2wk; CH ≥ 12 y: adult dose

14.3 Glaucoma Agents
14.3.1 Glaucoma Agents - Adrenergic Agonists

AE (dipivefrin): burning, mydriasis, blurred vision, follicular conjunctivitis
CI (dipivefrin): narrow angle glaucoma, hypersensitivity to dipivefrin

Dipivefrin	PRC B, Lact ?
Propine, Generics Sol/Gtt (oph) 0.1%	**Glaucoma:** 1 Gtt q12h

14.3.2 Glaucoma Agents – Alpha₂ Agonists

AE (apraclonidine): upper lid elevation, conjunctival blanching, mydriasis, irregular heart beat;
AE (brimonidine): lid retraction, headache, drowsiness, conjunctival blanching
CI (apraclonidine): hypersensitivity to apraclonidine or clonidine
CI (brimonidine): hypersensitivity to brimonidine, concomitant MAOI therapy

Apraclonidine	EHL 8h, PRC C, Lact ?
Iopidine *Sol/Gtt (oph)* 0.5%, 1%	**Glaucoma:** 1-2 Gtt (0.5%) tid; **perioperative IOP** ↑: 1 Gtt (1%) 1h prior to surgery, then 1 Gtt immediately after surgery

Brimonidine	EHL 3h, PRC B, Lact -
Alphagan *Sol/Gtt (oph)* 0.2%	**Glaucoma:** 1 Gtt tid

14.3.3 Glaucoma Agents – Beta Blockers

AE (beta blockers): eye: conjunctival irritation, dry eyes, decline of papillary blood supply; systemic: bronchospasm, bradycardia, hypotension, cardiac failure ↑
CI (beta blockers): cardiac insufficiency (NYHA III and IV), bradycardia, asthma

Betaxolol	EHL 12-22h, PRC C, Lact ?
Betoptic S *Susp/Gtt (oph)* 0.25% **Generics** *Sol/Gtt (oph)* 0.5%	**Glaucoma:** 1-2 Gtt bid

Levobunolol	EHL 6.1h, PRC C, Lact -
Betagan, Generics *Sol/Gtt (oph)* 0.25%, 0.5%	**Glaucoma:** 1-2 Gtt (0.5%) qd-bid or 1-2 Gtt (0.25%) bid

Timolol	EHL 4h, PRC C, Lact -
Apo-Timop *Sol/Gtt (oph)* 0.25%, 0.5% **Tim-AK** *Sol/Gtt (oph)* 0.5% **Timoptic** *Sol/Gtt (oph)* 0.25%, 0.5% **Timoptic-XE** *Sol (gel forming)/Gtt (oph)* 0.25%, 0.5% **Generics** *Sol/Gtt (oph)* 0.25%, 0.5%	**Glaucoma:** 1 Gtt (0.25 or 0.5%) bid or 1 Gtt of gel (0.25 or 0.5% Timoptic XE) qd

14.3.4 Glaucoma Agents – Carbonic Anhydrase Inhibitors

AE (acetazolamide): taste DO, paresthesia, metabolic acidosis, tinnitus;
AE (brinzolamide): blurred vision, bitter taste;
AE (dorzolamide): bitter taste, superficial punctate keratitis, blurred vision, ocular burning, photophobia, conjunctivitis;
CI (acetazolamide): hyponatremia/hypokalemia, severe hepatic disease, hyperchloremic acidosis, hypersens. to acetazolamide;
CI (brinzolamide, dorzolamide): hypersens. to product ingredients

Acetazolamide	EHL 4-8h, PRC C, Lact -
Diamox *Tab 250mg, Inj 500mg/vial, Cap sust. rel. 500mg* **Generics** *Tab 250mg*	**Glaucoma:** 250 mg PO qd-qid(immediate release) or 500 mg PO qd-bid (ext.rel); **acute glaucoma:** ini 250 mg IV q4h, then PO, or ini 500mg PO, then 125-250mg PO q4h; DARF: GFR (ml/ min) >50: q6h, 10-50: q12h, <10: contraind.

Brinzolamide	EHL 111d, PRC C, Lact -
Azopt *Susp/Gtt (oph) 1%*	**Glaucoma:** 1 Gtt tid; DARF: CrCl (ml/min) <30: contraind., caution in moderate RF

Dorzolamide	EHL 4mo, PRC C, Lact -
Trusopt *Sol/Gtt (oph) 2%*	**Glaucoma:** 1 Gtt tid; DARF: CrCl (ml/min) <30: contraind., caution in moderate RF

Dorzolamide + Timolol	PRC C, Lact -
Cosopt *Sol/Gtt (oph) 2% + 0.5%*	**Glaucoma:** 1 Gtt bid; DARF: CrCl (ml/min) <30: contraind., caution in moderate RF

14.3.5 Glaucoma Agents – Cholinergic Agonists

AE (cholinergics): conjunctival reddening, accommodation disturbances, transient myopia, spasms of ciliary muscle, (headache, aching eyes), iridocysts, retinal detachment, cataracts
AE (pilocarpine): blurred vision, difficulty in night vision, burning or itching of eyes
CI (cholinergics): malignant glaucoma, secondary glaucoma, iritis, corneal damage
CI (pilocarpine): hypersensitivity to pilocarpine products, acute iritis or glaucoma after cataract extraction, uncontrolled asthma

Pilocarpine	EHL 0.76-1.35h, PRC C, Lact ?
Diocarpine Sol (oph) 1%, 2%, 4% **Isopto Carpine** Sol (oph) 0.5%, 1%, 2%, 4%, 6% **Pilopine HS** Gel (oph) 4% **Generics** Sol (oph) 2%	**Glaucoma:** 1-2 Gtt up to tid-qid or ½ inch ribbon (4% gel) hs; for drug delivery system see Prod Info

14.3.6 Glaucoma Agents – Prostaglandin F₂ (Alpha) Analogues

AE (prostaglandin analogues): conjunctival hyperemia, growth of eyelashes, ocular pruritus, iris pigmentation, ocular irritation
CI (prostaglandin analogues): known hypersensitivity

Bimatoprost	EHL 45min, PRC C, Lact ?
Lumigan Sol/Gtt (oph) 0.03%	**Glaucoma:** 1 Gtt hs

Latanoprost	EHL 17min, PRC C, Lact ?
Xalatan Sol/Gtt (oph) 0.005%	**Glaucoma:** 1 Gtt hs

Travoprost	EHL no data, PRC C, Lact ?
Travatan Sol/Gtt (oph) 0.004%	**Glaucoma:** 1 Gtt hs

14.4 Mydriatics, Cycloplegics
14.4.1 Anticholinergics

AE (cyclopentolate): IOP↑, burning, photophobia, blurred vision, conjunctivitis;
AE (homatropine): stinging/burning, keratitis, IOP↑, eye pain; **AE** (tropicamide): ocular irritation, blurred vision;
CI (cyclopentolate): glaucoma, hypersensitivity to cyclopentolate products;
CI (homatropine): hypersensitivity to homatropine products, primary glaucoma
CI (tropicamide): narrow angle glaucoma, sensitivity to tropicamide

Atropine	PRC C, Lact ?
Isopto Atropine *Sol/Gtt (oph)* 1% **Generics** *Sol/Gtt* 1%, *Oint (oph)* 1%	**Anterior uveitis/postop mydriasis:** 1 Gtt (1–2% sol) up to tid or ¼ inch ribbon (1% oint) up to tid; mydriasis lasts 7–14d; **preoperative mydriasis/refraction:** 1 Gtt (1% sol) with 1 Gtt phenylephrine (2.5% or 10%) prior to surgery; **ciliary block glaucoma:** ini 1 Gtt (1–2% sol) with 1Gtt phenylephrine 10% tid-qid, red to maint 1Gtt 1– 2% sol qd–qod; **posterior synechiae:** 1 Gtt 2% alternately with phenylephrine 10% q5–10min x 5 applications each
Cyclopentolate	PRC C, Lact ?
Cyclogyl *Sol/Gtt (oph)* 1% **Diopentolate** *Sol/Gtt (oph)* 1% **Generics** *Sol/Gtt (oph)* 0.5%	**Refraction:** 1–2 Gtt (1–2%), rep prn in 5–10min, apply 45min prior to procedure; mydriasis lasts 6–24h
Homatropine	PRC C, Lact ?
Isopto Homatropine *Sol/Gtt (oph)* 2%, 5% **Generics** *Sol/Gtt (oph)* 2%	**Refraction:** 1–2 Gtt (sol 2%) or 1 Gtt (sol 5%) in eye(s) prior to procedure, rep prn q5–10min; **uveitis:** 1–2 Gtt (2– 5%), rep up to max q3–4h; mydriasis lasts 1–3d
Tropicamide	PRC N, Lact ?
Diotrope *Sol/Gtt (oph)* 0.5%, 1% **Mydriacyl** *Sol/Gtt (oph)* 0.5%, 1% **Generics** *Sol/Gtt (oph)* 1%	**Fundus exam:** 1–2 Gtt (0.5%) in eye(s) 15–20min prior to exam, rep prn q30min; mydriasis lasts 6h

14.4.2 Sympathomimetics

AE (phenylephrine): tachycardia, HTN, MI, SAH; **CI** (phenylephrine): hypersensitivity to phenylephrine products, narrow angle glaucoma, HTN, CAD, BPH

Phenylephrine	PRC C, Lact ?
Dionephrine Sol/Gtt (oph) 2.5% **Mydfrin** Sol/Gtt (oph) 2.5% **Generics** Sol/Gtt (oph) 2.5%, 10%	**Ophthalmologic exams:** 1-2 Gtt (2.5 or 10%) prior to procedure; **ocular surgery:** 1-2 Gtt (2.5 or 10%) prior to surgery; **glaucoma:** 1 Gtt (10%) qid with atropine; **uveitis:** 1-2 Gtt (2.5 or 10%) tid with atropine; **minor eye irritat.:**1-2 Gtt (0.12%) qid prn; **refraction:** 1 Gtt (2.5%) after atropine; mydriasis lasts 5h

14.5 Ocular Decongestants, Anti-Allergics
14.5.1 H$_1$-Receptor Antagonists

AE (levocabastine): ocular irritation, headache, drowsiness; **AE** (olopatadine): headache, ocular burning, dryness, cold syndrome, rhinopharyngitis, dysgeusia
CI (levocabastine): hypersensitivity to levocabastine products, soft contact lenses
CI (olopatadine): hypersensitivity to olopatadine

Levocabastine	EHL 33-40h, PRC C, Lact ?
Livostin Susp/Gtt (oph) 0.05%	**Seasonal allergic conjunctivitis:** 1 Gtt in each eye bid- qid x up to 2wk; **CH** ≥ 12 y: adult dose

Olopatadine	EHL 3h, PRC C, Lact ?
Patanol Sol/Gtt (oph) .1%	**Allergic conjunctivitis:** 1-2 Gtt bid in each eye within 6- 8h; **CH** >3 y: adult dose

14.5.2 H$_1$-Antagonist, Mast Cell Stabilizer

CI (ketotifen fumarate): hypersensitivity to ketotifen products or benzoate compounds

Ketotifen Fumarate	EHL 21h, PRC C, Lact ?
Zaditor Sol/Gtt (oph) 0.025%	**Allergic conjunctivitis:** 1 Gtt q8-12h in each eye; **CH** > 3 y: adult dose

14.5.3 Mast Cell Stabilizers

Cromolyn Sodium	EHL 80-90min, PRC B, Lact ?
Opticrom, Generics *Sol/Gtt (oph)* 2%	**Allergic ocular DO:** 1-2 Gtt in each eye 4-6 x/d; **CH** $\geq$ 4 y: adult dose
Lodoxamide Tromethamine	EHL 8.5h, PRC B, Lact ?
Alomide *Sol/Gtt (oph)* 0.1%	**Allergic ocular DO:** 1-2 Gtt qid x up to 3mo; **CH** $\geq$ 2 y: adult dose
Nedocromil	EHL 1.5-3.3h, PRC B, Lact ?
Alocril *Sol/Gtt (oph)* 2%	**Allergic conjunctivitis:** 1-2 Gtt bid; **CH** $\geq$ 3 y: adult dose

14.5.4 Sympathomimetics

AE (naphazoline): local mucosal irritation, HTN, CNS effects, tremor, eye irritation and redness; **CI** (naphazoline): hypersensitivity to naphazoline products, narrow angle glaucoma, hyperthyroidism, CAD, BPH, HTN

Naphazoline	PRC C, Lact ?
Naphcon Forte, Vasocon *Sol/Gtt (oph)* 0.1%	**Ocular vasoconstrictor/decongestant:** 1 Gtt q3-4h prn up to qid

14.5.5 Sympathomimetics + H$_1$-Receptor Antagonists

Naphazoline + Pheniramine	PRC C, Lact ?
Naphcon-A *Sol/Gtt (oph)* 0.025% + 0.3%	**Ocular decongestant:** 1-2 Gtt bid-qid prn; **CH** $\geq$ 6 y: adult dose

14.6 Local Anesthetics

AE: allergic reactions, corneal damage after long-term use

Proparacaine	PRC C, Lact ?
Alcaine, Diocaine *Sol/Gtt (oph)* 0.5%	**Local anesthetic:** 1-2 Gtt prior to procedure, rep q 5- 10min x 1-3 doses (suture or foreign body removal) or x 5-7 doses (cataract or glaucoma surgery)
Tetracaine	PRC C, Lact ?
Pontocaine, Generics *Sol/Gtt (oph)* 0.5%	**Local anesthetic:** 1-2 Gtt prior to procedure

14.7 Other Ophthalmologic Drugs

Artifical Tears	PRC N, Lact ?
Genteal *Gel (oph) Hydroxypropyl-methylcellulose* **Isopto Tears** *Sol/Gtt (oph) Hypromellose 1%* **Thera Tears** *Sol/Gtt (oph) Sodium Carboxymethyl Cellulose 0.25%* **Visine Advance True Tears** *Sol/Gtt (oph) Hypromellose 0.2% + Glycerine 0.2%* **Refresh Liquigel** *Sol/Gtt (oph) Sodium Carboxymethyl Cellulose 1%* **Tears Plus** *Polyvinyl alcohol 1.4%* **Tears Naturale Forte** *Sol/Gtt (oph) Hydroxypropyl methylcellulose 0.3% + Dextran 70 0.1% + Glycerine 0.2%* **Tears Naturale P.M.** *Lub White petrolatum, mineral oil, lanolin* **Visine Advance True Tears** *Sol/Gtt (oph) Hydroxypropyl methylcellulose + Glycerine* **Visine Contact Lens Eye Drops** *Sol/Gtt (oph) Hydroxypropylmethylcellulose + Glycerine* **Visine True Tears Eye Drops** *Sol/Gtt (oph) Polyethylene Glycol*	**Ophthalmic lubricant:** 1-2 Gtt tid-qid prn
Oxymetazoline	PRC C
Visine Workplace Eye Drops *Sol/Gtt (oph) 0.025%*	**Minor eye irritation:** ch>6 and adults: 1-2 gtts q6h PRN
Tetrahydrozoline	PRC C
Visine Original Eye Drops *Sol/Gtt (oph) 0.05%*	**Conjunctival congestion:** 1-2 gtts 2-4 times/d PRN
Tetrahydrozoline + Polyethylene Glycol	PRC C
Visine Cool Eye Drops *Sol/Gtt (oph) 0.05% + 1%*	**Minor eye irritation:** ch>6 and adults: 1-2 gtts q6h PR
Tetrahydrozoline + Zinc Sulfate	PRC C
Visine Allergy Eye Drops *Sol/Gtt (oph) 0.05% + 0.25%*	**Minor eye irritation:** 1-2 gtts q6h PRN

15. ENT

15.1 Antihistamines
15.1.1 Sedating Antihistamines

MA: competitive blockage of H1-receptors (see antihistamines →227, →265, →266)
AE (antihistamines): sedation, excitatory appearances (small children), dry mouth, glaucoma, micturition DO; **AE** (azatadine): drowsiness, epigastric distress, urinary retention or frequency; **AE** (cetirizine): drowsiness, fatigue (mild sedation), dry mouth, headache; **AE** (clemastine): sedation, shortness of breath; **AE** (chlorpheniramine): drowsiness, N/V; **AE** (diphenhydramine): dyskinesias, anaphylaxis, sedation; **AE** (hydroxyzine): xerostomia, drowsiness, headache;
CI (antihistamines): urinary retention, glaucoma;
CI (azatadine): hypersens. to azatadine/related antihistamines, use of MAOI, narrow-angle glaucoma or urinary retention; **CI** (cetirizine): hypersens. to cetirizine or hydroxyzine; **CI** (clemastine): hypersens. to clemastine, MAOI therapy, lower resp tract symptoms; **CI** (chlorpheniramine, dexchlorpheniramine): hypersens. to product ingredeints; **CI** (diphenhydramine): hypersens. to diphenhydramine, MAOI Tx, chicken pox, measles, blisters (topical use), topical use on eyes; **CI** (hydroxyzine): hypersens. to hydroxyzine

Azatadine	EHL 9h, PRC B, Lact ?
Optimine *Tab 1mg*	**Allergic rhinitis, urticaria:** 1-2mg PO bid; **CH** >12y: 1- 2mg PO bid; DARF not req

Cetirizine	EHL 7.4-9h, PRC B, Lact ?
Reactine *Tab 5mg, 10mg, 20 mg, Syr 5mg/5ml* **Generics** *Tab 5mg, 10mg*	**Allergic rhinitis, urticaria:** 5-10mg PO qd, max 20mg/d; **CH** 2-6y: 2.5mg PO qd, max 5mg/d, >6y: 5-10mg PO qd, max 10mg/d; DARF: GFR (ml/min): <30: max 5mg/d

Chlorpheniramine	EHL 20h, PRC B, Lact -
Novo-Pheniram *Syr 2.5g/5ml, Tab 4mg*	**Allergic rhinitis:** 4mg PO q4-6h; ext.rel 8mg PO q8-12h or 12mg PO q12h, max 24mg/d; **CH** 6-11y: 2mg PO q4- 6h, max 12mg/d, >12y: adult dose; DARF: not req

Clemastine	EHL 21h, PRC B, Lact -
Tavist *Tab 1mg*	**Allergic rhinitis, urticaria:** 1.34-2.68mg PO bid-tid, max 8.04mg/d; **CH** 6-12y: 0.5mg PO bid, max 6mg/d

Diphenhydramine	EHL 4-8h, PRC B, Lact -
Allerdryl Cap 25mg, 50mg **Allernix** Cap 25mg, 50mg, Elixir (oral) 12.5mg/5ml **Benadryl** Cap 25mg, 50mg, Cream 2%, Elixir (oral) 12.5mg/5ml, Liq (oral) 6.25mg/5ml, Tab (chew) 12.5mg **Nytol** Cap 25mg **Nytol Extra Strength** Cap 50mg **Simply Sleep** Cap 25mg **Unisom Extra Strength/Extra Strength Sleepgels** **Generics** Cap 25mg, 50mg, Elixir (oral) 2.5mg/ml, Inj 50mg/ml	**Allergic rhinitis, rhinorrhea:** 25-50mg PO/IV/IM q4-6h, max 0.4g/d; **motion sickness:** 25-50mg PO 30min before exposure, then prn q4-6h; **CH** 1.25mg PO qid, max 0.3g/d; **anaphylaxis , insomnia ,** DARF: GFR (ml/min) >50: q6h, 10-50: q6-12h, < 10: q12- 18h; see Prod Info
Hydroxyzine	EHL 3-20h, PRC C, Lact -
Atarax Syr 10mg/5ml, Inj 50mg/ml **Generics** Cap 10mg, 25mg, 50mg, Syr 10mg/5ml, Inj 50mg/ml	**Allergic reactions, pruritus:** 25-100mg PO/IM tid-qid; **CH** <6y: 50mg/d PO div tid-qid, >6y: 50-100mg/d PO div tid- qid

15.1.2 Nonsedating Antihistamines

MA, AE, CI (antihistamines): see antihistamines →227, →265, →266
AE (fexofenadine): nausea, dyspepsia, fatigue; **AE** (loratadine): sedation, dizziness, dry mouth, headache, nausea; **CI** (fexofenadine): hypersensitivity to fexofenadine; **CI** (loratadine): hypersensitivity to loratadine

Desloratadine	EHL 27h, PRC C, Lact ?
Aerius Tab 5mg	**Allergic rhinitis, urticaria:** 5mg PO qd; DARF: 5mg PO qod
Fexofenadine	EHL 14-18h, PRC C, Lact -
Allegra Tab 60mg	**Allergic rhinitis, urticaria:** 60mg PO bid or 180mg qd; **CH** 6-11y: 30mg PO bid, >12y: adult dose; DARF: 60mg PO qd
Loratadine	EHL 12-15h, PRC B, Lact ?
Claritin Tab 10mg, Tab (orally disint) 10mg, Syr 1mg/ml **Generics** Tab 10mg	**Allergic rhinitis, urticaria:** 10mg PO qd; **CH** 6-11y: adult dose; DARF: GFR (ml/min) <30: 10mg PO qod

Loratadine + Pseudoephedrine	PRC C, Lact +
Claritin Liberator *Cap ext. release 10mg + 240mg*	**Allergic rhinitis:** 1 cap PO qd

15.2 Nasal Preparations
15.2.1 Anticholinergics

AE: dry mouth, bitter taste, epistaxis, nasal dryness, nasal congestion
CI: hypersensitivity to ipratropium products

Ipratropium Bromide	EHL 1.6h (IV), PRC B, Lact ?
Atrovent *Spray (metered, nasal) 0.03% (0.021mg/spray), 0.06% (0.042mg/spray)* **Generics** *Spray (metered, nasal) 0.03% (0.021mg/spray)*	**Rhinorrhea associated with allergic rhinitis:** 2 sprays (0.03%) in each nostril bid-tid; **CH ≥ 6y:** adult dose; **rhinorrhea associated with common cold/vasomotor rhinitis:** 2 sprays (0.06%) in each nostril tid-qid; **CH ≥ 12y:** adult dose

15.2.2 Antihistamines, Mast Cell Stabilizers

MA/EF: see antihistamines →227, →265, →266

Cromolyn	EHL 22-25h, PRC C, Lact -
Generics *Spray (nasal) 1%, 2%*	**Allergic rhinitis:** 1 spray in each nostril q4-6h ; **CH ≥ 6y:** adult dose

15.2.3 Corticosteroids

AE (beclomethasone): adrenal suppression, candidiasis, nasopharyngeal irritation
AE (budesonide): nasal stinging, throat irritation, nasal dryness, epistaxis, headache
AE (flunisolide): nasal irritation, dysphonia, headache
AE (fluticasone): hoarseness, nasal burning/epistaxis, nasal congestion, pruritus/burning, eosinophilia
AE (mometasone): burning, atrophy, pruritus, headache
AE (triamcinolone): GI distress, fluid and electrolyte disturbances, HPA axis suppression, mild euphoria/depression
CI (beclomethasone, budesonide, flunisolide, fluticasone): hypersensitivity to product ingredients/corticosteroids, status asthmaticus or other acute episodes of asthma
CI (mometasone): hypersensitivity to mometasone or other corticosteroids
CI (triamcinolone): systemic fungal infections

Beclomethasone	EHL 3h, PRC C, Lact ?
Gen-Beclo AQ *Spray (metered, nasal)* 0.05mg/spray **Rivanase AQ** *Spray (metered, nasal)* 0.05mg/spray **Generics** *Spray (metered, nasal)* 0.05mg/spray	**Allergic rhinitis/nasal polyp PRO:** 1-2 spray(s) (0.042- 0.084mg) in each nostril bid; **CH** >12y: adult dose, 6-12y: 1 spray (0.042mg) in each nostril bid, max 0.084mg bid
Budesonide	EHL 2-3h PRC C, Lact ?
Rhinocort Aqua *Spray (metered, nasal)* 0.064mg/spray	**Allergic rhinitis:** 2 sprays in each nostril bid or 4 sprays qd; **CH** ≥ 6y: adult dose, max 4 sprays/d (0.032mg/spray) or 2 sprays/d (0.064mg/spray)
Flunisolide	EHL 1-2h, PRC C, Lact ?
Rhinalar, Generics *Spray (metered, nasal)* 0.025mg/spray	**Allergic rhinitis:** 2 sprays in each nostril bid, prn incr to 2 sprays in each nostril tid, max 8 sprays/nostril/d; **CH** 6-14y: 1 spray in each nostril tid or 2 sprays in each nostril bid, max 4 sprays/ nostril/d
Fluticasone	EHL 7.8h, PRC C, Lact ?
Flonase *Spray (metered, nasal)* 0.05mg/spray	**Allergic rhinitis:** 2 sprays in each nostril qd or 1 spray in each nostril bid, decr to 1 spray in each nostril qd when appropriate; **CH** >4y: 1-2 sprays in each nostril qd, max 2 sprays/nostril/d
Mometasone	EHL 5.8h, PRC C, Lact ?
Nasonex *Spray (metered, nasal)* 0.05mg/spray	**Allergic rhinitis:** 2 sprays in each nostril qd; **CH** ≥ 12y: adult dose, 3-11y: 1 spray in each nostril qd
Triamcinolone	EHL 2-3h PRC C, Lact ?
Nasacort AQ *Spray (met.nas.)* 0.055mg/spray	**Allergic rhinitis:** ini 2 sprays in each nostril bid, prn decr to 2 sprays/nostril qd, max 8 sprays/d; **CH** ≥ 12y: adult dose, 6-12y: 1-2 sprays in each nostril qd

15.2.4 Nasal (Topical) Decongestants

AE (sympathomimetic decongestants): reactive hyperemia, mucus membrane burning, dryness, tachycardia, BP↑. Long use: epithelial damage, chronic stuffy nose
AE (oxymetazoline): rebound congestion, mucosal irritation, CNS effects, tremors
AE (pseudoephedrine): restlessness, HTN, arrhythmias
CI (sympathomimetic decongestants): rhinitis sicca, severe coronary diseases
CI (oxymetazoline, phenylephrine): hypersensitivity to product ingredients, narrow angle glaucoma, hyperthyroidism, CAD, BPH, HTN
CI (pseudoephedrine): hypersensitivity to product ingredients or sympathomimetics, MAOI therapy, severe HTN/CAD

Oxymetazoline	EHL 5-8h, PRC C, Lact ?
Claritan Allergic Congestion Relief *Spray (nasal)* 0.05% **Claritan Eye Allergy Relief** *Sol (nasal)* 0.25mg/ml **Dristan Long Lasting** *Mist (nasal)* 0.05%, *Spray (nasal)* 0.05% **Drixoral** *Spray (nasal)* 0.05%	Nasal congestion: 2-3 sprays/Gtt (0.05%) in each nostril bid x 3d; CH ≥ 6y: adult dose, 2-5y: 2-3 Gtt (0.025%) in each nostril bid x 3d
Pseudoephedrine	EHL 9-16h PRC C, Lact ?
Balminil Decongestant *Syr* 30mg/ml **Contac Cold 12 Hour Relief Non Drowsy** *Cap (sust rel)* 120mg **Eltor 120** *Cap (sust rel)* 120mg **Pseudofrin** *Tab* 60mg **Sudafed Decongestant** *Tab* 30mg **Sudafed Decongestant Children's Chewable** *Tab (chew)* 15mg **Sudafed Decongestant Extra Strenght** *Tab* 60mg **Sudafed Decongestant 12 Hour** *Cap* 120mg	Nasal congestion: 60mg PO q4-6h or 120mg PO q12h (ext.rel) or 240mg PO qd (ext.rel), max 240mg/d; CH >12y: adult dose, 6-11y: 30mg PO q4-6h, max 120mg/d, 2-5y: 15mg PO q4-6h, max 60mg/d, 2-3y: 1.6ml; pediatric Gtt PO q4-6h: 12-23 mo: 1.2ml, 4-11 mo: 0.8ml, 0-3 mo: 0.4ml, max 4 doses/d
Xylometazoline	PRC C, Lact ?
Decongest *Sol* 0.1%	Nasal congestion: 1-3 Gtt/spray in each nostril q8-10h prn

15.2.5 Other Nasal Preparations

Framycetin + Phenylephrine + Gramicidin

Soframycin Nasal Spray *Spray (nasal)* 12.5 + 2.5 + 0.05mg/ml	***Nasal infection/congestion:*** 2 sprays in each nostril every 4 hours. Max 6 times per day
Saline Nasal Spray	EHLPRC A, Lact +
Generics *Spray (nasal)* 0.7%	**Nasal dryness:** 1-3 sprays/Gtt in each nostril prn

15.3 Ear Preparations
15.3.1 Antibacterial/Antifungal Combinations

AE (acetic acid): local stinging or burning
CI (acetic acid): hypersensitivity to acetic acid products, perforated tympanic membranes, vaccinia and varicella (steroid- containing ear drops)

Acetic Acid + Aluminium Acetate	PRC C, Lact ?
Generics *Sol/Gtt (otic)* 2% + 0.79%	**Otitis externa:** 4-6 Gtt in affected ear(s) q2-3h, keep moist (cotton plug) x 24h

15.3.2 Agents for Otitis Externa Prophylaxis

Aluminium Acetate + Benzethonium	PRC N, Lact ?
Buro-Sol *Sol/Gtt (otic)* 0.5% + 0.03%	**Otitis externa** (PRO): 4-5 Gtt in ears after swimming, bathing; **CH** adult dose

15.3.3 Antibacterial/Corticosteroid Combinations

Ciprofloxacin + Hydrocortisone	PRC C, Lact -
Cipro HC *Susp/Gtt (otic)* 0.2% + 1%	**Otitis externa:** 3 Gtt into affected ear(s) bid x 7d; **CH** ≥ 1y: adult dose
Hydrocortisone + Polymyxin + Neomycin	
Cortisporin *Sol/Gtt (oph/otic)* 10,000 U/ml + 3.5mg/ml + 10mg/ml	**Otitis externa:** 4 Gtt in affected ear(s) tid-qid; **CH** 3 Gtt in affected ear(s) tid-qid

15.3.4 Decongestant/Analgesic Combinations

Benzocaine + Antipyrine	PRC C, Lact ?
Auralgan *Sol (otic)* 14mg/ml + 54mg/ml	**Otitis media** (adjunct): 2-4 Gtt tid-qid or q1-2h prn; **cerumen removal:** 2-4 Gtt tid x 2-3d to detach cerumen, then prn for discomfort, insert moistened cotton plug (with sol)

15.3.5 Surfactants, Ceruminolytics

AE (cerumenex eardrops): localized dermatitis reactions, allergic contact dermatitis, skin ulcerations, burning and pain at the application site and skin rash
CI (carbamide peroxide): hypersensitivity to carbamide peroxide products, ear drainage or discharge, perforated tympanic membrane
CI (cerumenex eardrops): perforated tympanic membrane, otitis media, history of hypersensitivity to cerumenex eardrops or to any of its components

Triethanolamine	PRC C, Lact ?
Cerumenex *Sol/Gtt (otic)* 10%	**Cerumen removal:** fill ear canal with sol, insert cotton plug x 15-30min, then flush, max x 4d

15.4 Mouth and Lip Preparations
15.4.1 Antifungals

AE (clotrimazole): N/V, LFT's↑ (transient), contact dermatitis
AE (nystatin): diarrhea, vaginal irritation/pain, N/V, rash
CI (clotrimazole, nystatin): hypersensitivity to product ingredietns

Clotrimazole	EHL 3.5-5h, PRC C, Lact ?
Generics *lozenge (oral)* 10mg	**Oral candidiasis:** 1 troche dissolved slowly in mouth 5x/ d x 14d; **CH** ≥ 3y: adult dose; **prevention of oropharyngeal candidiasis in immunocompromised patients:** 1 troche dissolved slowly in mouth tid until end of chemotherapy/high-dose corticosteroids

Nystatin	PRC C, Lact +
Nilstat *Powder (oral) 100%, Tab 500,000 U, Susp 100,000 U/ml* **Nyaderm** *Susp 100,000 U/ml* **Generics** *Susp 100,000 U/ml*	**Thrush:** 5ml PO swish and swallow qid with ½ of dose in each cheek or 1-2 lozenges 4–5x/d, max 14d; **CH** 2ml PO swish and swallow qid with 1ml in each cheek or use a cotton sqab, premature and low birth weight infants: 0.5ml PO in each cheek qid or use a cotton squab

15.4.2 Other Mouth and Lip Preparations

AE (chlorhexidine gluconate): skin irritation, tooth staining, altered taste
CI (chlorhexidine gluconate): hypersensitivity to chlorhexidine products

Anetholtrithion	PRC C, Lact ?
Sialor *Tab 25mg*	**Xerostomia:** 25mg PO tid before meals
Benzocaine	PRC C, Lact ?
Anbesol *Gel 6.4%, 7.5%, 20%, Liq 6.5%, 20%* **Zilactin Baby, Zilactin-B** *Gel 10%*	**Mouth or lip pain:** apply q4-6h
Benzydamine	PRC C, Lact ?
Sun-Benz *Sol (oral) 0.15%* **Tantum** *Sol (oral) 0.15%* **Generics** *Sol (oral) 0.15%*	**Mouth or throat pain:** 15 mL PO gargled/ rinsed for 30sec. and spit q30min-6h
Chlorhexidine Gluconate	PRC B, Lact ?
Oro-Clense, Peridex, Generics *Sol (dental) 0.12%*	**Gingivitis:** apply 15ml x 30sec bid as oral rinse (qam and qpm after brushing teeth), expectorate after rinsing
Dequalinium	EHL n/a
Dequadin *Lozenges 0.25mg, Paint 0.5%*	**Mouth and throat infections:** 1 lozange PO q2-3h; **oral pain:** apply paint to area q2-3h
Hexetidine	EHL n/a
Steri/Sol *Liq 0.1%*	**Tonsilitis, pharyngitis, laryngitis, gingivitis, stomatitis, oral thrush, Vincent's angina:** swish and gargle 15ml for 30 sec. PO bid

Lidocaine	PRC C, Lact +
Zilactin-L *Liq* 2.5%	**Lip pain:** apply q1-2h
Lidocaine Viscous	PRC B, Lact +
Lidodan Viscous *Sol (top)* 2% **Xylocaine** *Sol (top)* 2%	**Mouth or lip pain:** 15ml topically or swish and spit q3h, max 8 doses/24h or 4.5mg/kg or max 300mg, use lowest effective dose, prn apply to small sore places with cotton-tipped applicator; **CH** >3y: 3.75-5ml topically or swish and spit up to q3h
Octyl Methoxycinnamate + Homosalate + Oxybenzone + Dimethicone + Menthol	
Zilactin-Lip *Balm* 7% + 4% + 3% + 1.5% + 0.5%	**Chapped lips:** apply tid-qid
Pilocarpine	PRC C, Lact ?
Salagen *Tab* 5mg	**Xerostomia:** ini 5mg PO tid-qid, max 30mg/d
Povidone-iodine	PRC D, Lact ?
Betadine *Mouth wash* 1%	Mouth wash
Triamcinolone Acetonide	PRC C, Lact ?
Kenalog in Orabase, Oracort *Paste* 0.1%	Apply bid-tid with finger, apply about 0.5cm of paste to the oral lesion

16. Urology

16.1 Bladder Agents

16.1.1 Antispasmodics (Parasympatholytics)

MA/EF (parasympatholytics): blockage of muscarine receptors, mainly direct action on smooth muscles (papaverine-like) ⇒ tonicity of smooth muscleso in GI + urinary tract
AE: sweat secretiono, dry mouth, tachycardia, accommodation DO, glaucoma
AE (hyoscyamine): dry mouth, urinary hesitancy, blurred vision, tachycardia, headache
AE (oxybutynin): tachycardia, anticholinergic EF, insomnia, somnolence, sexual dysfunction
AE (tolterodine): dry mouth, headache, dyspepsia, constipation, xerophthalmia
CI: glaucoma, urinary retention, tachyarrhythmia, GI stenosis, toxic megacolon, myasthenia gravis
CI (hyoscyamine): hypersensitivity to hyoscyamine products, glaucoma, intestinal obstruction, severe liver/renal disease
CI (oxybutynin): glaucoma, GI obstruction, obstructive uropathy, myasthenia gravis, colitis
CI (tolterodine): urinary/gastric retention, glaucoma, hypersensitivity to tolterodine

Hyoscyamine	EHL 3.5h, PRC C, Lact -
Levsin *Tab 0.125mg, Tab ext.rel. 0.125mg, Gtt 0.125mg/ml, Inj 0.5mg/ml*	**Bladder spasm:** 0.125-0.3mg PO qid; ext.rel.: 0.375- 0.75mg bid; max 1.5 g/d; **CH** 2-12y: 0.0625-0.125mg PO qid; ext.rel.: 0.375mg PO bid, >12y: 0.125-0.25mg PO qid; ext.rel.: see adults; **GI** →86
Oxybutynin	EHL 1.1-2.3h, PRC B, Lact ?
Ditropan *Syr 5mg/5ml, Tab 5mg* **Ditropan XL** *Tab ext.rel. 5mg, 10mg* **Oxybutyn** *Tab 5mg* **Oxytrol** *Patch 3.9mg/d* **Generics** *Syr 5mg/5ml, Tab 2.5mg, 5mg*	**Bladder spasm:** 5mg PO bid-tid, max 5mg PO qid; ext.rel.: 5-15mg PO qd, max 30mg PO qd; **CH** >5y: 5mg PO bid, max 5mg PO tid
Propantheline	EHL (biphasic) 57.9min, 2.93h, PRC C, Lact ?
Pro-Banthine *Tab 7.5mg, 15mg*	**Urinary incontinence, neurogenic bladder:** 15mg q4- 6h, max 90mg PO qid; GI, peptic ulcer
Tolterodine	EHL 1.9-3.7h, PRC C, Lact -
Detrol *Tab 1mg, 2mg* **Unidet** *Cap ext. release 2mg, 4mg*	**Overactive bladder:** 2mg PO bid; 1mg PO if reduced hepatic function

16.1.2 Bladder Spasm

AE (flavoxate): nervousness, headache, blurred vision, drowsiness, N/V
AE (prosed/DS): rapid pulse, flushing, blurred vision, dizziness, shortness of breath or troubled breathing, difficult micturition, acute urinary retention, dry mouth, N/V
AE (urised): generalized skin rash, dry mouth, flushing, difficulty in initiating micturition, rapid pulse, dizziness, blurring of vision, acute urinary retention
CI (flavoxate): intestinal obstruction, obstructive uropathy
CI (prosed/DS, urised): glaucoma, urinary bladder neck obstruction, pyloric or duodenal obstruction or cardiospasm, hypersensitivity to any of the ingredients

Flavoxate	EHL no data, PRC B, Lact ?
Urispas *Tab 200mg*	**Incontinence, bladder spasm:** 100-200mg PO tid-qid; **CH** >12y: see adults

16.1.3 Other Bladder Agents

AE (pentosan polysulfate): peripheral edema, headache, dizziness, nausea
AE (phenazopyridine): GI DO, headache, rash, hemolytic anemia, nephrotoxicity, hepatitis
CI (pentosan polysulfate): hypersensitivity to pentosan polysulfate sodium
CI (phenazopyridine): hypersensitivity to phenazopyridine, hepatitis, renal insufficiency

Pentosan Polysulfate	EHL 4.8h, PRC B, Lact ?
Elmiron *Cap 100mg*	**Interstitial cystitis:** 100mg PO tid
Phenazopyridine	EHL no data, PRC B, Lact ?
Phenazo *Tab 100mg, 200mg*	**Dysuria:** 200mg PO tid for 2d; ch 6-12y: 12mg/kg/d PO div tid for 2d

16.2   Erectile Dysfunction

MA/E (alprostadil): identical to prostaglandin E1 d vasodilation
MA/EF (sildenafil): specific phosphodiesterase inhibitor ⇒ relaxation of corpus cavernosal
smooth muscle cells ⇒ blood flow into cavernosal spaces ↑
MA/EF (yohimbine): alpha2-adrenergic blocker → erectogenic
AE (alprostadil): penile pain, neonatal apnea, bradycardia, fever
AE (sildenafil): headache, flushing, dyspepsia, abnormal vision, nasal congestion
AE (yohimbine): anxiety, nervousness, tremor, irritability, agitation, manic reactions,
bronchospasm, cough, antidiuresis, dizziness, headache, HTN, tachycardia, N/V, flushes
CI (alprostadil): priapism, hypersensitivity to alprostadil, neonatal respir. distress syndrome
CI (sildenafil): hypersensitivity to sildenafil, concurrent use of nitrates
CI (yohimbine): chronic inflammation of sexual organs, prostatitis, antidepressants,
tyramine-containing food, gastric/duodenal ulcers, hypersensitivity to yohimbine, children,
psychiatric patients, renal or liver disease

Alprostadil	EHL 5-10min, PRC X, Lact -
Caverject *Inj 20mcg/vial, Inj 10mcg/ml, 20mcg/ml* **Prostin VR** *Inj 500mcg/ml* **Generics** *Inj 0.5mg/ml*	**Erectile dysfunction:** 2.5mcg intracavernosal injection, incr prn stepwise by 2.5, 5, 10mcg to max 40mcg; 125- 250mcg intraurethral, incr decrease dose prn; max 1000mcg; max 2 uses in 24h
Sildenafil	EHL 4h, PRC B , Lact -
Viagra *Tab 25mg, 50mg, 100mg*	**Erectile dysfunction:** 50mg PO 0.5-4h before intercourse, incr prn to max 100mg PO; max 1dose/d; >65y: reduce dose
Tadalafil	EHL 17.5h, PRC B, Lact -
Cialis *Tab 10mg, 20mg*	**Erectile dysfunction:** 20mg PO prior to intercourse
Vardenafil	EHL 4-5h, PRC B, Lact -
Levitra *Tab 10mg, 20mg*	**Erectile dysfunction:** 5-20mg PO prior to intercourse
Yohimbine	EHL 0.6h, PRC N, Lact -
Yocon *Tab 5.4mg* **Generics** *Tab 2mg, 5.4mg, 6mg*	**Erectile dysfunction:** 5.4mg PO tid up to 10wk

16.3 Benign Prostatic Hyperplasia

16.3.1 Alpha-Reductase Inhibitors

MA/EF (finasteride): inhibition of the 5-α-reductase $\Rightarrow$ inhibition of transformation of testosterone into dihydrotestosterone $\Rightarrow$ prostatic hyperplasia $\downarrow$
AE (finasteride): sexual dysfunction, breast tenderness/enlargement
CI (finasteride): severe hepatic insufficiency, hypersensitivity to finasteride products

Dutasteride	EHL 5wk, PRC X, Lact +
Avodart *Cap 0.5mg*	**Benign prostatic hypertrophy:** 0.5mg PO qd

Finasteride	EHL 6h, PRC X, Lact -
Propecia *Tab 1mg* **Proscar** *Tab 5mg*	**Benign prostatic hypertrophy:** 5mg PO qd; DARF: not req

16.3.2 Peripheral Antiadrenergic Agents

MA/EF (tamsulosin, terazosin): selective blockage of α1-receptors in the smooth musculature of the prostate and the bladder neck $\Rightarrow$ urine flow$\downarrow$
AE (doxazosin): hypotension, dizziness, vertigo, headache; **AE** (tamsulosin, terazosin): dizziness, postural hypotension, headache, palpitations, retrograde ejaculation
CI (doxazosin): hypersensitivity to doxazosin products or other quinazolines
CI (tamsulosin, terazosin): postural dysregulation, severe hepatic insufficiency

Alfuzosin	
Xatral *Tab sust. release 10mg*	**Benign prostatic hypertrophy:** 10mg PO qd

Doxazosin	EHL 8.8-22hPRC C, Lact ?
Cardura *Tab 1mg, 2mg, 4mg* **Generics** *Tab 1mg, 2mg, 4mg*	**Benign prostatic hypertrophy:** ini 1mg PO qd, incr prn to max 8mg PO qd

Tamsulosin	EHL 9-13h, PRC B, Lact -
Flomax *Cap 0.4mg*	**Benign prostatic hypertrophy:** 0.4mg PO qd, incr prn after 2-4wk to 0.8mg PO qd; DARF: not req

Terazosin	EHL 9-12h, PRC C, Lact ?
Hytrin *Tab 1mg, 2mg, 5mg, 10mg* **Generics** *Tab 1mg, 2mg, 5mg, 10mg*	**Benign prostatic hypertrophy:** ini 1mg PO qd, incr prn to 2-10mg PO qd, max 20mg/d; DARF: not req

16.4 Prostate Cancer

MA/EF (bicalutamide, flutamide, nilutamide): competitive blocker of nuclear androgen receptors ⇒ action of androgens ↓; pure antiandrogen without gestagen-like effects
MA/EF (leuprolide, goserelin): GnRH agonist ⇒ gonadotropin secretion ↓, ovarian/testicular steroidogenesis ↓
AE (bicalutamide): hot flashes, diarrhea, pain
AE (flutamide): diarrhea, cystitis, rectal bleeding, hot flashes, liver injury
AE (goserelin): bone pain, hot flashes, gynecomastia, impotence, breakthrough bleeding
AE (leuprolide): amenorrhea, hot flashes, vaginal spotting, bone pain, N/V, edema
AE (nilutamide): hot flashes, gynecomastia, N/V, LFT ↑, blurred vision
CI (bicalutamide): hypersensitivity to bicalutamide products
CI (flutamide): hypersensitivity to flutamide products, severe hepatic impairment
CI (goserelin): hypersensitivity to goserelin products
CI (leuprolide): hypersensitivity to leuprolide products/GnRH agonists
CI (nilutamide): hypersensitivity to nilutamide, severe hepatic impairment, severe respiratory insufficiency

Bicalutamide	EHL 5.8d, PRC X, Lact ?
Casodex *Tab 50mg*	**Prostate CA:** 50mg PO qd
Flutamide	EHL 9.6h, PRC D, Lact ?
Euflex *Tab 250mg* **Generics** *Tab 250mg*	**Prostate CA:** 250mg PO tid
Goserelin	EHL 2.3-4.2h, PRC X, Lact -
Zoladex *Implants 3.6mg, 10.8mg*	**Prostate CA:** 3.6mg implant SC q4wk or 10.8mg implant SC q12wk
Leuprolide	EHL 3h, PRC X, Lact -
Eligard *Inj 10.2mg/syr, 28.2mg/syr* **Lupron** *Inj 5mg/ml* **Lupron Depot** *Inj 3.75mg/vial, 7.5mg/vial, 11.25mg/vial, 22.5mg/vial, 30mg/vial*	**Prostate CA:** 1mg SC qd or 7.5mg IM qmo or 22.5mg IM q3mo or 30mg IM q4mo; **implant:** 65mg SC q12mo
Nilutamide	EHL 38-59.1h, PRC C, Lact ?
Anandron *Tab 50mg*	**Prostate CA:** 300mg PO qd for 30d, then 150mg PO qd

16.5 Nephrolithiasis

MA/EF (allopurinol): inhibition of xanthine oxidase ⇒ uric acid formation ↓ ⇒ uricostatic
AE (acetoh. acid): N/V, headache; **AE** (allopurinol): pruritus, rash, allergic reactions, N/V, myelosuppression, leukopenia, hepatotoxicity, xanthic calculus; **AE** (K+ citrate): metabolic alkalosis, hyperkalemia, N/V, diarrhea; **CI** (acetoh. acid): serum creatinine > 2.5mg/dL, urine infected by non-urease-producing organism, patients amenable to surgery/antimicrobials; **CI** (allopurinol): allergy to allopurinol; **CI** (potassium citrate): severe renal impairment

Allopurinol	EHL 1-2h, PRC C, Lact ?
Zyloprim *Tab* 100mg, 200mg, 300mg **Novo-Purol** *Tab* 100mg, 200mg, 300mg **Generics** *Tab* 100mg, 200mg, 300mg	**Recurrent calcium oxalate stones:** 200-300mg PO qd; DARF: GFR (ml/min): 10-20: 200mg/ d; <10: 100mg/d
Potassium Citrate	EHL no data, PRC C, Lact ?
K-Lyte *Tab (efferv)* 25mEq **Polycitra-K** *Crystals* 30mEq/pkt, *Sol (oral)* 10mEq/5ml	**Nephrolithiasis:** 10-20mEq PO tid-qid, max 100mEq/d

16.6 Other Urologic Drugs

AE (bethan.): diarrhea, miosis, excessive lacrimation, flushing of skin;
AE (desm.): nausea, flushing, headache;
CI (bethan.): hyperthyroidism, peptic ulcer, asthma, bradycardia, hypotension, vasomotor instability, CAD, epilepsy, Parkinsonism, GI inflamm./spasms, peritonitis, vagotonia;
CI (desm.): hypersens. to desmopressin, ch < 3mo, Type IIB von Willebrand's

Bethanechol	EHL no data, PRC C, Lact ?
Duvoid *Tab* 10mg, 25mg, 50mg **Myotonachol** *Tab* 10mg, 25mg **Generics, pms** *Tab* 10mg, 25mg, 50mg	**Urinary retention:** 10-50mg PO tid-qid; 2.5-5mg SC tid- qid
Desmopressin	EHL IV 75.5min, PO 90-150min, PRC B, Lact ?
DDAVP *Tab* 0.1, 0.2mg, *Spray (nasal)* 0.01mg/Spray, *Inj* 0.004mg/ml **DDAVP Rhinyle Nasal Solution** pray 0.25mg/bot **Minirin** *Tab* 0.1mg **Octostim** *Spray (nasal)* 0.15mg/Spray, *Inj* 0.015mg/ml **Generics** *Spray (nasal)* 0.01mg/Spray	**Nocturnal enuresis:** >6y: ini 20mcg, intranasally hs, maint 10-40mcg; **diabetes insipidus; hemophilia A:**

17. Gynecology, Obstetrics

17.1 Sex Hormones, Hormone Drugs
17.1.1 Estrogens

MA/EF: sec. female sexual characteristics↑, proliferation of endometrium, liquefying of cervical mucus, protein anabolism, mineralocorticoid EF, Ca^{2+} resorption↑, Ca^{2+} uptake in bone↑;
AE: thrombosis, skin reactions, edema, glucose tolerance↓;
CI: hepatic DO, hormone dependent breast/uterus CA, previous thromboembolism, pancreatitis, previous HTN

Esterified Estrogens	EHL no data, PRC X, Lact -
Neo Estrone *Tab 0.3mg, 0.625mg, 1.25mg*	**Menopausal vasomotor symptoms:** 1.25mg PO qd, cyclically 3wk on/1wk off or contin. + progestin qd; **atrophic vaginitis:** 0.3-1.25mg PO qd, cyclically, if no response, >1.25mg/d; **female hypogonadism:** 2.5- 7.5mg PO qd div x 20d followed by a 10d rest period; rep until bleeding; **female castration, primary ovarian failure:** 1.25mg PO qd, cyclically; **breast CA palliation in certain patients:** 10mg PO tid ≥ 3mo; **PRO of postmenopausal osteoporosis:** 0.3-1.25mg PO qd, estrogen qd + progestin for last 10-12d of cycle
Estradiol	EHL 1h, PRC X, Lact -
Estrace *Tab 0.5mg, 1mg, 2mg*	**Menopausal vasomotor symptoms and atrophic vaginitis, female hypogonadism, female castration and primary ovarian failure:** 1-2mg PO qd, cyclically 3wk on/1wk off or continuous + progestin qd; **breast CA palliation in certain patients:** 10mg PO tid ≥ 3mo; **PRO of postmenopausal osteoporosis:** 0.5mg PO qd, cyclically 3 wk on/1 wk off or contin. with progestin qd, estrogen qd + progestin for last 10-12d of cycle; **atrophic vaginitis:** local application

Estradiol Transdermal System	EHL no data, PRC X, Lact -
Climara *Film (ext.rel, TD)* 0.05, 0.1mg/d **Estraderm** *Film (ext.rel, TD)* 0.025, 0.05, 0.1mg/d **Estradot** *Film (ext.rel, TD)* 0.0375, 0.05, 0.075, 0.1mg/d **Oesclim** *Film (ext.rel, TD)* 0.025, 0.05mg/d **Vivelle** *Film (ext.rel, TD)* 0.0375, 0.05, 0.075, 0.1mg/d	**Menopausal vasomotor symptoms and atrophic vaginitis, female hypogonadism, female castration and primary ovarian failure:** ini 0.025-0.05mg/d patch 1-2/wk, depending on the product, typical regimen: 3wk on and 1wk off or continuously + progestin qd, **postmenopausal osteoporosis** (PRO): 0.025 mg/d– 0.1mg/d patch
Estradiol Valerate	EHL no data, PRC X, Lact -
Generics *Inj* 10mg/ml	**Menopausal vasomotor symptoms and atrophic vaginitis, female hypogonadism, female castration and primary ovarian failure:** 10–20mg IM q4wk
Estrogens, Conjugated	EHL 4-18.5h, PRC X, Lact -
Premarin *Tab* 0.3mg, 0.625mg, 0.9mg, 1.25mg, *Crm (vag)* 0.625mg/g, *Inj* 25mg/vial **Generics** *Tab* 0.3mg, 0.625mg, 0.9mg, 1.25mg	**Abnormal uterine bleeding:** 25mg IV/IM q6-12h, **normalizing bleeding time in AV malformations and underlying renal impairment:** 30–70mg IV/PO qd until normal, estrogen qd + progestin for last 10-12d of cycle
Estrogens, Synthetic, Conjugated	EHL 4-18.5h, PRC X, Lact -
C.E.S. *Tab* 0.3mg, 0.625mg, 0.9mg, 1.25mg **Premarin** *Tab* 0.3mg, 0.625mg, 0.9mg, 1.25mg, *Crm (vag)* 0.625mg/g, *Inj* 25mg/vial **Generics** *Tab* 0.3mg, 0.625mg, 0.9mg, 1.25mg	**Menopausal vasomotor symptoms:** 0.625-1.25mg PO qd, cyclically 3wk on/1wk off or contin. + progestin qd; estrogen qd + progestin for last 10-12d of cycle
Estropipate	EHL no data, PRC X, Lact -
Ogen *Tab* 0.625mg, 1.25mg, 2.5mg	**Menopausal vasomotor symptoms, vulvar and vaginal atrophy:** 0.625-5mg PO qd cyclically 3wk on/ 1wk off or contin. + progestin qd; **female hypogonadism, female castration, primary ovarian failure:** 1.25-7.5mg PO qd cyclically 3wk on and 8-10d off; **PRO of osteoporosis:** 0.625mg PO qd x 25d/31d cycle; estrogen qd + progestin for the last 10-12d of the cycle

17.1.2 Selective Estrogen Receptor Modulators

MA/EF: bind on estrogen receptors ⇒ selective expression of estrogen regulating genes ⇒ bone density ↑, total + LDL cholesterol ↓; **AE:** hot flashes, leg cramps, higher risk of thromboembolic illnesses; **CI:** women of childbearing age, history of thromboembolism, hypersensitivity to raloxifene, severe hepatic/renal insufficiency, endometrial or breast CA

Raloxifene	EHL 27.7h, PRC X, Lact ?
Evista *Tab 60mg*	**Osteoporosis PRO/Tx:** 60mg PO qd; **breast CA PRO:** 60–120mg PO qd

17.1.3 Antiestrogens

MA/EF: (anastrozole, exemestane, letrozole): aromatase inhibition,
AE (aromatase inhibitors): hot flashes, nausea, fatigue, sweating, increased appetite,
CI (aromatase inhibitors): premenopausal, pregnancy, lactation
MA/EF (tamoxifen): blockage of peripheral estrogen receptors;
AE (tamoxifen): alopecia, bone pain, hot flashes, vaginal bleeding, cycle DO, hyperplasia of endometrium, N/V, hypercalcemia;
CI (tamoxifen): severe leuko- and thrombopenia, severe hypercalcemia

Anastrozole	EHL 50h, PRC D, Lact ?
Arimidex *Tab 1mg*	**Breast CA; adjuvant Tx (postmenopause):** 1mg PO qd

Exemestane	EHL 24h, PRC D, Lact ?
Aromasin *Tab 25mg*	**Breast CA; adjuvant Tx (postmenopause):** 25mg PO qd

Letrozole	EHL 2d, PRC C, Lact ?
Femara *Tab 2.5mg*	**Advanced or metastatic breast CA (postmenopause):** 2.5mg PO qd

Tamoxifen	EHL 5-7d, PRC D, Lact ?
Apo-Tamox *Tab 10mg, 20mg* Nolvadex *Tab 10mg, 20mg* Tamofen *Tab 10mg, 20mg* Generics *Tab 10mg, 20mg*	**Breast CA, adjuvant Tx/PRO in high-risk women:** 20mg PO qd x 5 y

17.1.4 Progestins

MA/EF: secretive transformation of endometrium, pregnancy maintenance, inhibition of ovulation, thickening of cervical mucus, body temperature ↑
AE: acne, hepatic dysfunction, edema, weight gain, nausea, headache, dysmenorrhea
CI: hepatic diseases, cholestasis, retained abort, vesicular mole

Levonorgestrel	EHL 11-45h, PRC X, Lact ?
Mirena *Intrauterine device (IUD) 52mg* **Norplant** *Implant 36mg* **Plan B** *Tab 0.75mg*	**Contraception:** implant complete system subdermal 8- 10cm above the elbow crease within 7d after onset of menses (Implant) or fundal insertion of IUD; **postcoital contraception:** 1 Tab PO, rep in 12h, Tx within 24-72h after sexual intercourse

Medroxyprogesterone Acetate	EHL 38-46 h, PRC D, Lact +
ratio-MPA *Tab 2.5mg, 5mg, 10mg* **Depo-Provera** *Inj 50mg/ml, 150mg/ml* **Gen-Medroxy** *Tab 2.5mg, 5mg, 10mg* **Novo-Medrone** *Tab 2.5mg, 5mg, 10mg* **Provera** *Tab 2.5mg, 5mg, 10mg, 100mg*	**Contraception:** 150mg IM q13wk, inj only during first 5d after onset of menses or within 5d postpartum if not breastfeeding or, if breastfeeding, at 6wk postpartum; **secondary amenorrhea:** 5-10mg PO qd x 5-10d; **abnormal uterine bleeding:** 5-10mg PO qd x 5-10d beginning on the 16th or 21st day of the cycle (after estrogen priming); **hormone replacement Tx to prevent endometrial hyperplasia:** 10mg PO qd for the last 12d mo, or 2.5-5mg PO qd continuously; **endometrial hyperplasia:** 10-30mg PO qd (long-term) or 40-100mg PO qd (short-term) or 500mg IM biw

Megestrol	EHL 13-105h, PRC D (Tab), X (Susp) Lact ?
Megace *Tab 40mg, 160mg, Susp 40mg/ml* **Generics** *Tab 40mg, 160mg*	**AIDS anorexia:** 800mg Susp PO qd; **palliative Tx of advanced CA of the breast:** Tab 40mg PO qid; **endometrial CA:** Tab 40-320mg/d in div doses; **endometrial hyperplasia:** 40-160mg PO qd x 3-4mo; **CA-associated anorexia/cachexia:** 80-160mg PO qid

Norethindrone	EHL 4-13h, PRC X, Lact -
Micronor *Tab 0.35mg*	**Amenorrhea, abnormal uterine bleeding:** 2.5-10mg PO qd x 5-10d during 2nd half of menstrual cycle; **endometriosis:** 5mg PO qd x 2wk, incr by 2.5mg q2wk to 15mg/d; **contraception:** (Micronor, Nor-qd) 1 Tab PO qd

Progesterone, micronized	EHL 16.8-18.3h, PRC X, Lact ?
Prometrium *Cap 100mg* Generics *Inj 50mg/ml*	**Hormone replacement Tx to prevent endometrial hyperplasia:** 200mg PO hs 12d/mo; **secondary amenorrhea:** 400mgPO hs x 10d; **hormone replacement Tx to prevent endometrial hyperplasia:** 100mg hs continuously

17.1.5 Hormone Replacement Combinations

Conjugated Estrogens + Medroxyprogesterone	PRC X, Lact -
Premplus *Tab 0.625mg + 5mg*	**Menopausal vasomotor symptoms, vulvar/vaginal atrophy, and PRO of postmenopausal osteoporosis:** 1 Tab containing estrogens PO qd d1–14, then 1 Tab containing estrogens/progestins PO qd d15–28 (Premphase); 1 Tab PO qd (Prempro)

Estradiol + Norethindrone	PRC X, Lact -
Estalis *Film (ext.rel, TD) (0.05mg + 0.14mg)/24h, (0.05mg + 0.25mg)/24h* Estracomb *Film (ext.rel, TD) (0.05mg + 0.25mg)/24h*	**Menopausal vasomotor symptoms, vulvar and vaginal atrophy, female hypogonadism, castration, primary ovarian failure, PRO of postmenopausal osteoporosis:** 2 patch/wk

Ethinyl Estradiol + Norethindrone	PRC X, Lact -
FemHRT *Tab 0.005mg + 1mg*	**Menopausal vasomotor symptoms, PRO of postmenopausal osteoporosis:** 1 Tab PO qd

17.2 Oral Contraceptives
17.2.1 Monophasics

MA (monophasics): administration of the same fixed amount of an estrogen-gestagen combination qd for 21 d ⇒ antigonadotropic effects ⇒ suppression of ovulation
AE/CI (monophasic): see triphasics →286

Desogestrel + Ethinyl Estradiol	PRC X, Lact -
Marvelon *Tab (21) 0.15mg + 0.03mg, Tab (21/7) 0.15mg + 0.03mg/plac* **Ortho-Cept** *Tab (21) 0.15mg + 0.03mg Tab (21/7) 0.15mg + 0.03mg/plac*	**Contraception:** 1 Tab PO qd
Ethinyl Estradiol + Ethynodiol	PRC X, Lact -
Demulen 30 *Tab (21) 0.03mg+2mg, Tab (21/7) 0.03mg+2mg/plac*	**Contraception:** 1 Tab PO qd
Mestranol + Norethindrone	PRC X, Lact -
Ortho-Novum 1/50 *Tab (21, 21/7) 0.05mg + 1mg/plac*	**Contraception:** 1 Tab PO qd
Ethinyl Estradiol + Levonorgestrel	PRC X, Lact -
Alesse *Tab (21, 21/7) 0.02mg + 0.1mg/plac* **Min-Orval** *Tab (21, 21/7) 0.03mg + 0.15mg/plac*	**Contraception:** 1 Tab PO qd; **postcoital contraception:** 0.1mg ethinyl estradiol + 0.5mg levonorgestrel or 5 Tab Alesse or 4 Tab Min-Orval, rep each in 12h within 72h after sexual intercourse
Ethinyl Estradiol + Norelgestromin	PRC X, Lact +
Evra *Film (ext.rel, TD) 0.75 + 6mg/d*	**Contraception:** apply 1 patch qd x 21 d then no patch for 7 d, repeat cycle
Ethinyl Estradiol + Norethindrone	PRC X, Lact -
Brevicon 0.5/35 *Tab 0.035mg + 0.5mg,* **Brevicon 1/35** *Tab 0.035mg + 1mg* **Loestrin 1.5/30** *Tab 0.03mg + 1.5mg* **Minestrin 1/20** *Tab 0.02mg + 1mg* **Ortho 1/35** *Tab 0.035mg + 1mg* **Ortho 0.5/35** *Tab 0.035mg + 0.5mg* **Select 1/35** *Tab 0.035mg + 1mg*	**Contraception:** 1 Tab PO qd

Ethinyl Estradiol + Norgestimate	PRC X, Lact -
Cyclen *Tab* 0.035mg + 0.25mg	**Contraception:** 1 Tab PO qd
Ethinyl Estradiol + Norgestrel	PRC X, Lact -
Ovral *Tab (21, 21/7)* 0.05mg + 0.25mg/plac	**Contraception:** 1 Tab PO qd; **postcoital contraception:** 2 Tab Ovral or 4 Tab Lo/ Ovral, rep each in 12h

17.2.2 Biphasics

MA (biphasic): first half of menstrual cycle: estrogen-only, or combination with low-dose gestagen; second half of menstrual cycle: regular estrogen-gestagen combination ⇒ inhibition of ovulation; **AE/CI** (biphasic): see triphasics →286

Ethinyl Estradiol + Norethindrone	PRC X, Lact -
Synphasic *Tab (10/11)* 0.035mg + 0.5mg/0.035mg + 1mg, *Tab (10/ 11/7)* 0.035mg + 0.5mg/0.035mg + 1mg/plac	**Contraception:** 1 Tab PO qd

17.2.3 Triphasics

MA: 3 phases with different estrogen + gestagen combination ⇒ inhibition of ovulation
AE (estrogen-gestagen combinations): seborrhea, acne, dizziness, headache, N/V, breast tenderness, depression, vaginal candidiasis, thrombotic events
CI (estrogen-gestagen combinations): hepatic dysfunction, cholestasis, hepatic tumors, hormone-dependent malignant tumors, past or present history of thrombosis

Ethinyl Estradiol + Levonorgestrel	PRC X, Lact -
Triphasil, Triquilar *Tab (6/5/10)* 0.03mg + 0.05mg/0.04mg + 0.075mg/0.03mg + 0.125mg, *Tab(6/5/10/7)* 0.03mg + 0.05mg/0.04mg + 0.075mg/0.03mg + 0.125mg/plac	**Contraception:** 1 tab PO qd
Ethinyl Estradiol + Norethindrone	PRC X, Lact -
Ortho 7/7/7 *Tab (7/7/7)* 0.035mg + 0.5mg/0.035mg + 0.75mg/0.035mg + 1mg	**Contraception:** 1 Tab PO qd
Ethinyl Estradiol + Norgestimate	PRC X, Lact -
Tri-Cyclen *Tab (7/7/7)* 0.035mg + 0.18mg/0.035mg + 0.215mg/0.035mg + 0.25mg	**Contraception, adult acne** (ortho tri-cyclen): 1 Tab PO qd

17.2.4 Progestin Only Contraceptives (Minipill)

MA: low-dose gestagen-only administration qd for 28 d ⇒ no inhibition (suppression) of ovulation, but cervical mucus viscosity ↑ ; **AE:** irregular menstrual cycles, intracyclic menstrual bleeding; **CI:** serious hepatic dysfunction

Norethindrone	EHL 4-13h, PRC X, Lact -
Micronor *Tab 0.35mg*	**Contracept.:** (Micronor, Nor-qd) 1 Tab PO qd

17.3 GnRH Agonists

MA/EF: high doses of gonadotropin releasing hormones ⇒ complete down regulation of pituitary receptors ⇒ production of sex hormones sinks to castration levels;
AE (goserelin): bone pain, hot flashes, gynecomastia, impotence, breakthrough bleeding;
AE (leuprolide): hot flashes, vaginal hemorrhage, bone pain, N/V, peripheral edema;
AE (nafarelin): acne, hot flashes, irregular menstrual bleeding, breast enlargement;
CI (goserelin): hypersensitiv. to goserelin; **CI (leuprolide):** hypersensitivity to leuprolide / GnRH agonists; **CI (nafarelin):** undiagnosed vaginal bleeding, hypersensitivity to nafarelin

Ganirelix Acetate	EHL 12.8h (1x), 16.2h (multiple), PRC X, Lact -
Orgalutran *Inj 250mcg/0.5ml*	**Infertility:** 250mcg SC qd during early to mid follicular phase, continue Tx qd until day of hCG administration

Goserelin	EHL 2.3h (female), PRC X, Lact -
Zoladex *Implant System 3.6mg/syringe, 10.8mg/syringe*	**Endometriosis:** 3.6mg implant SC q28d x 6mo or 10.8mg implant SC q12wk x 6mo; **palliative Tx of breast CA:** 3.6mg implant SC q28d; **endometrial thinning prior to ablat. for dysfunction. uterine bleeding:** 3.6mg SC 4wk preop or 3.6mg SC q4wk x 2, followed by surgery in 2–4wk

Leuprolide	EHL 3h, PRC X, Lact -
Lupron *Inj 5mg/ml* Lupron Depot *Inj 3.75mg/vial, 7.5mg/vial, 11.25mg/vial, 22.5mg/vial, 30mg/vial*	**Endometriosis/uterine leiomyomata (fibroids):** 3.75mg IM q mo or 11.25mg IM q3mox6mo (endometriosis) or x3mo fibroids); **central precocious puberty:** Inj: 50mcg/kg/d SC, incr by 10mcg/kg/d until total down regulation, Inj depot: 0.3mg/kg/4wk IM, incr by 3.75mg q4wk until adeq. down regulation

Nafarelin	EHL 2.7 h, PRC X, Lact -
Synarel *Spray 2mg/ml*	**Endometriosis:** 200mcg spray into one nostril q am, the other nostril q pm x 6mo, incr prn to 4 x 200mcg/d; **central precocious puberty:** 2 sprays into each nostril q am + qpm, incr prn to 1,800mcg/d

17.4 Fertility Drugs
17.4.1 Gonadotropins

AE (chorionic gonadotropin): headache, irritability, precocious puberty, gynecomastia, injection site pain;
AE (menotropins): adnexal torsion (with ovarian enlargement), ovarian cysts, flu-like symptoms, pulmonary/vascular complications;
CI (chorionic gonadotropin): precocious puberty, prostatic CA, other androgen dependent neoplasia, hypersens. to chorionic gonadotropin; epilepsy, migraine, asthma, cardiac/renal disease;
CI (menotropins): vaginal/intracranial bleeding, adrenal/thyroid DO, ovarian cysts or enlargement, primary ovarian failure, pituitary tumor, primary testicular failure

| Chorionic Gonadotropins, hCG
EHL 5.6h, PRC X, Lact ?

Pregnyl *Inj 10,000 U/vial*
Profasi HP *Inj 10,000 U/vial*

Follitropins, FSH
EHL 17-44h, PRC X, Lact ?

Gonal-F *Inj 75 U, 150 U/vial, 1200 U/vial*
Puregon *Inj 50, 100 U/vial*

Menotropins, FSH/LH
EHL 2.2-2.9h, PRC X, Lact ?

Humegon *Inj 75+75 U/vial* | **Induction of ovulation and pregnancy:** ini with menotropins 75U FSH/LH IM qd x 7-12d, then 5,000-10,000 U single shot of hCG IM the day after last menotropin dose, rep prn for 2 more cycles, if evidence for ovulation, incr mentropin dose prn to max 150U FSH/LH; **induction of spermatogenesis in male hypogonadotropic hypogonadism:** 75U FSH/LH IM 3x/wk, prior to administration of menotropins, hCG 5000 U IM 3x/wk until adequate serum testosterone levels and masculinization is achieved, then ini 75U FSH/LH IM 3x/ wk, reduce hCG to 2000 U 2 x/wk, continue for ≥ 4mo, incr prn to 150U FSH/LH |

17.4.2 Ovulatory Stimulants

AE (clomiphene): blurred vision, ovarian enlargement, vasomotor flushing, abdominal pain
CI (clomiphene): uncontrolled thyroid or adrenal dysfunction, liver disease, abnormal uterine bleeding, ovarian cysts, organic intracranial lesion

Clomiphene	EHL 5d, PRC D, Lact ?
Clomid *Tab 50mg* **Serophene** *Tab 50mg*	**Ovulation induction:** 50mg x 5d, ini at any time if no history of recent uterine bleeding, otherwise ini at 5th d of cycle, prn incr to 100mg x 5d in ≥ 30d, max 3 Tx

Gonadorelin	
Lutrepulse *Inj 3.2mg/10ml*	**Ovulation induction:** 1-20mcg SC/IV

17.5 Myometrial Relaxants

AE (indomethacin): headache, GI distress
AE (magnesium): flushing, hypotension, muscle weakness
AE (nifedipine): peripheral edema, headache, dizziness, tachycardia
AE (terbutaline): tremor, tachycardia, headache, nausea, palpitations
CI (indomethacin): hypersensitivity to the drug, asthma, history of recent rectal bleeding or proctitis, allergic reactions to ASA or other anti-inflammatories
CI (magnesium): 2hr preceding delivery, heart block
CI (nifedipine): hypersensitivity to nifedipine or other CCBs, symptomatic hypotension, persistent dermatologic reactions, CHF
CI (terbutaline): hypersensitivity to terbutaline products

Indomethacin	EHL 4.5h, PRC X, Lact -
Novo-Methacin *Cap 25mg, 50mg, Supp 50mg, 100mg* **Nu-Indo** *Cap 25mg, 50mg* **Rhodacine** *Supp 50mg, 100mg* **Generics** *Cap 25mg, 50mg, Supp 50mg, 100mg*	**Preterm labor** (2nd-3rd line): ini 50-100mg PO/PR, then 5mg PO/PR q6-12-48h; **primary dysmenorrhea:** 25mg PO tid-qid; **patent ductus arteriosus:** neonates <48h: 1st dose 0.2mg/kg, 2nd dose 0.1mg/kg, 3rd dose 0.1mg/ kg, 2-7d: 1st dose 0.2mg/kg, 2nd dose 0.2mg/kg, 3rd dose 0.2mg/kg, >7d: 1st dose 0.2mg/kg, 2nd dose 0.25mg/kg, 3rd dose 0.25mg/kg

Magnesium Sulfate	EHL no data, PRC A, Lact +
Generics *Inj 500mg/ml*	**Seizure prevention in preeclampsia or eclampsia:** 1- 4g IV x 2-4min, 5g in 250ml D5W IV inf, max 3ml/min or 4-5g of 50% sol IM q4h prn; **premature labor:** 6g IVx 20min, then 2-3g/h titrat. to ↓ contract.; DARF: required monitor serum level, maint urine output 100ml/4h

Nifedipine	EHL 49-137min (pregnancy), PRC C, Lact +
Adalat XL *Tab ext.rel 20mg, 30mg, 60mg* Apo, Nu-Nifed *Cap 5mg, 10mg* Apo-Nifed PA *Tab ext. rel. 10mg, 20mg* Novo-Nifedin *Cap 5mg, 10mg* Generics *Tab ext.rel 10mg, 20mg*	**Preterm labor:** ini 10mg PO/SL q20-30min, max 40mg in 1st h of Tx, if successful, maint 10-20mg PO q4-6h or 60- 160mg ext. rel PO qd; DARF: not required

Terbutaline	EHL 11-26 h, PRC B, Lact +
Bricanyl Tablets *Tab 2.5mg, 5mg*	**Preterm labor:** 0.25mg SC q30min up to 1mg/4h or 2.5- 10mcg/min IV, incr slowly to max 17.5-30mcg/min or 2.5- 5mg PO q4-6h

17.6 Labor Induction, Cervical Ripening

MA (oxytocin): contraction of uterine smooth muscle, promotion of milk ejection by stimulation of smooth muscle contraction in the mammary glan;
AE (dinoprostone): GI effects, back pain, fetal HR abnormality;
AE (misoprostol): diarrhea, abdominal pain;
AE (oxytocin): arrhythmias, subarachnoid hemorrhage, hypotension;
CI (dinoprostone): cardiac/pulmonary/renal/hepatic disease, hypersensitivity to dinoprostone products, history cesarean section/ traumatic delivery , cephalopelvic disproportion, fetal distress;
CI (misoprostol): hypersensitivity to misoprostol or prostaglandins;
CI (oxytocin): signific. cephalopelvic disproportion, unfavorable fetal positions, fetal distress, hypertonic uterus, when vaginal delivery is contraindicated, hypersensitivity to oxytocin, severe toxemia

Carbetocin	
Duratocin *Inj 100mcg/vial*	**Prevention of uterine atony:** 100mcg IV

Dinoprostone	EHL 2.5-5min, PRC X (C for cerv. ripen.), Lact ?
Cervidil *Insert ext.rel (vaginal) 10mg* **Prepidil** *Gel (endocervical) 0.5mg/syringe* **Prostin E2** *Tab 0.5mg, Gel (endocervical) 1mg/syringe, 2mg/syringe*	**Cervical ripening:** gel: 1 syringe via catheter placed into cervical canal below the internal os, rep prn q6h, max 3 doses. insert: 1 insert in the posterior fornix of the vagina
Ergonovine Maleate	PRC X, Lact ?
Generics *Inj 0.25mg/ml*	**Prevention of uterine atony:** 200mcg IV/IM
Misoprostol	EHL rapid, PRC X, Lact -
Generics *Tab 0.1mg, 0.2mg*	**Cervical ripening/labor induction:** 25–100mcg oral tablet intravaginally q3-4h, max 500mcg/24h or 50mcg PO q4h, max 6 doses or 200mcg PO q6-8h, max 2 doses
Oxytocin	EHL 3-5min, PRC X, Lact -, nasal spray +
Generics *Inj 10 U/ml*	**Induction/stimulation of labor:** 10U in 1000ml NS, 1- 2mU/min IV as continuous inf (6-12ml/h), incr by 1-2 mU/ min q30min until a contraction pattern is established, max 20mU/min; **promotion of milk ejection:** 1 spray in one nostril 2min prior to nursing during 1st wk of puerperium

17.7 Uterotonics

AE (carboprost): emesis/diarrhea, paresthesia, fever/chills, dystonia, breast tenderness
AE (methylergonovine): HTN, N/V, dizziness, palpitations, severe headache, hallucinations
CI (carboprost): hypersensitivity to prostaglandin, acute pelvic inflammatory disease
CI (methylergonovine): hypersensitivity to methylergonovine products, HTN/toxemia

Carboprost	EHL no data, PRC C, Lact ?
Hemabate *Inj 0.25mg/ml*	**Refractory post-partum uterine bleeding:** 250mcg IM, rep prn q15-90min, max 2mg

see Oxytocin →291

17.8 Vaginal Preparations
17.8.1 Antibacterials

Clindamycin Phosphate	EHL 1.5-5h, PRC B, Lact +
Dalacin *Crm (vag)* 2%	**Bacterialvaginosis:** 1 applicatorful (approx. 100mg clindamycin phosphate in 5g cream) intravaginally hs x 7d or one supp qhs x 3d

Metronidazole, local and systemic	EHL 6-11 h, PRC B/X (1st trimester), Lact ?
Flagyl *Cap* 500mg, *Crm (vag)* 10%, *Supp (vag)* 500mg MetroCream *Crm (top)* 0.75% MetroGel *Gel (top)* 0.75% Nidagel *Gel (vag)* 7.5mg/g Noritate *Crm (top)* 1% Generics *Tab* 250mg *Inj* 5mg/ml	**Bacterial vaginosis** (local): 1 applicatorful (approx. 37.5mg metronidazole/5g) vag hs or bid x 5d; **bacterial vaginosis** (systemic): Flagyl ER: 750mg PO qd x 7d, other oral Tab: 500mg PO bid x 7d, in pregnancy (not 1st trimester): 250 mg PO tid x 7d; **trichomoniasis:** 2g PO single dose or 250mg PO tid x 1wk or 375-500mg PO bid x 1wk, treat sex partners, too; **Giardia:** 250 mg PO tid x 5-7d; **pelvic inflammatory disease:** 500mg PO bid + ofloxacin 400mg PO bid x 14d; DARF: GFR (ml/min) >10: 100%, <10: 50%

17.8.2 Antifungals

AE (clotrimazole, nystatin, terconazole, tioconazole; topical): vaginal irritation/pain
CI (butoconazole, clotrimazole, miconazole, nystatin, terconazole): hypersensitivity to product ingredients
CI (tioconazole): hypersensitivity to tioconazole or miconazole products

Clotrimazole	EHL 3.5-5h, PRC B, Lact ?
Canesten *Crm* 1%, 2%, 10% **Canesten Insert Combi-Pak** *Supp (vag)* 200mg + *Crm* 1%, *Supp (vag)* 500mg + *Crm* 1% **Canesten Cream Combi-Pak** *Crm appl.* 500mg + *Crm* 1% Clotrimaderm *Crm (vag)* 1%, 2%	**Local Tx of vulvovaginal candidiasis:** 1 applicatorful 1% cream hs x 7d or 1 applicatorful 2% cream hs x 3d or 100mg Tab (vag) hs x 7d or 200mg Tab (vag) hs x 3d or 500mg Tab (vag) x 1, prn top cream for external symptoms bid x 7d

Econazole	PRC C, Lact ?
Ecostatin *Supp (vag) 150mg*	**Vaginal candidiasis:** 150mg vag qd x 3d
Fluconazole	EHL 30h, PRC C, Lact -
Diflucan *Tab 50mg,100mg, Cap 150mg, Susp 50mg/5ml, Inj 2mg/ml* **Generics** *Tab 50mg,100mg, Cap 150mg*	**vaginal candidiasis:** 150mg PO single dose
Miconazole	EHL 24 h, PRC C, Lact ?
Micatin *Crm 2%, Spray 2%* **Micazole** *Crm (vag) 2%* **Monistat** *Crm (vag) 2%, Supp (vag) 100mg, Supp (vag) 400mg, 1200mg* **Monistat 3** *Crm (vag) 4% applicators (total of 3)* **Monistat Derm** *Crm (top) 2%* **Monistat Dual-Pak** *Supp (vag) 100mg + Crm 2%, Supp (vag) 400mg + Crm 2%, Supp (vag) 1200mg + Crm 2%*	**Vulvovaginal candidiasis:** 1 applicatorful 2% cream vag hs x 7d or 100mg supp vag hs x7d or 200mg supp vag hs x 3d or 1200mg vag insert hs x 1, top cream for external symptoms bid x 7d
Nystatin	EHL not absorbed, PRC C, Lact ?
Candistatin *Crm 100,000 U/g* **Nilstat** *Powder 1 billion U/bottle, Crm 100,000 U/g, Oint 100,000U/g, Crm (vag) 100,000 U/g, Tab (vag) 100,000 U* **Nyaderm** *Crm 100,000 U/g, Oint 100,000 U/g, Crm (vag) 25,000 U/g*	**Local Tx of vulvovaginal candidiasis:** 100,000 U Tab vag hs x 2 wk, treat external lesions with cream
Terconazole	EHL 6.9 h, PRC C, Lact -
Terazol *Crm (vag) 0.4%, 0.8%, Supp (vag) 80mg* **Terazol Dual-Pack** *Supp (vag) 80mg + Crm (vag) 0.8%*	**Local Tx of vulvovaginal candidiasis:** 1 applicatorful 0.4% cream vag hs x 7d or 1 applicatorful 0.8% cream vag hs x 3d or 80mg supp vag hs x 3d
Tioconazole	EHL not absorbed, PRC C, Lact -
GyneCure Tandempak *Oint (vag) 6.5% + Crm (vag) 1%, Supp (vag) 300mg + Crm (vag) 1%*	**Local Tx of vulvovaginal candidiasis:** 1 applicator ful (approx. 4.6 g) vag hs x 1

17.8.3 Postmenopausal Vaginal Preparations

Estradiol Vaginal Ring	EHL no data, PRC X, Lact -
Estring *Insert (ext.rel, vag) 0.0075mg/24h*	**Menopausal atrophic vaginitis:** insert into upper 1/3 of vaginal vault, replace after 90d

Estradiol Vaginal Tablet	EHL no data, PRC X, Lact -
Oestrilin *Supp (vag) 0.25mg* **Vagifem** *Tab (vag) 25 mcg*	**Menopausal atrophic vaginitis:** ini 1 Tab (vag) qd x 2wk, maint 1 Tab (vag) 2x/wk

Estrogen Gel/Cream	PRC X, Lact ?
Estrogel *Gel (vag) 0.06%* **Neo Estrone** *Crm (vag) 1mg/g* **Oestrilin** *Crm (vag) 1mg/g* **Premarin** *Crm (vag, conjugated estrogens) 0.625mg/g*	**Atrophic vaginitis/kraurosis vulvae:** Estrogel: 2.5g intravaginally qd cyclically, 3wk on and 1 wk off, Premarin: 0.5-2g intravaginally qd cyclically, 3wk on and 1 wk off,

17.8.4 Other Vaginal Preparations

Progesterone Gel	EHL no data, PRC NR Lact ?
Crinone *Gel (vag) 8%*	**Progesterone supplementation in assisted reproduction technology:** 90mg progesterone (gel 8%) vag qd; **progesterone replacement in assisted reproduction technology:** 90mg progesterone (gel 8%) vag bid; **secondary amenorrhea:** progesterone (gel 4%) vag qod x 6 doses, prn gel 8% qod x 6 doses; **contraception:** fundal insertion of progestasert IUD

17.9 Other Gynecologic, Obstetric Drugs

AE (clonidine): CNS depression, orthostasis, localized reactions, dry mouth;
AE (danazol): hepatic dysfunction, weight gain, acne, menstrual disturbances;
AE (RHO Immune Globulin): chills, headache, intravascular hemolysis;
CI (clonidine): hypersensitivity to clonidine products, conduction defects, bleeding DO, injection site infection;
CI (danazol): undiagnosed abnormal vaginal bleeding, hepatic/renal/cardiac dysfunction;
CI (RHO Immune Globulin): hypersensitivity to human globulin B, Rho(D)/D(U) positive patients, Rho(D) negative patients sensitized to Rho(D)/D(U) antigens neonates, IgA deficiency

Clonidine	EHL 12 - 16 h, PRC C, Lact ?
Catapres Tab 0.1mg, 0.2mg **Dixarit** Tab 0.025mg **Generics** Tab 0.1mg, 0.2mg	**Menopausal flushing:** 0.1-0.4mg/d PO div bid-tid or TD 0.1mg/d (1 patch qwk)
Danazol	EHL 4.5h, PRC X, Lact ?
Cyclomen Cap 50mg, 100mg, 200mg	**Endometriosis:** ini 400mg PO bid, then decr to a dose sufficient to maintain amenorrhea x 3-6mo, max 9mo; **fibrocystic breast disease:** 100-200mg PO bid x 4- 6mo; **menorrhagia:** 100-400mg PO qd x 3mo; DARF: contraind. in RF
Doxylamine + Pyridoxine	
Diclectin Tab del. rel. 10mg + 10mg	**Nausea of pregnancy:** 2 Tab PO qhs and 1 Tab PO bid PRN
Rho(D) Immune Globuline	PRC C, Lact ?
BayRho-D Full Dose Inj 300mcg/vial **WinRho SDF** Inj 120mcg/vial, 300mcg/vial, 1000mcg/vial	**PRO of isoimmunization in Rh-negative women following spontaneous or induced abortion or termination of ectopic pregnancy** ≧12 wk gestation: 50mcg (Microdose) IM; **PRO of maternal sensitization ot the Rh factor in pregnancy/after childbirth:** 300mcg IM if fetal packed RBC volume that entered mother's blood due to fetomaternal hemorrhage <15ml (30ml of whole blood), if >15ml, admin 600mcg IM

18.   Toxicology

18.1   Drugs, Antidotes

Acetylcysteine	EHL 2.27h, PRC B, Lact ?
Mucomyst *Sol (inhal)* 20% Parvolex *Sol (inhal)* 200mg/ml Generics *Inj* 200mg/ml	**Acetaminophen toxicity:** loading dose 140mg/kg PO or NG as soon as possible, then 70mg/kg q4h x 17 doses, prn mix in water; IV use: pyrogen-free IV; acetylcysteine is available only through participating poison centers; **CH** adult dose
Atropine	EHL 4h, PRC C, Lact ?
Generics *Inj* 0.4, 0.6mg/ml	**Organophosphate poisoning:** 2-5 mg IV, rep prn q10- 30min; **CH** 0.05mg/kg IV, rep prn q10-30min
Charcoal	PRC B, Lact +
Charcodote (in sorbitol) *Liquid (oral)* 200mg/ml Charcodote aqueous (in water) *Liquid (oral)* 200mg/ml Charcodote TFS *Liquid (oral)* 200mg + 200mg (sorbitol)/ml	**Gut decontamination:** 25-100g (0.5-1g/kg or 10 times the amount of poison ingested) PO or NG as soon as possible, rep prn q4h; **CH** >1y: adult dose
Deferoxamine	EHL 3-6 h, PRC C, Lact ?
Desferal *Inj* 500mg/vial, 2g/vial Desferrioxamine Mesilate *Inj* 500mg/vial Generics *Inj* 500mg/vial	**Chronic iron overload:** 500mg-1,000mg IM qd and 2g IV inf (max 15mg/kg/h) with each unit of blood or 1-2g SC qd (20-40mg/kg/d) x 8-24h via contin. inf pump; **acute iron toxicity:** ini 1g IM, then 500mg IM q4h x 2 doses, rep prn 500mg IM q4-12h, max 6g/24h; IV route (only in patients with CVS collapse): ini 1g slowly IV (max 15mg/ kg/h), then 500mg x 4h for 2 doses at max rate of 125mg/ h, prn subsequent doses of 500mg x 4-12h at max rate of 125mg/h; DARF: contraind. unless undergoing dialysis
Digoxin Immune Fab	EHL 15-20h, PRC C, Lact ?
Digibind *Inj* 38mg/vial	**Digoxin intoxication:** single large dose intoxication: of vials= (total digital body load in mg/0.5) IV; based on steady-state concentrations: adult: of vials= ((serum digoxin in nmol/L x 0.781 x wt. in kg)/100) IV; **CH** of vials = ((serum digoxin in nmol/L x 0.765 x wt. in kg)/1000) IV

Dimercaprol	EHL very short (no exact data), PRC N, Lact ?
BAL in oil *Inj 100mg/ml*	**Arsenic/gold poisoning, mild:** 2.5mg/kg deeply IM 4x/d x 2d, bid on d3, then qd x 10d or until recovery; **arsenic/gold poisoning, severe:** 3mg/kg deeply IM q4h x 2d, qid on d3, bid x 10d or until recovery; **mercury poisoning:** ini 5mg/kg, then 2.5mg/kg qd-bid x 10d; **acute lead encephalopathy:** 4mg/kg q4h x 2-7d, after 1st dose, combined Tx with edetate calcium disodium at separate site; **lead poisoning, mild:** ini 4mg/kg, then 3mg/kg q4h x 2-7d; DARF: req

Edetate Calcium Disodium	EHL 1.4-3h, PRC C, Lact -
Calcium Disodium Versenate *Inj 200mg/ml*	**Lead poisoning:** rec dosage for blood lead level >20mcg/deciliter and <70mcg/deciliter: 1g/m²/d IM x 8-12h x 5d, then interrupt Tx x 2-4d, then rep prn 5-day course of Tx, max 75mg/kg/d, mix for IM use 1ml of inj concentrate with 1ml lidocaine or procaine 1%; DARF: CrCl (mg/deciliter) 2-3: 50% q24h x 5d, rep prn qmo, 3-4: 50% q48h x 3 doses, rep prn qmo, >4: 50% qwk, rep prn qmo

Ethanol	EHL 0.232mg/(ml x h), PRC N, Lact -
Ethanol	**Methanol poisoning:** if acidosis, visual changes, blood MeOH level >25mg/deciliter, ini loading dose 10ml/kg of 10% ethanol in D5W x 20-30min, maint 1-2ml/kg/h, maint blood ethanol level 100-150mg/deciliter

Flumazenil	EHL 41-79min, PRC C, Lact ?
Anexate *Inj 0.1mg/ml* **Generics** *Inj 0.1mg/ml*	**Benzodiazepine sedation reversal:** 0.2mg IV x 15sec, after 30sec prn 0.2mg q1min, max 1mg total dose, usual dose 0.6-1mg; **benzodiazepine overdose reversal:** 0.2mg IV x 30sec, after 30sec prn 0.3mg, then prn 0.5mg q1min, max 3mg total dose; DARF: not required

Fomepizole	EHL 5h (oral), PRC C, Lact ?
Antizol *Inj 1g/ml*	**Methanol/Ethylene glycol toxicity:** ini loading dose 15mg/kg slowly IV x 30min, then 10mg/kg slowly IV q12h x 4 doses, then 15mg/kg slowly IV q12h, then until ethylene glycol concentrations <20mg/deciliter or ini 15mg/kg PO, in 12h 5mg/kg PO, then 10mg/kg PO q12h ethylene glycol plasma levels =0; DARF: consider additional dialysis

Ipecac Syrup	PRC C, Lact ?
Generics *Syr*	**Induction of emesis:** 15-30ml PO, then 3-4 glasses of water, rep if vomiting does not occur within 20-30min; **CH** 1-12y: 15ml, then 1-2 glasses of water, rep if vomiting does not occur within 20-30min

Methylene Blue	PRC C, Lact ?
Generics *Inj 50mg/5ml*	**Methemoglobinemia (drug induced):** (1-2mg/kg IV 0.1- 0.2ml/kg of 1% sol) x 5min, do not use in cyanide poisoning; DARF: use with caution in severe RF

Penicillamine	EHL 1-7.5h, PRC D, Lact -
Cuprimine *Cap 125mg, 250mg* **Depen** *Tab 250mg*	**Wilson's disease:** 750mg-1.5g/d resulting incupriuresis of 2mg/d, adjust dosage based on urinary copper analysis and determination of free copper in the serum; **lead poisoning:** 1-1.5g/d x 1-2mo given 2h before or 3h after meals; DARF: GFR (ml/min) <50%: avoid drug

Pralidoxime	EHL 1.23h, PRC C, Lact ?
Protopam *Inj 1g/vial*	**Organophosphate toxicity (severe):** 1-2g IV in 100ml saline x 15-30min or IV at max rate of 200mg/min or as a 5% sol in water IV x >5min, rep prn in 1h 1g IV, then prn continuous IV inf at rate of 500mg/h; DARF: required (no exact data available)

Sodium Thiosulfate	PRC C, Lact ?
Generics *Inj 2.5g/10ml*	**Cyanide poisoning:** 12.5g IV at a rate of 0.625-1.25g/min; **CH** 412.5mg/kg or 7g/square meter body surface area IV at a rate of 0.625-1.25 g/min

Sorbitol	PRC N, Lact +
Generics *Sol (oral) 70%*	**Laxative:** 30-150ml (70% sol) PO or 120ml (25-30% sol) PR; **CH** 2-11y 2ml/kg (70% sol) PO or 30-60 ml (25- 30% sol) PR

May 2005

Su	1	
Mo	2	
Tu	3	
We	4	
Th	5	
Fr	6	
Sa	7	
Su	8	Mother's Day
Mo	9	
Tu	10	
We	11	
Th	12	
Fr	13	
Sa	14	
Su	15	
Mo	16	
Tu	17	
We	18	
Th	19	
Fr	20	
Sa	21	
Su	22	
Mo	23	Victoria Day
Tu	24	
We	25	
Th	26	
Fr	27	
Sa	28	
Su	29	
Mo	30	
Tu	31	

June 2005

We	1	
Th	2	
Fr	3	
Sa	4	
Su	5	
Mo	6	
Tu	7	
We	8	
Th	9	
Fr	10	
Sa	11	
Su	12	
Mo	13	
Tu	14	
We	15	
Th	16	
Fr	17	
Sa	18	
Su	19	Father's Day
Mo	20	
Tu	21	Summer Solstice
We	22	
Th	23	
Fr	24	St. Jean-Baptiste-Day (Quebec)
Sa	25	
Su	26	
Mo	27	
Tu	28	
We	29	
Th	30	

July 2005

Fr	1	Canada Day
Sa	2	
Su	3	
Mo	4	
Tu	5	
We	6	
Th	7	
Fr	8	
Sa	9	
Su	10	
Mo	11	
Tu	12	
We	13	
Th	14	
Fr	15	
Sa	16	
Su	17	
Mo	18	
Tu	19	
We	20	
Th	21	
Fr	22	
Sa	23	
Su	24	
Mo	25	
Tu	26	
We	27	
Th	28	
Fr	29	
Sa	30	
Su	31	

August 2005

Mo	1	Civic Holiday
Tu	2	
We	3	
Th	4	
Fr	5	
Sa	6	
Su	7	
Mo	8	
Tu	9	
We	10	
Th	11	
Fr	12	
Sa	13	
Su	14	
Mo	15	
Tu	16	
We	17	
Th	18	
Fr	19	
Sa	20	
Su	21	
Mo	22	
Tu	23	
We	24	
Th	25	
Fr	26	
Sa	27	
Su	28	
Mo	29	
Tu	30	
We	31	

September 2005

Th	1	
Fr	2	
Sa	3	
Su	4	
Mo	5	Labour Day
Tu	6	
We	7	
Th	8	
Fr	9	
Sa	10	
Su	11	
Mo	12	
Tu	13	
We	14	
Th	15	
Fr	16	
Sa	17	
Su	18	
Mo	19	
Tu	20	
We	21	
Th	22	Fall Equinox
Fr	23	
Sa	24	
Su	25	
Mo	26	
Tu	27	
We	28	
Th	29	
Fr	30	

October 2005

Sa	1	
Su	2	
Mo	3	
Tu	4	Jewish New Year
We	5	
Th	6	
Fr	7	
Sa	8	
Su	9	
Mo	10	Thanksgiving Day
Tu	11	
We	12	
Th	13	Yom Kippur
Fr	14	
Sa	15	
Su	16	
Mo	17	
Tu	18	
We	19	
Th	20	
Fr	21	
Sa	22	
Su	23	
Mo	24	
Tu	25	
We	26	
Th	27	
Fr	28	
Sa	29	
Su	30	Daylight Saving Time Ends
Mo	31	Halloween

November 2005

Tu	1	
We	2	
Th	3	
Fr	4	
Sa	5	
Su	6	
Mo	7	
Tu	8	
We	9	
Th	10	
Fr	11	Remembrance Day
Sa	12	
Su	13	
Mo	14	
Tu	15	
We	16	
Th	17	
Fr	18	
Sa	19	
Su	20	
Mo	21	
Tu	22	
We	23	
Th	24	
Fr	25	
Sa	26	
Su	27	
Mo	28	
Tu	29	
We	30	

December 2005

Th	1	
Fr	2	
Sa	3	
Su	4	
Mo	5	
Tu	6	
We	7	
Th	8	
Fr	9	
Sa	10	
Su	11	
Mo	12	
Tu	13	
We	14	
Th	15	
Fr	16	
Sa	17	
Su	18	
Mo	19	
Tu	20	
We	21	Winter Solstice
Th	22	
Fr	23	
Sa	24	Christmas Eve
Su	25	Christmas Day
Mo	26	Boxing Day, Hanukkah
Tu	27	
We	28	
Th	29	
Fr	30	
Sa	31	New Year's Eve

January 2006

Su	1	New Year's Day
Mo	2	
Tu	3	
We	4	
Th	5	
Fr	6	
Sa	7	
Su	8	
Mo	9	
Tu	10	
We	11	
Th	12	
Fr	13	
Sa	14	
Su	15	
Mo	16	
Tu	17	
We	18	
Th	19	
Fr	20	
Sa	21	
Su	22	
Mo	23	
Tu	24	
We	25	
Th	26	
Fr	27	
Sa	28	
Su	29	
Mo	30	
Tu	31	

February 2006

We	1	
Th	2	
Fr	3	
Sa	4	
Su	5	
Mo	6	
Tu	7	
We	8	
Th	9	
Fr	10	
Sa	11	
Su	12	
Mo	13	
Tu	14	Valentine's Day
We	15	National Flag of Canada Day
Th	16	
Fr	17	
Sa	18	
Su	19	
Mo	20	Family Day (Alberta)
Tu	21	
We	22	
Th	23	
Fr	24	
Sa	25	
Su	26	
Mo	27	
Tu	28	

March 2006

We	1	Ash Wednesday
Th	2	
Fr	3	
Sa	4	
Su	5	
Mo	6	
Tu	7	
We	8	
Th	9	
Fr	10	
Sa	11	
Su	12	
Mo	13	Commonwealth Day
Tu	14	
We	15	
Th	16	
Fr	17	St. Patrick's Day
Sa	18	
Su	19	
Mo	20	Spring Equinox
Tu	21	
We	22	
Th	23	
Fr	24	
Sa	25	
So	26	
Mo	27	
Tu	28	
We	29	
Th	30	
Fr	31	

April 2006

Sa	1	
Su	2	Daylight Saving Time Begins
Mo	3	
Tu	4	
We	5	
Th	6	
Fr	7	
Sa	8	
Su	9	Palm Sunday
Mo	10	
Tu	11	
We	12	
Th	13	Jewish Passover
Fr	14	Good Friday
Sa	15	
Su	16	Easter Sunday
Mo	17	Easter Monday
Tu	18	
We	19	
Th	20	
Fr	21	
Sa	22	
Su	23	Orthodox Easter Sunday
Mo	24	
Tu	25	
We	26	
Th	27	
Fr	28	
Sa	29	
Su	30	

May 2006

Mo	1	
Tu	2	
We	3	
Th	4	
Fr	5	
Sa	6	
Su	7	
Mo	8	
Tu	9	
We	10	
Th	11	
Fr	12	
Sa	13	
Su	14	Mother's Day
Mo	15	
Tu	16	
We	17	
Th	18	
Fr	19	
Sa	20	
Su	21	
Mo	22	Victoria Day
Tu	23	
We	24	
Th	25	
Fr	26	
Sa	27	
Su	28	
Mo	29	
Tu	30	
We	31	

June 2006

Th	1	
Fr	2	
Sa	3	
Su	4	
Mo	5	
Tu	6	
We	7	
Th	8	
Fr	9	
Sa	10	
Su	11	
Mo	12	
Tu	13	
We	14	
Th	15	
Fr	16	
Sa	17	
Su	18	Father's Day
Mo	19	
Tu	20	
We	21	Summer Solstice
Th	22	
Fr	23	
Sa	24	St. Jean-Baptiste-Day (Quebec)
Su	25	
Mo	26	
Tu	27	
We	28	
Th	29	
Fr	30	

July 2006

Sa	1	Canada Day
Su	2	
Mo	3	
Tu	4	
We	5	
Th	6	
Fr	7	
Sa	8	
Su	9	
Mo	10	
Tu	11	
We	12	
Th	13	
Fr	14	
Sa	15	
Su	16	
Mo	17	
Tu	18	
We	19	
Th	20	
Fr	21	
Sa	22	
Su	23	
Mo	24	
Tu	25	
We	26	
Th	27	
Fr	28	
Sa	29	
Su	30	
Mo	31	

August 2006

Tu	1	
We	2	
Th	3	
Fr	4	
Sa	5	
Su	6	
Mo	7	Civic Holiday
Tu	8	
We	9	
Th	10	
Fr	11	
Sa	12	
Su	13	
Mo	14	
Tu	15	
We	16	
Th	17	
Fr	18	
Sa	19	
Su	20	
Mo	21	
Tu	22	
We	23	
Th	24	
Fr	25	
Sa	26	
Su	27	
Mo	28	
Tu	29	
We	30	
Th	31	

September 2006

Fr	1	
Sa	2	
Su	3	
Mo	4	Labour Day
Tu	5	
We	6	
Th	7	
Fr	8	
Sa	9	
Su	10	
Mo	11	
Tu	12	
We	13	
Th	14	
Fr	15	
Sa	16	
Su	17	
Mo	18	
Tu	19	
We	20	
Th	21	
Fr	22	
Sa	23	Fall Equinox, Jewish New Year
Su	24	
Mo	25	
Tu	26	
We	27	
Th	28	
Fr	29	
Sa	30	

October 2006

Su	1	
Mo	2	Yom Kippur
Tu	3	
We	4	
Th	5	
Fr	6	
Sa	7	
Su	8	
Mo	9	Thanksgiving Day
Tu	10	
We	11	
Th	12	
Fr	13	
Sa	14	
Su	15	
Mo	16	
Tu	17	
We	18	
Th	19	
Fr	20	
Sa	21	
Su	22	
Mo	23	
Tu	24	
We	25	
Th	26	
Fr	27	
Sa	28	
Su	29	Daylight Saving Time Ends
Mo	30	
Tu	31	Halloween

November 2006

We	1	
Th	2	
Fr	3	
Sa	4	
Su	5	
Mo	6	
Tu	7	
We	8	
Th	9	
Fr	10	
Sa	11	Remembrance Day
Su	12	
Mo	13	
Tu	14	
We	15	
Th	16	
Fr	17	
Sa	18	
Su	19	
Mo	20	
Tu	21	
We	22	
Th	23	
Fr	24	
Sa	25	
Su	26	
Mo	27	
Tu	28	
We	29	
Th	30	

December 2006

Fr	1	
Sa	2	
Su	3	
Mo	4	
Tu	5	
We	6	
Th	7	
Fr	8	
Sa	9	
Su	10	
Mo	11	
Tu	12	
We	13	
Th	14	
Fr	15	
Sa	16	Hanukkah
Su	17	
Mo	18	
Tu	19	
We	20	
Th	21	
Fr	22	Winter Solstice
Sa	23	
Su	24	Christmas Eve
Mo	25	Christmas Day
Tu	26	Boxing Day
We	27	
Th	28	
Fr	29	
Sa	30	
So	31	New Year's Eve

January 2007

Mo	1	New Year's Day
Tu	2	
We	3	
Th	4	
Fr	5	
Sa	6	
Su	7	
Mo	8	
Tu	9	
We	10	
Th	11	
Fr	12	
Sa	13	
Su	14	
Mo	15	
Tu	16	
We	17	
Th	18	
Fr	19	
Sa	20	
Su	21	
Mo	22	
Tu	23	
We	24	
Th	25	
Fr	26	
Sa	27	
Su	28	
Mo	29	
Tu	30	
We	31	

February 2007

Th	1	
Fr	2	
Sa	3	
Su	4	
Mo	5	
Tu	6	
We	7	
Th	8	
Fr	9	
Sa	10	
Su	11	
Mo	12	
Tu	13	
We	14	Valentine's Day
Th	15	National Flag of Canada Day
Fr	16	
Sa	17	
Su	18	
Mo	19	Family Day (Alberta)
Tu	20	
We	21	Ash Wednesday
Th	22	
Fr	23	
Sa	24	
Su	25	
Mo	26	
Tu	27	
We	28	

March 2007

Th	1	
Fr	2	
Sa	3	
Su	4	
Mo	5	
Tu	6	
We	7	
Th	8	
Fr	9	
Sa	10	
Su	11	
Mo	12	Commonwealth Day
Tu	13	
We	14	
Th	15	
Fr	16	
Sa	17	St. Patrick's Day
Su	18	
Mo	19	
Tu	20	
We	21	Spring Equinox
Th	22	
Fr	23	
Sa	24	
Su	25	
Mo	26	
Tu	27	
We	28	
Th	29	
Fr	30	
Sa	31	

April 2007

Su	1	Palm Sunday, Daylight Saving Time Begins
Mo	2	
Tu	3	Jewish Passover
We	4	
Th	5	
Fr	6	Good Friday
Sa	7	
Su	8	Easter Sunday, Orthodox Easter Sunday
Mo	9	Easter Monday
Tu	10	
We	11	
Th	12	
Fr	13	
Sa	14	
Su	15	
Mo	16	
Tu	17	
We	18	
Th	19	
Fr	20	
Sa	21	
Su	22	
Mo	23	
Tu	24	
We	25	
Th	26	
Fr	27	
Sa	28	
Su	29	
Mo	30	

May 2007

Tu	1	
We	2	
Th	3	
Fr	4	
Sa	5	
Su	6	
Mo	7	
Tu	8	
We	9	
Th	10	
Fr	11	
Sa	12	
Su	13	Mother's Day
Mo	14	
Tu	15	
We	16	
Th	17	
Fr	18	
Sa	19	
Su	20	
Mo	21	Victoria Day
Tu	22	
We	23	
Th	24	
Fr	25	
Sa	26	
Su	27	
Mo	28	
Tu	29	
We	30	
Th	31	

June 2007

Fr	1	
Sa	2	
Su	3	
Mo	4	
Tu	5	
We	6	
Th	7	
Fr	8	
Sa	9	
Su	10	
Mo	11	
Tu	12	
We	13	
Th	14	
Fr	15	
Sa	16	
Su	17	Father's Day
Mo	18	
Tu	19	
We	20	
Th	21	Summer Solstice
Fr	22	
Sa	23	
Su	24	St. Jean-Baptiste-Day (Quebec)
Mo	25	
Tu	26	
We	27	
Th	28	
Fr	29	
Sa	30	

July 2007

Su	1	Canada Day
Mo	2	
Tu	3	
We	4	
Th	5	
Fr	6	
Sa	7	
Su	8	
Mo	9	
Tu	10	
We	11	
Th	12	
Fr	13	
Sa	14	
Su	15	
Mo	16	
Tu	17	
We	18	
Th	19	
Fr	20	
Sa	21	
Su	22	
Mo	23	
Tu	24	
We	25	
Th	26	
Fr	27	
Sa	28	
Su	29	
Mo	30	
Tu	31	

August 2007

We	1	
Th	2	
Fr	3	
Sa	4	
Su	5	
Mo	6	Civic Holiday
Tu	7	
We	8	
Th	9	
Fr	10	
Sa	11	
Su	12	
Mo	13	
Tu	14	
We	15	
Th	16	
Fr	17	
Sa	18	
Su	19	
Mo	20	
Tu	21	
We	22	
Th	23	
Fr	24	
Sa	25	
Su	26	
Mo	27	
Tu	28	
We	29	
Th	30	
Fr	31	

September 2007

Sa	1	
Su	2	
Mo	3	Labour Day
Tu	4	
We	5	
Th	6	
Fr	7	
Sa	8	
Su	9	
Mo	10	
Tu	11	
We	12	
Th	13	Jewish New Year
Fr	14	
Sa	15	
Su	16	
Mo	17	
Tu	18	
We	19	
Th	20	
Fr	21	
Sa	22	Yom Kippur
Su	23	Fall Equinox
Mo	24	
Tu	25	
We	26	
Th	27	
Fr	28	
Sa	29	
Su	30	

October 2007

Mo	1	
Tu	2	
We	3	
Th	4	
Fr	5	
Sa	6	
Su	7	
Mo	8	Thanksgiving Day
Tu	9	
We	10	
Th	11	
Fr	12	
Sa	13	
Su	14	
Mo	15	
Tu	16	
We	17	
Th	18	
Fr	19	
Sa	20	
Su	21	
Mo	22	
Tu	23	
We	24	
Th	25	
Fr	26	
Sa	27	
Su	28	Daylight Saving Time Ends
Mo	29	
Tu	30	
We	31	Halloween

November 2007

Th	1	
Fr	2	
Sa	3	
Su	4	
Mo	5	
Tu	6	
We	7	
Th	8	
Fr	9	
Sa	10	
Su	11	Remembrance Day
Mo	12	
Tu	13	
We	14	
Th	15	
Fr	16	
Sa	17	
Su	18	
Mo	19	
Tu	20	
We	21	
Th	22	
Fr	23	
Sa	24	
Su	25	
Mo	26	
Tu	27	
We	28	
Th	29	
Fr	30	

December 2007

Sa	1	
Su	2	
Mo	3	
Tu	4	
We	5	Hanukkah
Th	6	
Fr	7	
Sa	8	
Su	9	
Mo	10	
Tu	11	
We	12	
Th	13	
Fr	14	
Sa	15	
Su	16	
Mo	17	
Tu	18	
We	19	
Th	20	
Fr	21	
Sa	22	Winter Solstice
Su	23	
Mo	24	Christmas Eve
Tu	25	Christmas Day
We	26	Boxing Day
Th	27	
Fr	28	
Sa	29	
Su	30	
Mo	31	New Year's Eve

315

January 2008

Tu	1	New Year's Day
We	2	
Th	3	
Fr	4	
Sa	5	
Su	6	
Mo	7	
Tu	8	
We	9	
Th	10	
Fr	11	
Sa	12	
Su	13	
Mo	14	
Tu	15	
We	16	
Th	17	
Fr	18	
Sa	19	
Su	20	
Mo	21	
Tu	22	
We	23	
Th	24	
Fr	25	
Sa	26	
Su	27	
Mo	28	
Tu	29	
We	30	
Th	31	

February 2008

Frh	1	
Sa	2	
Su	3	
Mo	4	
Tu	5	
We	6	Ash Wednesday
Th	7	
Fr	8	
Sa	9	
Su	10	
Mo	11	
Tu	12	
We	13	
Th	14	Valentine's Day
Fr	15	National Flag of Canada Day
Sa	16	
Su	17	
Mo	18	Family Day (Alberta)
Tu	19	
We	20	
Th	21	
Fr	22	
Sa	23	
Su	24	
Mo	25	
Tu	26	
We	27	
Th	28	
Fr	29	

316 Appendix

Poison Control Centers

ALBERTA
Poison and Drug Information Services,
Foothills General Hospital,
1403-29th St. N.W.
Calgary, AB. T2N 2T9
1-800-332-1414;
(403) 670-1414 local;
(403) 670-1472 (fax)

BRITISH COLUMBIA
B.C. Drug and Poison Information Centre,
St. Paul's Hospital,
1081 Burrard St.,
Vancouver, BC V6Z 1Y6
1-800-567-8911;
(604) 682-5050 local;
(604) 631-5262 (fax);
E-mail: daws@dpk.bc ca

MANITOBA
Provincial Poison Information Centre,
Children's Hospital Health Sciences Centre
840 Sherbrook St.,
Winnipeg, MB R3A 1S1
(204) 787-2591 emergency inquiries;
(204) 787-2444 general inquiries;
(204) 787-4807 (fax)

NEW BRUNSWICK
Poison Control Centre,
The Moncton Hospital,
135 McBeath Ave.,
Moncton, NB E1C 6Z8
(506) 857-5555 emergency inquiries;
(506) 857-5353 general;
(506) 857-5360 (fax)

Emergency Department,
Saint John Regional Hospital,
P.O.Box 2100;
Saint John, NB E2L 4L2
(506) 648-6222 local;
(506) 648-6901 (fax)

NEWFOUNDLAND
Provincial Poison Control Centre,
The Dr. Charles A. Janeway Child Health Centre,
710 Janeway Place,
St. John's, NF A1A 1R8;
(709) 722-1110

NORTHWEST TERRITORIES
Emergency Department,
Stanton Yellowknife Hospital,
P.O.Box 10,
Yellowknife, NT X1A 2N1
(867) 669-4100

NOVA SCOTIA
Poison Control Centre,
The Izaak Walton Killam Children's Hospital,
P.O.Box 3070,
Halifax, NS B3J 3G9
(902) 428-8161 local;
(902) 428-3213 (fax);
1-800-565-8161 toll free from P.E.I

ONTARIO
Ontario Regional Poison Information Centre
Children's Hospital of Eastern Ontario,
401 Smyth Road,
Ottawa, ON K1H 8L1
1-800-267-1373 toll-free Ontario;
(613) 737-1100 emergency inquiries;
(613) 737-2320 general inquiries;
(613) 738-4862 (fax)

Ontario Regional Poison Information Centre,
The Hospital for Sick Children,
555 University Ave.,
Toronto, ON M5G 1X8
1-800-268-9017 toll-free;
(416) 598-5900 local;
(416) 813-7489 (fax)

PRINCE EDWARD ISLAND
Poison Control Centre,
The Izaak Walton Killam Children's Hospital,
P.O.Box 3070,
Halifax, NS B3J 3G9
1-800-565-8161 toll free from P.E.I

QUÉBEC
Centre antipoison du Québec,
Le Centre Hospitalier de l'Université Laval
2705 boul. Laurier,
Sainte-Foy, PQ G1V 4G2
1-800-463-5060;
(418) 656-8090;
(418) 654-2747 (fax)

SASKATCHEWAN
Emergency Department,
Regina General Hospital,
1440 14th Ave.,
Regina, SK S4P 0W5;
1-800-667-4545
(306)359-4545;
(306)359-4357(fax)

Emergency Department,
Royal University Hospital,
Saskatoon, SK S7N 0X0
1-800-363-7474;
(306) 966-1010;
(306) 966-1011 (fax)

YUKON TERRITORY
Emergency Department,
Whitehorse General Hospital,
5 Hospital Road, Whitehorse, YT Y1A 3H7
(403) 667-8726;
(403) 667-2471 (fax)

Bibliography

1. Arana GW, Hyman SE, Rosebaum JF, ed: Handbook of Psychiatric Drug Therapy, edn 4. Philadelphia: Lippincott Williams & Wilkins, 2000.

2. Bartlett JD, Jaanus SD, ed: Clinical Ocular Pharmacology, edn 4. Woburn: Butterworth-Heinemann, 2001.

3. Bauer LA, ed: Applied Clinical Pharmacokinetics, edn 1. New York: McGraw-Hill, 2001.

4. Bezchlibnyk-Butler KZ, ed: Clinical Handbook of Psychotropic Drugs, edn 11. Seattle, Hogrefe and Huber, 2001.

5. Billups NF, Billups SM, ed: American Drug Index 2001, edn 45. Philadelphia: Facts & Comparisons, 2001.

6. Braunwald E, Fauci AS, Kasper DL, Hauser SL, Longo DL, Jameson JL, ed: Harrison's Principles of Internal Medicine, edn 15. New York: Lippincott Williams & Wilkins, 2001.

7. Canadian Immunization Guide. Sixth Edition, http://www.hc-sc.gc.ca/, Health Canada, 2002.

8. Colbert BJ, Mason BJ, ed: Integrated Cardiopulmonary Pharmacology, edn 1. Upper Saddle River: Prentice Hall, 2001.

9. Compendium of Pharmaceuticals and Specialties, Thirty-sixth Edition. Canadian Pharmacists Association, 2001.

10. Compendium of Pharmaceuticals and Specialties. Thirty-seventh Edition. Canadian Pharmacists Association, 2002.

11. Compendium of Pharmaceuticals and Specialties. Thirty-eight Edition. Canadian Pharmacists Association, 2003.

12. Compendium of Pharmaceuticals and Specialties. Thirty-nine Edition. Canadian Pharmacists Association, 2004.

13. Compendium of Pharmaceuticals and Specialties. Fortieth Edition. Canadian Pharmacists Association, 2005.

14. Drug Product Database, http://www.hc-sc.gc.ca/hpb/drugs-dpd/, Health Canada.

15. Electronic Orange Book, http://www.fda.gov/cder/ob/, FDA, 2001.

16. Gibaldi M, ed: Drug Therapy, 2000: A Critical Review of Therapeutics, edn 1. New York: McGraw-Hill, 2000.

17. Joel G, Hardman LE, ed: Goodman & Gilman's The Pharmacological Basis of Therapeutics, edn 10. New York: McGraw-Hill, 2001.

18. Russ A, Nudo CG, Canadian Drug Pocket, first edition: Borm Bruckmeier Publishing, 2004.

19. Mycek MJ, Harvey RA, Champe PC, ed: Lippincott's Illustrated Reviews: Pharmacology: Special Millennium Update, edn 2. Philadelphia: Lippincott Williams & Wilkins, 2000.

20. Physician's Desk Reference 2001 (Library Edition), edn 55. Oradell: Physician's Desk Reference, 2001.

21. Reese RE, Betts RF, Gumustop B, ed: Handbook of Antibiotics, edn 3. Philadelphia: Lippincott Williams & Wilkins, 2000.

22. Skolnick P, ed: Antidepressants: New Pharmacological Strategies; edn 1. Totowa: Humana Press, 1997.

23. Wolverton SE, ed: Comprehensive Dermatologic Drug Therapy, edn 1. London: Saunders, 2001

Important Formulas

A–a O_2 gradient
= $(Fi_{O_2}\% / 100) \times (P_{atm} - 47\,mmHg) - (Pa_{CO_2} / 0.8) - Pa_{O_2}$
(all units in mmHg)

Anion gap
= $(Na^+ + K^+) - (Cl^- + [HCO_3^-])$
(all units mmol/L)

BSA (m^2)
= $\sqrt{height(cm) \times weight(kg)/60}$
(Mosteller. NEJM 1987; 317:109)

Lean Body Weight (men)
= $(1.10 \times weight(kg)) - 128 \, (weight^2 / (100 \times height(m))^2)$
Lean Body Weight (women)
= $(1.07 \times weight(kg)) - 148 \, (weight^2 / (100 \times height(m))^2)$

Ideal Body Weight (men)
= $50 + 2.3 \, (height(in) - 60)$
Ideal Body Weight (women)
= $45.5 + 2.3 \, (height(in) - 60$

Body Mass Index
= $Weight(kg) / Height(m)^2$

Estimated Creatinine Clearance (CrCl ml/min)
= $[[140 - age(yr)] \times weight(kg)] / [72 \times serum\,Cr(mg/dL)]$
(multiply by 0.85 for women); Cr: $\mu mol/l = 88.4 \times mg/dl$

Fractional Excretion of Sodium (FE_{Na})
= $(U_{Na} \times P_{Cr}) / (P_{Na} \times U_{Cr}) \times 100$

Serum Osmolality
= $(2 \times (Na^+ + K^+)) + (BUN) + (glucose)$
(all units mmol/L)

Notes

Index

Numerics

A

- typhoid fever 164
- varicella 163
- yellow fever 163
Immunoglobulins 164
Immunosuppressants 170
Immunosuppressives 166
Immunosupression 164
Imodium 80
Imogam 165
Imovax 163
Impetigo 237
Imuran 170
Inactivated Poliomyelitis Vaccine (IPV) 163
Incontinence
- urinary 274, 275
Indapamide 33
Inderal 15, 22, 202
Inderal LA 22, 202
Indinavir 151
Indomethacin 175, 176, 289
Indotec 176
Infarction
- myocardial 14, 20, 21, 22, 52, 53
Infection
- anaerobic 135
- anaerobic bacterial 140
- bone 125, 126, 127, 136
- campylobacter jejuni 132
- chlamydia 132
- CMV 144
- endocarditis 134
- genitourinary tract 121
- gram-negative 133
- HIV 148, 149, 150, 151
- intra-abdominal 122, 126, 127, 128, 129
- joint 125, 126
- life-threatening 127
- meningococcal 142
- MRSA 129
- mycobacterium avium 141
- mycoplasma pneumoniae 132

- nongonococcal urethritis 132
- ocular 253, 254, 255
- pneumocystis 143, 155, 156
- respiratory syncytial virus 147
- respiratory tract 121, 122, 125, 127, 128, 132
- sepsis 125
- severe fungal 152
- severe UTI 128
- skin 121, 122, 124, 125, 127, 128, 237
- soft tissue 124
- staphylococcal 120, 129
- streptococcal 129
- urinary tract 122
- UTI 125, 127, 128, 135, 138, 139, 141
- varicella zoster 144
Infergen 146
Infertility 287
Inflammatory disease 105, 106
Infliximab 88, 89
Influenza
- A 145
- Drugs 145
- Immunization 162
Influenza Vaccine 162
Infufer 96
Inhibace 23
Inhibace Plus 25
Inhibitors 29
- adrenergic 29
Innohep 51
Insect bites 247
Insomnia 197, 227, 229
Insufficiency
- adrenal 105, 106
Insulin
- Aspart 110
- Glargine 111
- Lente 111
- Lispro 110, 111
- Lispro-protamine 111
- NPH 111

- Regular 110, 111
- Ultralente 111
Insulins 110
- biphasic 111
- long-acting 111
- short-acting 110
Intal 67
Integrilin 54
Interferon 146
Interferon
- alfa 2a 146
- alfa 2b 146
- alfa-2b 146
- alfacon-1 146
- beta 1a 146
- beta 1b 146
Interferons 146
Interstitial cystitis 275
Intolerance
- lactose 85
Intoxication
- arsenic 297
- benzodiazepine 297
- ethylene glycol 297
- gold 297
- iron 296
- lead 297, 298
- magnesium 93
- methanol 297
- organophosphate 296, 298
Intrinsic
- sympathomimetic activity 22
Intron A 146
Intropin 10
Invirase 152
Iodine 38, 114, 155, 273
Iodoquinol 155
Ionamin 113
Ions 92
Iopidine 258
Ipecac Syrup 298
Ipol 163
Ipratropium 63, 65, 267
Ipratropium Bromide 65, 267
Irbesartan 26

Iron 96
- deficiency 96
- poisoning 296
Iron Dextran 96
Iron Sucrose 96
Irritable bowel syndrome 88
ISA 22
Ischemic stroke 52, 55
Isocaine 12, 191
Isocaine (with levonordefrin) 12, 191
Isoniazid 101, 141, 142
Isoproterenol 38, 40, 61
Isoptin 16, 28
Isoptin SR 28
Isopto Atropine 261
Isopto Carpine 260
Isopto Homatropine 261
Isopto Tears 264
Isosorbide Dinitrate 36
Isosorbide-5-Mononitrate 36
Isotamine 142
Isotretinoin 235, 236
Isotrex 237
Itching 247
Itraconazole 152, 153
Ivcegam Immuno 165
Ivermectin 155

J

Japanese encephalitis
- Immunization 163
Japanese Encephalitis Vaccine 162, 163
JE-Vax 163

K

K-10 92
Kaletra 151
Kaopectate 80
Kaposi's sarcoma 251
Kayexalate 100
K-Dur 92
Kemadrin 204

M

M.O.S. Sulfate 181
Maalox 76, 77
Macrobid 138
Macrodantin 138
Macrolides 131
Mafenide 236, 237
Maglucate 95
Magnesium 94
Magnesium
- Carbonate + Alginic acid 77
- Chloride 94
- Citrate 78
- Glucoheptonate 95
- Gluconate 95
- Hydroxide 76, 79
- Oxide 95
- Sulfate 12, 95, 290
Magnesium Hydroxide 76
Magnesium intoxication 93
Magnesium sulfate 12, 95, 290
Magnonat 94
Majeptil 222
Malaria 158
Malarone 158
Mandelamine 138
Manerix 215
Mania 194, 196
- acute 219
Mannitol 207
MAOI 215
Maprotiline 214
Marcaine 191
Marinol 83
Marvelon 285
Mast Cell Stabilizers 67
Maternal antepartum 105
Mavik 24
Maxalt 200
Maxipime 128
Maxitrol 257
Measles + Mumps + Rubella Vaccine (MMR) 159
Mebendazole 155
Meclizine 210

Medrol 13, 106
Medroxyprogesterone 283, 284
- Acetate 283
Mefenamic Acid 177
Mefloquine 157, 158
Megace 283
Megaloblastic anemia 103
Megestrol 283
Meglitinides 108
Mellaril 222
Meloxicam 177
Meningitec 160
Meningitis 121, 125, 127
- meningococcal 119
Meningococcal
- Immunization 160
Meningococcal Polysaccharide Vaccine 160
Menjugate 160
Menopausal
- flushing 295
- vasomotor symptoms 280, 281, 284
Menotropins 117, 288
Meperidine 180, 215
Mepivacaine 12, 190, 191
Meprobamate 209
Mepron 155
Mequinol 252
Meridia 113
Meropenem 129
Merrem 129
Mesalamine 84
Mesasal 84
M-Eslon 181
Mesoridazine 221
Mestinon 208
Mestranol 285
Mestranol + Norethindrone 285
Metabolic acidosis 16
Metadol 180, 231
Metaxalone 208
Metformin 109, 110
Methacholine 71
Methadone 180, 231
Methanol
- poisoning 297

Methazolamide 35
Methemoglobinemia 298
Methenamine 138
- Hippurate 138
- Mandelate 138
Methimazole 115
Methocarbamol 178, 179, 208, 209, 210
Methotrexate 170
Methotrimeprazine 222
Methoxacet Extra Strength 178
Methoxisal 179
Methsuximide 197
Methylcellulose 79, 264
Methyldopa 29, 35
Methylene Blue 298
Methylergonovine 291
Methylphenidate 232, 233
Methylprednisolone 13, 106
Methysergide 201
Metoclopramide 13, 83
Metolazone 33
Metoprolol 21
MetroCream 237, 292
MetroGel 237, 292
Metronidazole 75, 118, 140, 151, 155, 156, 237, 292
Mevacor 45
Mexiletine 37, 41
Mezlocillin 118
Miacalcin 99
Micanol 243
Micardis 24
Micatin 238, 293
Micazole 293
Miconazole 238, 292, 293
Micro-K 92
Micronor 284, 287
Midazolam 150, 152, 186
Midodrine 18
Migraine 22, 202
- prophylaxis 194
- therapy 200
Migranal 201
Milk ejection
- promotion 291

Milrinone 43
Mineral Oil 79
Minerals 92
Minestrin 1/20 285
Minipill 287
Minipress 30
Minirin 59, 117, 279
Minitran 37
Minocin 130
Minocycline 130
Minor eye irritation 264
Min-Orval 285
Minox 249
Minoxidil 31, 32, 249
Mirapex 205
Mirena 283
Mirtazapine 218
Misoprostol 75, 175, 290, 291
Mivacron 190
Mivacurium 189, 190
Mobicox 177
Moclobemide 215
Modafinil 232, 233
Modecate 224
Mogadon 197
Mometasone 246, 267, 268
- Furoate 246
Monistat 238, 293
Monistat 3 293
Monitan 20
Monoamine Oxidase
- Inhibitors 215
Monocor 20
Monophasics 285
Monopril 23
Montelukast 66
Monurol 141
Morphine 13, 179, 181, 187
Morphine 181
Morphine Sulfate 181
Motion sickness 82, 210, 266
Mouth preparations 291
Moxifloxacin 137
MS contin 181
MSD Enteric Coated ASA 172

S   **343**

ECG pocket

PDA Software by Börm Bruckmeier

Drug pocket for PDA   The new drug list
  clear structure organized by major drug categories and indications

Drug Therapy pocket for PDA
  therapy schemes for all major diseases

ICD-9-CM pocket for PDA
  all official codes, > 32,000 index entries, > 136,000 cross-references

Medical Abbreviations pocket for PDA
  over 10,000 abbreviations and acronyms

ECG pocket for PDA
  handy reference for identifying
  the most important ECG findings

**Differential Diagnosis
pocket** for PDA
  over 800 lists of symptoms,
  signs and abnormal findings

Medical Abbreviations pocket
🏠 Abb | Txt | Sym | 🗓 🗒 ◀ | ?
• **Index by Abbreviation**
• **Index by Text**
• **Search for Symbol**
• My Bookmarks
• About
• Help

Homeopathy pocket for PDA
  extensive descriptions of more
  than 100 homeopathic remedies

Medical Spanish pocket for PDA
  essential tool for communicating with Spanish-speaking patients

Medical Spanish Dictionary pocket for PDA
  over 40,000 entries, English-Spanish and Spanish-English

Medical Spanish pocket PLUS for PDA
  includes contents of Medical Spanish pocket for PDA as well as
  Medical Spanish Dictionary pocket for PDA

coming soon: Normal Values pocket for PDA
  all important normal reference laboratory values

Table of Contents, Text samples, PDA demo files... www. **media4u** .com

Neurology pocketcard Set

Neurology pocketcard is a clearly organized set of two plastic cards providing all the important information on:

- Neurological examination
- Dermatomes
- Innervations and clinical findings of ocular muscles
- Topodiagnostic relevance of ocular movement disorders
- Clinically relevant muscles and their innervation
- Mini Mental State Test
- Glasgow Coma Scale
- Procedure for patients with impaired consciousness of unclear origin
- Vascular territories of the cerebral hemispheres
- Intracranial cerebral vessels
- Cerebrospinal fluid (CSF), CSF serum ratio

ISBN 1-59103-021-8
US $ 6,95

Neurology pocketcards represent a must-have companion for every medical professional.

Börm
Bruckmeier
Verlag

www.media4u.com

Börm Bruckmeier Publishing
PO Box 388
Ashland, OH 44805

Börm
Bruckmeier
Publishing

Phone: 888-322-6657
Fax: 419-281-6883

Name		E-mail	
Address			
City		State	Zip

Subtotal

Sales Tax, add only for: CA 8%; OH 6.25%   + **Sales Tax**

Shipping & Handling for US address: + **S & H**
UPS Standard: 10% of subtotal with a minimum of $5.00
UPS 2nd Day Air: 20% of subtotal with a minimum of $8.00

= **Total**

Credit Card: ❏ Visa ❏ Mastercard ❏ Amex ❏ Discover
Card Number

Exp. Date   Signature

For foreign orders, quantity rebate, optional shipping and payment please inquire:
service@media4u.com

Books and Pocketcards also available at...   www.**media4u**.com

Börm Bruckmeier Products

pockets

	COPIES		PRICE/COPIES		PRICE
Anatomy pocket		x	US $ 14.95	=	
Canadian Drug pocket		x	US $ 14.95	=	
Differential Diagnosis pocket		x	US $ 14.95	=	
Drug pocket 2005		x	US $ 12.95	=	
Drug pocket plus 2005		x	US $ 24.95	=	
Drug Therapy pocket 2003-2004		x	US $ 14.95	=	
ECG pocket		x	US $ 12.95	=	
EMS pocket		x	US $ 14.95	=	
Homeopathy pocket		x	US $ 14.95	=	
Medical Abbreviations pocket		x	US $ 12.95	=	
Medical Classifications pocket		x	US $ 14.95	=	
Medical Spanish pocket		x	US $ 12.95	=	
Medical Spanish Dictionary pocket		x	US $ 14.95	=	
Medical Spanish pocket plus		x	US $ 22.95	=	
Normal Values pocket		x	US $ 12.95	=	
Respiratory pocket		x	US $ 14.95	=	

pocketcards

	COPIES		PRICE/COPIES		PRICE
Antibiotics pocketcard 2005		x	US $ 3.95	=	
Antifungals pocketcard		x	US $ 3.95	=	
BLS/ALS pocketcard		x	US $ 3.95	=	
ECG pocketcard		x	US $ 3.95	=	
ECG Evaluation pocketcard		x	US $ 3.95	=	
ECG Ruler pocketcard		x	US $ 3.95	=	
ECG pocketcard Set (3)		x	US $ 9.95	=	
Emergency Drugs pocketcard		x	US $ 3.95	=	
H&P pocketcard		x	US $ 3.95	=	
Medical Abbreviations pocketcard Set (2)		x	US $ 6.95	=	
Medical Spanish pocketcard		x	US $ 3.95	=	
Neurology pocketcard (2)		x	US $ 6.95	=	
Normal Values pocketcard		x	US $ 3.95	=	
Periodic Table pocketcard		x	US $ 3.95	=	

	= Subtotal	

Books and Pocketcards also available at...   www.media4u.com